BSAVA Manual of
Canine and Feline
Advanced Veterinary Nursing

Second edition

Editors:

Alasdair Hotston Moore
MA VetMB CertSAC CertVR CertSAS MRCVS
Department of Clinical Veterinary Science, University of Bristol,
Langford House, Langford, Bristol BS40 5DU

and

Suzanne Rudd
DipAVN(Medical) VN
Department of Clinical Veterinary Science, University of Bristol,
Langford House, Langford, Bristol BS40 5DU

Published by:

British Small Animal Veterinary Association
Woodrow House, 1 Telford Way, Waterwells Business Park,
Quedgeley, Gloucester GL2 2AB

A Company Limited by Guarantee in England.
Registered Company No. 2837793.
Registered as a Charity.

Reprinted 2015

Other veterinary nursing titles from BSAVA:

Manual of Exotic Pet and Wildlife Nursing
Manual of Practical Animal Care
Manual of Practical Veterinary Nursing
Textbook of Veterinary Nursing (formerly Jones's Animal Nursing)

Other titles in the BSAVA Manuals series:

Manual of Canine & Feline Abdominal Imaging
Manual of Canine & Feline Abdominal Surgery
Manual of Canine & Feline Anaesthesia and Analgesia
Manual of Canine & Feline Behavioural Medicine
Manual of Canine & Feline Cardiorespiratory Medicine
Manual of Canine & Feline Clinical Pathology
Manual of Canine & Feline Dentistry
Manual of Canine & Feline Dermatology
Manual of Canine & Feline Emergency and Critical Care
Manual of Canine & Feline Endocrinology
Manual of Canine & Feline Endoscopy and Endosurgery
Manual of Canine & Feline Fracture Repair and Management
Manual of Canine & Feline Gastroenterology
Manual of Canine & Feline Haematology and Transfusion Medicine
Manual of Canine & Feline Head, Neck and Thoracic Surgery
Manual of Canine & Feline Musculoskeletal Disorders
Manual of Canine & Feline Musculoskeletal Imaging
Manual of Canine & Feline Nephrology and Urology
Manual of Canine & Feline Neurology
Manual of Canine & Feline Oncology
Manual of Canine & Feline Ophthalmology
Manual of Canine & Feline Radiography and Radiology: A Foundation Manual
Manual of Canine & Feline Rehabilitation, Supportive and Palliative Care:
   Case Studies in Patient Management
Manual of Canine & Feline Reproduction and Neonatology
Manual of Canine & Feline Surgical Principles: A Foundation Manual
Manual of Canine & Feline Thoracic Imaging
Manual of Canine & Feline Ultrasonography
Manual of Canine & Feline Wound Management and Reconstruction
Manual of Canine Practice: A Foundation Manual
Manual of Exotic Pets: A Foundation Manual
Manual of Feline Practice: A Foundation Manual
Manual of Ornamental Fish
Manual of Psittacine Birds
Manual of Rabbit Medicine
Manual of Rabbit Surgery, Dentistry and Imaging
Manual of Raptors, Pigeons and Passerine Birds
Manual of Reptiles
Manual of Rodents and Ferrets
Manual of Small Animal Practice Management and Development
Manual of Wildlife Casualties

**For further information on these and all BSAVA publications, please visit our website:
www.bsava.com**

Contents

List of contributors   v

Foreword   vii

Preface   viii

1   **Advanced nursing practice**   1
Andrea Jeffery

2   **Advanced medical nursing**   9
Gerry Polton and Liz Branscombe

3   **Clinical nutrition**   54
Rachel Lumbis and Daniel L. Chan

4   **Physiotherapy and rehabilitation**   72
Brian J. Sharp

5   **Management of the critical care unit**   103
Belinda Andrews-Jones and Amanda Boag

6   **Advanced fluid therapy**   114
Paula Hotston Moore and Jo Murrell

7   **Advanced anaesthesia and analgesia**   128
Kathy Challis and Chris Seymour

8   **Advanced surgical nursing**   145
Alison Young and Mickey Tivers

9   **Dentistry**   175
Lisa Milella and Maureen Helm

10 **Endoscopy**   195
    Emma Barty and Philip Lhermette

11 **Advanced imaging**   220
    Lindsay Crane and Esther Barrett

12 **Clinical pathology in practice**   250
    Mark Pinches

13 **Practice administration**   286
    Sarah C. Hibbert

14 **Nursing clinics**   302
    Hayley L. McLeod

15 **Behaviour**   313
    Trudi Atkinson and Francesca Riccomini

Appendix: Conversion tables   329

Index   330

Contributors

Belinda Andrews-Jones VTS(ECC) DipAVN(Surgical) VN
The Royal Veterinary College, Hawkshead Lane, North Mymms, Hatfield, Hertfordshire AL9 7TA

Trudi Atkinson DipAS(CABC) CCAB VN
Bradford-on-Avon, Wiltshire

Esther Barrett MA VetMB DipECVDI DVDI MRCVS
Department of Clinical Veterinary Science, University of Bristol, Langford House, Langford, Bristol BS40 5DU

Emma Barty HND(VNS) RVN
Elands Veterinary Clinic, Station Road, Dunton Green, Sevenoaks, Kent TN13 2XA

Amanda Boag MA VetMB DipACVIM DipACVECC FHEA MRCVS
The Royal Veterinary College, Hawkshead Lane, North Mymms, Hatfield, Hertfordshire AL9 7TA

Liz Branscombe DipAVN(Surgical) RVN
Davies Veterinary Specialists, Manor Farm Business Park, Higham Gobion, Hertfordshire SG5 3HR

Kathy Challis DipAVN(Surgical) VN
Department of Clinical Veterinary Medicine, University of Cambridge, Madingley Road, Cambridge CB3 0ES

Daniel L. Chan DVM DipACVECC DipACVN MRCVS
The Royal Veterinary College, Hawkshead Lane, North Mymms, Hatfield, Hertfordshire AL9 7TA

Lindsay Crane VN
Department of Clinical Veterinary Science, University of Bristol, Langford House, Langford, Bristol BS40 5DU

Maureen Helm Cert Dentistry VN
Denbies View Veterinary Centre, Westcott Road, Dorking, Surrey RH4 3DP

Sarah C. Hibbert MBA CMgr CVPM
Avonvale Veterinary Practice Ltd, Ratley Lodge, Ratley, Banbury OX15 6DT

Paula Hotston Moore CertEd VN
Department of Clinical Veterinary Science, University of Bristol, Langford House, Langford, Bristol, BS40 5DU

Andrea Jeffery MSc DipAVN(Surgical) CertEd RVN
Department of Clinical Veterinary Science, University of Bristol, Langford House, Langford, Bristol BS40 5DU

Philip Lhermette BSc (Hons) CBiol MIBiol BVetMed MRCVS
Elands Veterinary Clinic, Station Road, Dunton Green, Sevenoaks, Kent TN13 2XA

Rachel Lumbis BSc (Hons) CertSAN VN
The Royal Veterinary College, Hawkshead Lane, North Mymms, Hatfield, Hertfordshire AL9 7TA

Hayley L. McLeod BSc (Hons) RVN
Branshaw View, 41 Laycock Lane, Near Keighley, West Yorkshire BD22 0PH

Lisa Milella BVSc MRCVS
The Veterinary Dental Surgery, 53 Parvis Road, Byfleet, Surrey KT14 7AA

Jo Murrell BVSc (Hons) PhD DipECVAA MRCVS
Department of Clinical Veterinary Science, University of Bristol, Langford House, Langford, Bristol BS40 5DU

Mark Pinches BVSc MSc DipRCpath DipECVCP MRCVS
5 Hartley Green, Bollington, Cheshire SK10 5JF

Gerry Polton MA VetMB MSc (Clin Onc) MRCVS
Davies Veterinary Specialists, Manor Farm Business Park, Higham Gobion, Hitchin, Hertfordshire SG5 3HR

Francesca Riccomini BSc (Hons) BVetMet DipAS (CABC) CCAB DipArch MRCVS
34 Brook Road, Twickenham, Middlesex TW1 1JE

Chris Seymour MA VetMD DVA MRCVS
Department of Veterinary Medicine, University of Cambridge, Madingley Road, Cambridge CB3 0ES

Brian J. Sharp MSc(VetPhys) BSc(Phys) BSc(Biol) PGCE PGDipHealthEd MCSP HPC Reg ACPAT
The Royal Veterinary College, Hawkshead Lane, North Mymms, Hatfield, Hertfordshire AL9 7TA

Mickey Tivers BVSc CertSAS MRCVS
The Royal Veterinary College, Hawkshead Lane, North Mymms, Hatfield, Hertfordshire AL9 7TA

Alison Young DipAVN(Surgical) RVN
The Royal Veterinary College, Hawkshead Lane, North Mymms, Hatfield, Hertfordshire AL9 7TA

Foreword

Veterinary nurses are increasingly aware of the need for up-to-date knowledge so that they can develop their professional skills whilst working within the constraints and limitations of both professional and employment law. The approach taken with this second edition of Advanced Veterinary Nursing is however a practical one.

The *BSAVA Manual of Canine and Feline Advanced Veterinary Nursing, second edition* has maintained the high BSAVA standards established in other Manuals and with the previous edition, and it has been updated and extended to take account of developments within the profession and in practice.

The editors and authors have also ably drawn out the implications for veterinary nurses, exposing the important issues and identifying the key points that need to underpin accountable veterinary nursing practice. The Manual presents an exhilarating visual and literary perspective of the different aspects of veterinary nursing, serving as an invaluable source of knowledge for qualified veterinary nurses and those undertaking a diploma or degree.

Significant changes within the veterinary nursing profession have taken place since the previous edition of this Manual was published. More guidance on regulation has emerged from the Royal College of Veterinary Surgeons (RCVS), which will aid veterinary nurses so that they can understand the changing context within their area of work.

Chapter 1 on Advanced veterinary nursing practice provides an excellent insight into how the profession has evolved and the emerging career opportunities. This book is a 'must have' for anyone who wants to advance their veterinary nursing practice.

Barbara Cooper Hon Assoc RCVS CertEd Lic IPD DTM VN
College of Animal Welfare
July 2008

Preface

Veterinary nursing has progressed rapidly over the last 20 years. With the recent development of self-regulation, veterinary nurses are being recognized in their own right and taking further steps forward as true professionals. The veterinary nursing qualification now opens many doors to further careers and qualifications, ensuring the 'glorified cleaner' image is a thing of the past. Along with veterinary science, veterinary nursing is developing, our knowledge is increasing and standards of nursing care are becoming more advanced.

As editors we decided that to build upon the first edition of the *BSAVA Manual of Advanced Veterinary Nursing*, we would approach a number of veterinary nurses to be the main authors for many of the chapters: after all, they have first-hand experience of what is important for a veterinary nurse to know. Many veterinary surgeons with an area of expertise have also been involved to ensure that the developments in veterinary science are shared amongst all within the profession. We also wanted to look at areas within veterinary nursing that had made significant developments. Physiotherapy, behaviour and the introduction of nurse-led clinics are just three of the major advances within the veterinary nursing profession.

In line with the advanced nursing diplomas, we wanted to create a Manual that would be useful for both the surgical and medical aspects of the course. However, it became apparent that covering the whole of, for example, medical nursing would be a Manual in itself; therefore, we hope this Manual will interlink with many of the BSAVA veterinary Manuals already produced. With many veterinary nurses now pursuing careers in a specific stream, such as anaesthesia, and gaining post-qualification certificates, e.g. in nutrition, we wanted to ensure that information at an advanced level was included.

The Manual has a canine and feline focus. Cats are now accepted as a species in their own right and need different requirements and nursing techniques to that of the dog. We have tried to incorporate more of these differences to promote this recognition.

Finally, we wanted this Manual not only to be useful academically but to be a valuable source of practical information. Within the series of veterinary nursing manuals, this book is intended to appeal to qualified veterinary nurses and those in the final years of undergraduate programmes, as well as to student nurses. We hope it will be useful for those preparing for exams, a source of reference for others, and an inspiration to those wishing to advance the art and science of veterinary nursing.

We have very much enjoyed working on this Manual and would like to thank the authors for their hard work and understanding. We would also like to give special thanks to our colleagues at Langford and to Marion Jowett, Nicola Lloyd and Ben Dales at BSAVA Publications for all their support and guidance.

Alasdair Hotston Moore
Suzanne Rudd

June 2008

Advanced nursing practice

Andrea Jeffery

This chapter is designed to give information on:

- The development of veterinary nursing
- The current structure of qualifications available to veterinary nurses
- Career paths for veterinary nurses
- Nursing practice and nursing models

Historical overview of the profession

Veterinary nursing is a relatively young profession compared with human-centred nursing. The latter has a history that goes back to the late nineteenth century and Florence Nightingale, who is 'considered the founder of nursing and the first nursing theorist' (Sibson, 2005). The original veterinary nursing training scheme began in 1961 with a 2-year training period that resulted in the first registered animal nursing auxiliaries (RANAs) working in practice in 1963. It was 2 years later, in 1965, that the British Veterinary Nursing Association (BVNA) was established. It was not until 1984, almost 20 years later, that a RANA could begin using the title 'Veterinary Nurse', as a result of a change in legislation with regard to the word 'nurse'.

The National Vocational Qualification (NVQ) system for veterinary nursing was established by the Royal College of Veterinary Surgeons (RCVS) in 2000 for both small animal and equine nurse training. This system of training incorporated a taught component (the syllabus) and a practical component (the national occupational standards). Unlike other NVQ qualifications, which are gained through continual assessment, it was decided that independent external written and practical examinations would still be held because of the nature of the qualification and the role of the veterinary nurse once qualified.

The RCVS is associated with veterinary nursing through its various functions:

- The maintenance of the Register and the List of veterinary nurses
- The award of the veterinary nursing NVQ and Vocationally Related Qualifications (VRQs)
- The award of veterinary nursing certificates and diplomas
- Non-statutory regulation of veterinary nurses.

Professional development

The advent of the NVQ system brought the need for qualified staff within veterinary practice to train as assessors. This has helped to improve the employability of veterinary nurses who, if they gain the qualification, are sought after by training practices (TPs). The two further qualifications that can be gained and used by veterinary nurses within the NVQ system are those of internal verifier and external verifier. A second career development stream for veterinary nurses within practice is that of veterinary practice management. The Veterinary Practice Management Association (VPMA) offers a recognized accredited certificate within this area; the Certificate in Veterinary Practice Management (CVPM) is a qualification that recognizes proficiency in administrative and management tasks. According to the VPMA, 'the qualification was established in 1995 and is designed to be immediately relevant to managers and employers in the veterinary sector and to indicate that the successful candidate has the appropriate knowledge, experience and expertise to be an effective manager'.

There have been short courses and congresses available to qualified veterinary nurses for many years, along with the Certificate in Education awarded by both further education (FE) and higher education (HE) institutions. The Advanced Diploma in Veterinary Nursing began in the early 1990s and was delivered as a distance learning programme by the BVNA and examined by the RCVS. It was not until 1998, however, that the first undergraduate programme for veterinary nurses was established.

There is a wide range of types and levels of professional development that veterinary nurses can pursue (Figure 1.1). When a course such as the Diploma in Advanced Veterinary Nursing or a Certificate in Education is offered to veterinary nurses through a higher education institution (HEI), each of the modules studied for will have 'credit weighting'

attached to them; these are transferable credit points and can be cumulative. A veterinary nurse can take the credit points forward to any other HEI and use them to form part of a BSc (Hons) in veterinary nursing, this could then be followed by a masters qualification (MSc or MEd) and a doctorate (PhD). This system is known as 'Accredited Prior Learning' (APL). A university will look at an individual's APL and decide how many credit points they have and what level within a university course structure they have attained. The veterinary nurse can then take their credit points forward and use them to broaden their depth and breadth of education.

It is important for veterinary nurses who wish to undertake HE to have a guide to the qualifications awarded by universities, and the descriptors in Figure 1.2 help to explain the different levels.

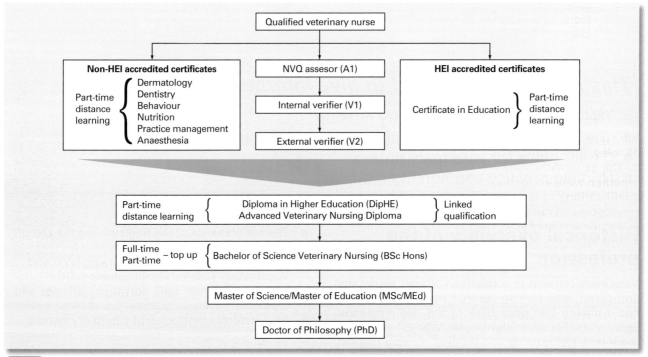

1.1   Possible educational progression within veterinary nursing.

Qualification	Comments
Certificate level *First step towards higher education (HE) qualification*	The holder will: ■ Have a sound knowledge of the basic concepts of a subject ■ Have learned to take different approaches to solving problems ■ Be able to communicate accurately
Intermediate level *Includes ordinary (non-honours) degrees, foundation degrees, diplomas in HE and other higher diplomas*	The holder will: ■ Have developed a sound understanding of the principles in field of study ■ Be able to apply those principles more widely ■ Be able to evaluate the appropriateness of different problem-solving approaches
Honours level *Honours degrees and also professional 'conversion' courses* *Usually 3 years if taken full-time*	The holder will: ■ Have developed an understanding of a complex body of knowledge, some at the current boundaries of the academic discipline ■ Have developed analytical techniques and problem-solving skills ■ Have developed an ability to evaluate evidence, arguments and assumptions, reach sound judgements and communicate effectively

1.2   Quality Assurance Agency (QAA) framework for higher education qualifications (January 2001). (continues) ▶

Qualification	Comments
Masters level *Awarded after completion of taught courses, programmes of research, or both* *Equivalent to 1 year of full-time study*	Much of the study will have been at, or informed by, the forefront of an academic or professional discipline The holder will: ■ Have shown originality in the application of knowledge ■ Understand how the boundaries of knowledge are advanced through research ■ Deal with complex issues both systematically and creatively ■ Show originality in tackling and solving problems
Doctoral *Awarded on the basis of original research* *Equivalent to 3 years of full-time study*	Doctorates are awarded for the creation and interpretation of knowledge that extends the forefront of a discipline, usually through original research The holder will: ■ Be able to conceptualize, design and implement projects for the generation of significant knowledge and/or understanding

1.2 (continued) Quality Assurance Agency (QAA) framework for higher education qualifications (January 2001).

Developing roles of the veterinary nurse

After qualification, veterinary nurses can fill a number of roles, both within the profession and related to it. The experience they have of veterinary practice, together with an increasing number of additional qualifications (see later), make them attractive to employers in a number of areas. In addition, changes in the ownership of veterinary practices have allowed veterinary nurses to own equity in practices and exercise influence over these businesses. Traditionally, practices were partnerships and only veterinary surgeons could be partners within them. However, limited companies and other structures can now provide veterinary services and veterinary nurses can be directors of these businesses.

Within practices and veterinary institutions, veterinary nurses fill roles extending beyond the traditional technical support for veterinary surgeons. Veterinary nurses experienced in clinical practice, and often with additional qualifications, are well placed to offer specialized nursing care (for example, in the critical care unit, during patient rehabilitation, supporting anaesthetic services, and performing minor surgery or radiography) (Figures 1.3 to 1.5). The changing education of student veterinary nurses has also led to many experienced veterinary nurses completing the training required to act as assessors and internal verifiers within the NVQ scheme (Figure 1.6).

The skills of the profession are also recognized through appointment to positions with administrative and management responsibilities, for example, as a senior veterinary nurse within the practice or as practice manager. Many practices have also recognized the value of veterinary nurses at the client interface, through the provision of nurse-led clinics for management of weight loss, pet behaviour and dental care. All of these are possible within the confines of legislation restricting the practice of veterinary surgery (including the act of diagnosis and the privilege to prescribe medication) to veterinary surgeons.

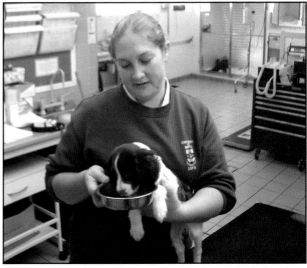

1.3 Veterinary nurse working in a specialized critical care unit. A puppy with a vascular ring anomaly is receiving postural feeding postoperatively.

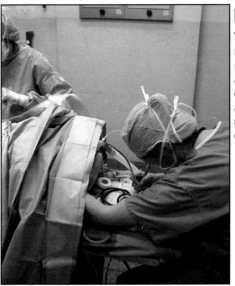

1.4 Veterinary nurse monitoring anaesthesia during abdominal surgery of a dog.

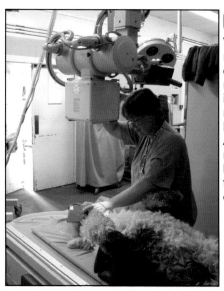

1.5 Veterinary nurse employed as radiographer in a veterinary referral hospital. An intraoral radiograph is being taken to investigate oral neoplasia.

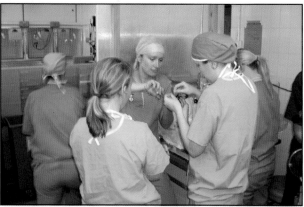

1.6 Experienced surgical nurse working with student veterinary nurses during resuscitation of puppies following a Caesarean section.

Outside clinical practice, veterinary nurses are widely employed in commerce. Their skills and experience are valuable in the marketing of veterinary drugs, diets, consumables and equipment to the profession. They also are employed by pet insurance companies to liaise with veterinary practices and to assess claims. Many experienced veterinary nurses acquire skills in teaching and are appointed in FE and HE to teach and train students in allied careers (animal care, veterinary nursing and veterinary surgery). Businesses that employ veterinary nurses also frequently ask them to visit veterinary practices not only to promote their products but also to provide continuing education to practice personnel.

Influence of the RCVS Veterinary Nursing syllabus and National Occupational Standards on nursing practice

The RCVS Veterinary Nursing Awarding Body published a revised syllabus in 2006 that reflected a changing emphasis within the educational framework of a profession moving towards self-regulation.

The aim of this change was three-fold:

- To ensure that student veterinary nurses were introduced to a problem-solving approach to their nursing
- To ensure that student veterinary nurses developed skills in independent learning
- To introduce student veterinary nurses to the professional as well as the legal obligations of a veterinary nurse.

This was a critical move away from a previously didactic and prescriptive way of educating veterinary nurses and something that college lecturers have embraced through a change in teaching styles and lesson structure.

The language used within the syllabus to describe the understanding required by student veterinary nurses was changed and within level 2 of the award a unit was introduced for the first time entitled 'Relationships and accountability in veterinary nursing practice'. The purpose of this area of learning was to educate students about their own professional accountability, along with identifying commonly occurring ethical issues that may arise in veterinary practice and how to manage ethical problems.

A number of key features of the previous syllabi remained within this new unit (VNT1), including communication skills. However, the education that student veterinary nurses have received since 2006 ensures that they have the ability to outline the legal and professional regulatory frameworks in which veterinary nurses worked prior to and following the introduction of self-regulation in September 2007.

One other key change that took place within the 2006 syllabus related to the move away from the medical model traditionally used when teaching veterinary nurses. According to the medical model the patient is a complex set of anatomical parts and physiological systems (Aggleton and Chalmers, 2000). The medical model emphasizes anatomical, physiological and biochemical malfunction as the causes of ill health and by doing so encourages a *disease-oriented* approach of the veterinary nurse to the patient. It is this disease-oriented approach that has influenced the way in which veterinary nurses have been educated historically; however, the revised syllabus has influenced a change in direction within nursing education to ensure that veterinary nurses have a more individualized, holistic, patient-oriented approach to care. This can be seen in the change in emphasis of the title and content of the anatomy and physiology unit 'Applied functional anatomy for veterinary nursing practice', which in the revised syllabus requires the student to receive an introduction to the link between the healthy and the unhealthy animal.

Within human-centred nursing the use of care pathways and models of nursing has been an accepted part of nursing practice since 1980 (Sibson, 2005). It was disenchantment with the medical model that was the main reason for the development of nursing theories and models of nursing within human-centred nursing. Nurses believed that the medical model was not a focus for their discipline. There were a number of other influences, including:

- The advent of university-educated nurses
- The quest for professional recognition
- The increase in the numbers of nurses with MSc and PhD degrees.

All of these factors now influence the veterinary nursing profession, and their key effect is to focus on a 'patient-centred approach' that provides a 'holistic' nursing approach to patient care, rather than the use of a 'medical model' that encourages a disease-oriented approach to the patient.

The introduction of unit VNT7 (Application of Veterinary Nursing Care) produced a landmark change in the way in which diseases are taught within veterinary nursing education. Student veterinary nurses should no longer be provided with lists of disease processes and clinical signs. With the skills learnt through applying the theories of the nursing process and models of nursing, the students will be educated in the planning of care for patients with commonly encountered conditions, such as circulatory disorders. This should not detract from the importance of knowing what the condition is and how it occurs, and cross references are made to the 'Applied functional anatomy for veterinary nursing practice' unit to ensure that students can see the link between the anatomy and physiology of the healthy animal and those of the sick animal. However, the emphasis of modern veterinary nurse education is on how the patient will be nursed and why. By educating student veterinary nurses to focus on the patient with the disease rather than the disease itself, they can draw up an individualized plan of care via a structured framework. By the systematic recording of this decision-making process, veterinary nurses will be producing a documented evidence base for their veterinary nursing practice. This provides a mechanism by which to move nursing away from a list of tasks to be carried out (the 'task-oriented approach') to thinking about individual patients and their needs and applying the nursing process, which is the *thinking* and *doing* approach that veterinary nurses use in their work (Wilkinson, 1996).

Student veterinary nurses will also be taught how to develop and write care plans for patients who are undergoing a range of veterinary interventions, such as fluid therapy, wound management and tube feeding. These care plans are developed within the framework of two human-centred nursing models: that of Roper, Logan and Tierney (2000) and the Orem model (Cavanagh, 1991) (see also the *BSAVA Manual of Practical Veterinary Nursing* and *BSAVA Textbook of Veterinary Nursing, 4th edition*). Both of these models have strong research bases. This change in nursing practice will help to develop autonomous veterinary nurse practitioners working alongside veterinary surgeons.

In order for a detailed care plan to be written, it is vital that a nursing assessment of the patient takes place upon admission. The information obtained is formally recorded as it will become the basis of the care plan. Documented care plans are a vital part of nursing as they ensure continuity in the care of patients (i.e. each veterinary nurse responsible for the patient will deliver the same level of care for that patient). In 2007 the Nursing and Midwifery Council (NMC) produced a document called Guidelines for Records and Record Keeping. This provides clear guidance for human-centred nurses on how records, including care plans, should be documented. The summary below is adapted from that document and provides a good basis for care plans for veterinary nursing patients until more detailed guidance is developed by the veterinary nursing profession itself.

The Summary of NMC Guidelines for Records and Record Keeping (2007) recommends that records should:

- Be factual, consistent and accurate, and written so that the meaning is clear
- Be made as soon as possible after an event has occurred, providing current information on the care and condition of the patient
- Be made clearly and in such a manner that the text cannot be erased or deleted without a record of the change
- Be made in such a manner that any alterations or additions are dated, timed and signed, or clearly attributed to a named person in an identifiable role in such a way that the original entry can still be read clearly
- Be accurately dated, timed and signed, with a signature printed alongside the first entry where this is a written entry, and attributed to a named person in an identifiable role for electronic records
- Not include abbreviations, jargon, meaningless phrases, irrelevant speculation and offensive subject statements. (The author believes that additional consideration should be given to the use of terminology and/or abbreviations, which should be consistent within the profession to prevent the risk of misinterpretation between professionals. It is also the author's view that the accurate recording of numbers and measurements is of particular importance, e.g. the dosage of a tablet should be recorded as '250 mg' and the patient's respiratory rate recorded as '22 breaths/minute' and not left just as a number of which the unit is not apparent)
- Be readable when photocopied or scanned
- Be made, wherever possible, with the involvement of the patient/client. (Author's note: this is not possible with a veterinary patient and involvement of the client will depend on individual practice policy and the wishes of the veterinary surgeon responsible for the case)
- Be recorded in terms that the client can understand
- Be consecutive
- Identify risks and/or problems that have arisen and the action taken to rectify them
- Provide clear evidence of the care planned, the decision made, the care delivered and the information shared.

The nursing process

Carrying out the nursing process ensures that veterinary nurses have a systematic approach to the delivery of care to every patient they nurse (Chandler *et al.*, 2007) (Figure 1.7).

Patient details:	12-month-old neutered male, Domestic Short-hair cat			
Reason for admission:	Fractured jaw			
Date and time:				

Universal self-care requisites	Self-care abilities	Self-care limitations	Patient actions	Nursing actions
Maintain intake of air	Breathes without difficulty	Unable to groom/clean therefore food sticks to nose	Breathes well when nostrils clear	Ensure nostrils remain clear during and after feeding Assess respiratory adequacy
Maintain intake of water	Can put mouth down to water bowl and lap water	Difficulty in drinking from a high-sided bowl	Drinking Swallowing	Provide water in a shallow bowl Keep a fluid balance chart Observe for signs of dehydration
Maintain intake of food	Can put mouth down to food bowl	Unable to prehend food	Can swallow when food in mouth	Ensure food is in manageable form Assist with feeding Maintain a record of food eaten
Manage elimination	All	Normally urinates outside in soil	Use litter tray to urinate and defecate	Provide litter tray containing soil Keep a record of urinary/faecal output
Balance activity and rest	Is able to rest and sleep	Unable to have free access	Walk around kennel Rest and sleep on Vetbed	Provide a large kennel Provide an environment for rest/sleep when required
Balance solitude and social integration	Is able to communicate through body language	Unable to purr or meow due to fracture Unable to communicate with brother		Provide regular nursing attention Organize for family, including children to visit
Prevention of hazards to life, well being and functioning	Possesses pain sensation Can hear and see	Cannot maintain safety of environment		Monitor vital signs and assess patient for changes in physical and psychological condition
Normalcy	Is able to communicate through body language	Unable to vocalize	Interact with staff, family and other animals	Provide an environment in which he feels at ease

1.7 The application of a nursing care plan (Orem model). (Reproduced from the *BSAVA Textbook of Veterinary Nursing, 4th edition*)

Assessment

Assessment will clearly establish the individual needs of the patient. It is only once a patient assessment has been performed that effective care can be given.

1. Collect the information needed from your own observations and information from the client and other team members.
2. Collate the information systematically and write it down.
3. Review the collated information.
4. Identify actual and potential nursing problems.
5. Identify priorities among the problems.

Planning

Once all the information has been gathered during the assessment phase, the next part of the nursing process is the planning stage. This is where the veterinary nurse plans what they are going to do about the nursing problems that have been identified. The aims are:

- To solve identified actual problems
- To prevent identified potential problems becoming actual ones
- To alleviate those problems that cannot be solved
- To help the patient/client cope positively with those problems that cannot be solved or alleviated
- To prevent recurrence of a treated problem
- To help the patient to be as comfortable as possible even when death is inevitable.

Setting goals

A goal has to be set for each actual and potential problem, and a distinction should be made between short-term and long-term goals. It is important that any goals set should be stated in terms of outcomes that are able to be observed, measured or tested so that effective evaluation can then be carried out. For example, a Persian cat wearing an Elizabethan collar has an *actual problem* of not being able to groom and a *potential problem* of matts developing in the fur due to this. A *short-term goal* would be to groom the cat twice daily with a wide-toothed comb. A *long-term goal* would be to remove the collar in order for the cat to groom itself.

Nursing plan

A plan is composed of all the proposed nursing interventions needed to achieve the goals. The plan should be written in enough detail that any veterinary nurse reading it would understand and be able to reliably implement it.

Implementation

Implementing the nursing plan is the 'doing' stage of the nursing process, otherwise known as the 'nursing intervention'. It is important that veterinary nurses make it clear what decision-making has taken place to justify the nursing intervention. All of this information should be clearly and indelibly recorded on the care plan.

Evaluation

Evaluation is a vital part of the nursing process; it is difficult to justify planning and implementing nursing interventions if the outcomes cannot be shown to have benefited either the patient or the client in some way.

Evaluation is a difficult thing to do. Ideally the evaluation will show that all the nursing goals have been achieved, but if this is not the case the following questions need to be asked:

- Have the goals you set for the patient been partially achieved?
- Is more information from the veterinary surgeon or the client needed to decide the next step in the nursing care?
- Is a specific problem unchanged and should the nursing intervention be changed or stopped?
- Is there a worsening of the problem and should the goal and nursing intervention be reviewed?
- Was the goal inappropriate when first set?
- Does the goal require interventions from other members of the veterinary team, e.g. veterinary surgeon or physiotherapist?

By asking these questions, a re-evaluation of the patient takes place that leads to a revision of the original nursing plan to address the issues that have become apparent during the evaluation. The changes that are required are recorded on the care plan and the whole process begins again.

Veterinary nursing – a self-regulated profession

In September 2007 a landmark event took place which the author believes moved veterinary nursing forwards towards a full professional identity. Following consultation with all members of the veterinary nursing profession and other interested parties (e.g. the BVNA and the British Small Animal Veterinary Association (BSAVA)), and after a 9-month period of awareness raising, the veterinary nursing profession opted for self-regulation. Statutory regulation will not be possible until there is a change to the Veterinary Surgeons Act of 1966. By becoming self-regulated the veterinary nursing profession provides an assurance to the public of the standard of behaviour and professional skill that should be expected of a regulated veterinary nurse.

The features of any profession, and therefore those expected of registered veterinary nurses, are an assured standard of training and qualification, a code of professional conduct, a commitment to maintain competence, and sanctions for those who knowingly transgress. The reason that the RCVS Veterinary Nurses Council believed that self-regulation should be put in place was that the RCVS veterinary nurses List gave no assurance of conduct to the public. Those on the RCVS veterinary nurses List do not have any requirement to remain competent, and therefore a veterinary nurse who qualified 15 years ago and who had not been employed as a veterinary nurse for several years could return to work with no professional requirement to refresh. There are also no sanctions for misconduct for those on the List.

As of 1 September 2007 all veterinary nurses who qualified and were listed after 1 January 2003 were automatically transferred on to the veterinary nurses Register, at which point they became known as Registered Veterinary Nurses (RVNs). In doing so they are required to adhere to the *RCVS Guide to Professional Conduct for Veterinary Nurses*. Veterinary nurses who were listed and/or qualified before 1 January 2003 were also formally invited to join the new Register voluntarily in September 2007. Once the move is made on to the Register a registered veterinary nurse cannot change their mind and move back on to the unregulated List; it is in effect a one-way street. Veterinary nurses who qualified before January 2003 and who wish to remain on the List will be able to do so and still be able to practise as veterinary nurses and undertake procedures identified in Schedule 3 of the Veterinary Surgeons Act 1966. However, the public have no reassurance that they are up-to-date in their clinical practice, nor do the listed veterinary nurses have to adhere to the *Guide to Professional Conduct*.

There was a planned lead-in period of 3 years (2007–2010) in order for the profession to become accustomed to self-regulation before the system became fully operational. The Register was set up in 'shadow form' in September 2007 but becomes 'live' in 2010, at which point veterinary nurses are likely to be subject to a preliminary investigation and possible disciplinary action if they have been found 'guilty of serious professional misconduct or if they have a criminal conviction which renders them unfit for practice, such as theft or a drugs related offence' (RCVS, 2007).

The RCVS believes that, as with other regulated professions, the benefits for those who enter the Register include:

- On a personal level, respect from other professionals, such as veterinary surgeons, who follow their own guides to professional conduct

7

- A strengthened position from which to develop a career structure within the workplace and increased status, which will be recognized by clients
- On a national level it is believed that by becoming regulated veterinary nursing will be strengthened in its development as a discipline in its own right and distinct from veterinary surgery.

The *Guide to Professional Conduct for Veterinary Nurses* was designed, for ease of use, using the same layout as that applied to veterinary surgeons, and it was hoped that during the initial phase of self-regulation registered veterinary nurses could speak to veterinary surgeons in the knowledge that they would be familiar with the layout. Sally Bowden and Dot Creighton (both veterinary nurses) were instrumental in the development of the *Guide* and it was their work that produced the 'Ten guiding principles', which are the anchor point upon which all other aspects are based and set out the professional behaviour expected of a veterinary nurse.

One of the requirements of the *Guide* is for any veterinary nurse who is on the Register to 'continue their professional education by keeping up-to-date with the general developments in veterinary nursing, particularly in their area of professional activity and must maintain a record'.

Continuing professional development

Registered veterinary nurses are required to undertake a minimum of 15 hours of continuing professional development (CPD) annually, or 45 hours over a 3-year period. The RCVS purposefully built in a degree of flexibility as it was recognized that a veterinary nurse may not achieve 15 hours in any particular year but may do 30 hours in one year and none in another. It was also recognized that most veterinary nurses would do much more than this already and would continue to do so. The CPD card for registered veterinary nurses clearly defines the type of professional development that can be counted:

- Self-directed and workplace learning, including informal distance learning
- Working towards an accredited qualification and/or participating in formal distance learning programmes
- Attending courses, conferences and other external meetings.

It is stipulated on the CPD card that 'undocumented private study' should not account for any more than 5 of the 15 hours in one year.

Returning to work after a break

Veterinary nurses who qualified before January 2003 and who return to practice after a break of 5 years or more are given a choice by the RCVS either to return to the unregulated List or to join the Register. Those who elect to join the new Register are required to produce evidence to demonstrate a period of at least 17 weeks (4 months) of supervised clinical practice. The aim of this period is for the veterinary nurse who has been out of work to update or refresh themselves, not to undertake a retraining programme.

References and further reading

Aggleton P and Chalmers H (2000) *Nursing Models and Nursing Practice, 2nd edn.* Palgrave Macmillan, Basingstoke

Cavanagh SJ (1991) *Orem's Model in Action, 3rd edn.* Palgrave Macmillan, Basingstoke

Chandler S, Seymour J and Jeffery A (2007) General nursing, the nursing process and nursing models. In: *BSAVA Textbook of Veterinary Nursing, 4th edn,* ed. D Lane *et al.,* pp. 246–279. BSAVA Publications, Gloucester

Roper N, Logan W and Tierney A (2000) *The Roper, Logan and Tierney Model of Nursing.* Churchill Livingstone, Edinburgh

Scott-Park F (2007) An introduction to veterinary practice. In: *BSAVA Manual of Practical Animal Care,* ed. P Hotston-Moore and A Hughes, pp. 1–13. BSAVA Publications, Gloucester

Sibson L (2005) The Nursing Process. In: *Compendium of Clinical Skills for Student Nurses,* ed. I Peate, 19–36. John Wiley and Sons, London

Wilkinson J (1996) *Nursing Process – a critical thinking approach.* Addison–Wesley Publishing Company, USA

Useful websites

Nursing and Midwifery Council
www.nmc-org.uk

Quality Assurance Agency for Higher Education
www.qaa.ac.uk

Royal College of Veterinary Surgeons
www.rcvs.org.uk

Veterinary Practice Management Association
www.vpma.co.uk

2

Advanced medical nursing

Gerry Polton and Liz Branscombe

This chapter is designed to give information on:

- Advanced concepts in medical nursing
- The application of the nursing process to these patients
- The principles and practice of veterinary oncology

Introduction

This chapter provides information on medical nursing at a level beyond that expected of the newly qualified veterinary nurse. The nursing process (see Chapter 1) is emphasized throughout this chapter. This approach is particularly useful for patients with medical conditions which are multifactorial.

Triage and examination of the patient

It is necessary for veterinary nurses to be able to accurately evaluate the stability of new admissions and existing patients in their care. A triage examination briefly reviews each body system in order of importance to highlight abnormal signs and devise a treatment plan. Following triage, a full clinical examination (secondary survey) is carried out on the stable patient (see *BSAVA Manual of Practical Veterinary Nursing* for further information).

Nursing the patient with non-specific clinical signs

Animals are frequently presented with non-specific clinical signs (Figure 2.1). These signs are reported in a substantial majority of patients with medical illness but in some cases diagnostic investigations prove unrewarding (or are declined). Nursing patients with non-specific malaise of undetermined cause can be extremely challenging.

Clinical sign	Differential diagnoses
Pyrexia/hyperthermia	Infection: bacterial; viral; other. Consider occult sites of infection: renal; biliary; peritoneal; uterine; tracking foreign body Inflammation: immune-mediated disease, haemolysis, polyarthritis, meningitis Neoplasia: lymphoma; intra-abdominal or intrathoracic mass(es) Heat stroke Respiratory obstruction Anxiety/pain

2.1 Non-specific clinical signs and potential underlying causes. (continues) ▶

Clinical sign	Differential diagnoses
Hypothermia	Hypovolaemia: shock; haemorrhage; hypoproteinaemia; Addison's disease Systemic inflammatory response: septicaemia; peritonitis; pyothorax Malnutrition: anorexia/inappetence Pain, particularly visceral distension Neurological disease Gastrointestinal disease: foreign body; torsion; perforation Error in measurement
Pain	Infection: bacterial; viral; other. Consider occult sites of infection: renal; biliary; peritoneal; uterine; tracking foreign body Inflammation: immune-mediated disease, polyarthritis, meningitis, nephritis, hepatitis Organ distension: neoplasia; luminal obstruction (urinary tract, biliary) Trauma
Polyphagia	Endocrinopathy: diabetes mellitus; hyperthyroidism Increased energy consumption: altered management; increased exercise; reduced ambient temperature Reduced energy utilization: gastrointestinal disease
Decreased appetite	Inability to eat: oral lesion; neurological disease; megaoesophagus Reluctance to eat: pain (see above); oesophagitis; gastritis; pyrexia (see above); reduced palatability; anxiety Nausea: gastrointestinal disease; toxaemia due to renal, enteric, systemic, uterine disease; drug administration; central nervous system disease Neoplasia Reduced energy consumption: hypothyroidism; altered management
Polydipsia	Increased fluid losses: renal disease; gastrointestinal disease; diabetes mellitus/insipidus; hypercalcaemia Increased thirst: primary/psychogenic polydipsia; altered diet
Increased bodyweight	Increased food intake: corticosteroid administration, Cushing's disease, altered palatability Reduced energy consumption: hypothyroidism; reduced exercise Fluid retention: ascites; oedema Failure to eliminate: megacolon; urinary retention Correction of prior fluid deficit Pregnancy
Decreased bodyweight	Reduced appetite (see above) Increased energy consumption: hyperthyroidism; diabetes mellitus Cachectic states: neoplasia; cardiac disease
Altered exercise	Reduced enthusiasm for exercise: pain (see above); pyrexia (see above); nausea; gastrointestinal disease; toxaemia due to renal, enteric, systemic, uterine disease; drug administration Reduced ability to exercise: cardiovascular disease; respiratory disease; anaemia; hypovolaemia; orthopaedic disease; neurological disease; corticosteroid administration; Cushing's disease

2.1 (continued) Non-specific clinical signs and potential underlying causes.

Diagnostic procedures

Patients with non-specific clinical signs can be challenging to investigate, not least because the practitioner is not directed to a specific problem or body system. In any decision-making process about which investigative procedures to perform, consideration must be given to the likely yield of that investigation balanced against the possible cost to the owner and patient. Cost in this context covers not only the financial implications but also the potential health risks of investigation and emotional disturbance for the owner or patient. The potential benefit of achieving a diagnosis must also be considered: mild disease does not warrant aggressive investigation, but grave disease does. Routine diagnostic procedures that might be employed include:

- Repeated physical examination
- Haematology including manual blood smear
- Biochemistry
- Manual urine microscopy
- Thoracic and abdominal radiography
- Abdominal ultrasonography.

Nursing considerations

When a diagnosis remains elusive, one of the most valuable tools is to repeatedly examine the patient. Nursing observations are critical in these cases for two reasons: to optimize nursing care and so that further subjective and objective data can be obtained. These continuing observations may result in the list of differential diagnoses being narrowed or may even allow a definitive diagnosis to finally be made.

Pyrexic and hyperthermic patients

Since pyrexia represents a physiological response to disease, interfering with this process could potentially perpetuate the underlying complaint. However, severely elevated body temperature can be dangerous in its own right and intervention may be necessary in cases considered to be severely pyrexic, despite the conceptual basis against this. Hyperthermia is managed by physical rather than pharmaceutical methods. Cellular processes fail as proteins begin to unravel at temperatures of 42°C. The central nervous system (CNS) specifically is injured by more modest increases in temperature. For these reasons, physical therapeutic methods are employed when the patient's core temperature reaches 40–41°C:

- The patient can be placed in a cool or air-conditioned room
- Ventilation can be improved, particularly if the patient is in a humid environment. A fan can be placed near the patient
- The patient can be covered with wet towels, which can be replaced as indicated
- A cold bath or shower can be used
- A cool water enema can be used.

Theoretically, rapid infusion of cooled intravenous fluids can be used to reduce body temperature; however, this carries a significant risk of complications. Infusion of fluids at room temperature and at conventional rates has a modest effect on patient temperature and cannot be relied upon as a sole method of cooling.

Pharmaceutical methods of controlling pyrexia include the administration of corticosteroids or non-steroidal anti-inflammatory drugs (NSAIDs). Particular consideration should be given to the patient's hydration status as it is often compromised in these cases; under such circumstances administration of anti-inflammatory drugs can lead to severe renal or gastric consequences.

Patients with an elevated body temperature can respond very quickly to cooling methods, resulting at times in hypothermia. A target body temperature of 39–39.5°C is recommended. Temperature must be monitored frequently to avoid excessive cooling.

Nursing the recumbent patient

There are a number of causes of recumbency but the nursing considerations for the care of these patients are primarily the same (Figure 2.2).

Nursing the patient with cardiovascular disease

Presenting complaints

Patients with moderate cardiac disease are classically presented due to exercise intolerance or collapse. Other presenting complaints include ill-thrift in animals with congenital anomalies, cough and signs of thromboembolic disease, such as stroke-like clinical signs, cold pulseless extremities and sudden unexplained cyanosis or other respiratory compromise.

Severe cardiac disease or cardiac failure is defined as an intrinsic inability of the heart to perfuse tissues adequately (at normal cardiac filling pressure). As a consequence, compensatory mechanisms are employed to increase cardiac filling pressure (Figure 2.3). This reduces the compensatory reserve available to the cardiovascular system. An unwanted consequence of this increase in filling pressure is the development of free fluid (pleural fluid or ascites) and oedema due to an increase in capillary pressure (and reduced osmolality due to fluid retention). Pulmonary oedema in particular results in reduced lung compliance, limited gaseous exchange and reduced oxygenation of haemoglobin, compounding the hypoxic effects of a failing circulation.

Actual problems	Potential problems	Nursing plan
Inability to mobilize	Decubitus ulcers, hypostatic pneumonia, stiff joints, muscle contracture	Assisted walking, coupage, turning, padded non-retentive bedding, physiotherapy (see Chapter 4)
Tachypnoea, restlessness or discomfort	Hyperthermia	Regular assessment of analgesic requirements
Loss of voluntary urination or incontinence	Bladder atony, urine scald	Bladder management: indwelling urinary catheter or assist patient outside for urination; use non-retentive bedding
Inability to eat and drink unaided or unable to reach food	Dehydration, poor nutrition leading to delayed healing	Tempt, hand-feed, encourage fluid intake, intravenous fluid therapy, record food intake, consider tube feeding
Inability to maintain body temperature	Hypothermia, thermal burns from inappropriate warming techniques	Patient warming (warm air) and temperature monitoring
Inability to groom and clean	Matted coat, pyoderma	Daily grooming/bath

2.2 Nursing plan for the recumbent patient. (NB this is not a comprehensive list; specific causes of recumbency or intercurrent disease may pose risks for other potential problems.)

Organ or tissue	Manner of blood pressure control
Heart	Stroke volume and heart rate
Arterioles	Diameter determines resistance to blood flow
Veins	Storage function (capacitance) allows prompt increase of circulating blood volume in response to neurohormonal stimuli
Autonomic nervous system	Sympathetic and parasympathetic stimulation of receptors to affect heart rate, stroke volume and blood vessel diameter
Kidney	Control of circulating fluid volume, monitoring blood pressure at the macula densa, renin release, aldosterone action
Lung	The respiratory cycle is associated with pressure changes in the thoracic vessels, with an increase in arterial pressure with each inspiration The lungs are also the site of conversion of angiotensin I to angiotensin II, which affects aldosterone function in kidneys and directly acts on arterioles to increase blood pressure
Aortic and carotid baroreceptors	Pressure (baro-) receptors in the aorta and carotid arteries sense and modulate autonomic control of blood pressure
Right atrium	In response to detection of increased circulating volume, atrial natriuretic peptide hormone is produced and affects sodium excretion
Hypothalamus	Osmoreceptors assess the tonicity of the circulating plasma and release antidiuretic hormone to retain pure water if tonicity is elevated
Adrenal gland	Adrenaline produced stimulating receptors in heart and vessels increasing stroke volume, heart rate and reducing vessel diameter
Blood	The thickness (viscosity) of blood influences blood pressure as greater pressure is required to distribute blood of increased viscosity
Skeletal muscle	Contraction of skeletal muscle compresses thin-walled veins and enhances forward movement of venous blood. This increases the volume of blood returned to the heart and stroke volume

2.3 Body systems involved in the maintenance of blood pressure.

Hypertension, in the absence of other clinical signs of an underlying disease, frequently presents with vision deficits due to retinal haemorrhage or detachment. Hypertension should be suspected in cases of renal disease, hyperthyroidism and Cushing's disease (hyperadrenocorticism) as well as less common conditions such as polycythaemia and phaeochromocytoma.

Diagnostic procedures

Electrocardiography

Electrocardiography is performed for two reasons:

- As a monitoring aid
- As a diagnostic tool in the evaluation of cardiovascular status.

An electrocardiogram (ECG) depicts the electrical activity of the heart but does not give information regarding the mechanical function of the heart or the severity of disease. Other diagnostic techniques (i.e. radiography and echocardiography) must be used in conjunction with electrocardiography to evaluate cardiac function. Diagnostic ECGs are carried out preferably on conscious non-sedated patients and the resulting trace recorded on paper for analysis.

Each part of the ECG complex arises from a particular area of the heart. The *P wave* is generated by atrial depolarization, the *QRS complex* is generated by ventricular depolarization, and the *T wave* is generated by ventricular repolarization. A pair of electrodes is called a lead; they may be either monopolar or bipolar. Bipolar leads consist of a positive and a negative electrode. Three active cables are placed on the patient's limbs (the fourth 'earths' the patient). A lead selector switch on the ECG machine selects different combinations of electrodes:

- To record lead I the machine makes the right forelimb electrode negative and the left forelimb electrode positive
- To record lead II the machine makes the right forelimb negative and the left hindlimb positive
- To record lead III the machine makes the left forelimb negative and the left hindlimb positive.

A wave of depolarization travelling towards a positive electrode will result in a positive deflection being recorded; a wave of depolarization travelling towards a negative electrode will result in a negative deflection being recorded.

An ECG shows:

- Heart rate
- Heart rhythm
- Presence or absence of dysrhythmias
- Evidence of metabolic or electrolyte abnormalities that affect the myocardium (e.g. hyper- or hypokalaemia)
- Evidence of abnormalities in cardiac chamber size.

Indications for electrocardiography

- Preoperative screening.
- During anaesthetic monitoring.
- Investigation of cardiac murmurs.
- Evaluation of dysrhythmias.
- Cardiomegaly.
- Acute onset of dyspnoea or cyanosis.
- Shock.
- Investigation of suspected electrolyte disturbances and systemic disease.
- Drug therapy (e.g. digoxin, lidocaine) monitoring.

Obtaining an ECG

The procedure for obtaining an ECG is detailed in Figure 2.4.

---

1. Place patient on a dry insulated surface.
2. Use standard positioning if this is not too distressing for the patient.
3. Attach one electrode on each limb in the standard configuration (Einthoven's limb lead system): on the forelimbs just above or below the olecranon; and on the hindlimbs just above or below the stifle. Electrodes can be stainless steel crocodile clips or adhesive patches (adhesive patch electrodes are best for long-term monitoring). Electrode jelly is used with clips to improve skin contact. Surgical spirit may be used but needs regular application as it evaporates.
   - Red lead – right forelimb.
   - Yellow lead – left forelimb.
   - Green lead – left hindlimb.
   - Black lead – right hindlimb.

   Do not allow the electrodes to contact each other, and keep the patient as still as possible during the procedure.
4. Record 5–10 complexes of leads I, II, III, aVr, aVl and aVf at paper speed 25 mm/second.
5. Record a rhythm strip of lead II at paper speed 50 mm/second.
6. Run a longer rhythm strip at a slower speed if possible when checking for dysrhythmia.
7. Record patient details, date, position and any drugs administered for reference.
8. Make a note of the paper speed, calibration (cm:mV) and whether filters were used.

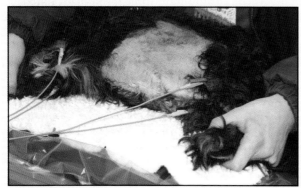

Standard positioning for a diagnostic ECG. The dog is restrained in right lateral recumbency with the limbs extended.

2.4 How to obtain an electrocardiogram (ECG).

Interpretation

Assessment of the trace quality

Artefacts on an ECG trace may be due to electrical interference. This should be minimized by:

- Ensuring there is good electrode contact
- Checking that the electrodes are not corroded or dirty
- Ensuring the equipment is 'earthed' and that other electrical equipment is turned off
- Not touching the electrodes and ensuring the limbs are held apart
- Moving the power leads away from the patient.

Patient-related artefacts (usually due to movement) should be reduced by:

- Working in a quiet area to reduce stress
- Placing the animal on a comfortable surface
- Filing down the teeth on the crocodile clips or using adhesive electrodes to minimize discomfort
- Sedation to reduce movement artefacts from rapid respiration/panting or muscle tremors, although this is not ideal.

Assessment of the heart rate from the trace

The number of complexes in 6 seconds should be counted and then multiplied by 10. Maximum and minimum rates should be obtained if the rate varies.

Assessment of the rhythm from the trace

When assessing the heart rhythm on an ECG, the key questions to address are:

- Is the rhythm regular or irregular?
- If irregular, is it regularly so or irregularly irregular?
- Is there a P wave for every QRS complex and is there a QRS complex for every P wave?
- Are all the P waves alike?
- Are all the QRS complexes alike? A normal complex is called the *sinus complex* (i.e. P wave, QRS complex and T wave).

Examples of ECG traces are given in Figure 2.5.

Sinus rhythm

Heartbeats that originate from the sinoatrial (SA) node make a rhythm called the *sinus rhythm*. A normal sinus rhythm will have a regular rate and rhythm.

- ***Sinus arrhythmia* is when the rate varies regularly due to changes in autonomic tone associated with respiration. This can be normal in the dog but not in the cat.**
- ***Sinus tachycardia* is where the rate is faster than normal; this may be caused by fear, pain, hypovolaemia or drug therapy (e.g. atropine).**
- ***Sinus bradycardia* is where the rate is slower than normal; this may be a normal rate for a fit animal or giant-breed dog. It could also be due to increased vagal tone, hypothermia, hypoxia, hyperkalaemia or hypothyroidism.**

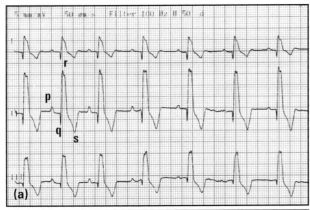

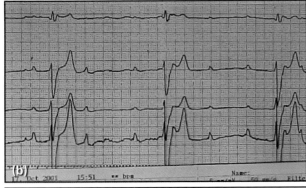

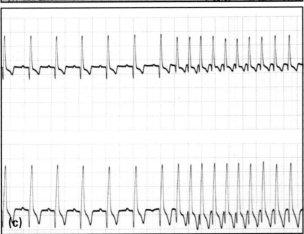

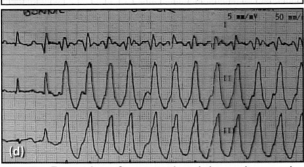

2.5 Examples of a normal and three abnormal ECG traces. **(a)** Normal ECG. Note the synchronous P waves and QRS complexes. Note also the consistency between complexes. **(b)** Third-degree atrioventricular block. Note the asynchrony between the P waves and QRS complexes. Note also the abnormal broad appearance of the QRS complexes. **(c)** Supraventricular tachycardia starts half-way along the trace. Note the rapid heart rate with normal QRS complex appearance.
(d) Ventricular tachycardia after two sinus beats. Note the rapid heart rate with abnormal broad QRS complexes.

Holter monitoring

In cases where episodic weakness or syncope is a clinical sign, it may not be possible to detect abnormalities during a routine cardiac examination. In these cases, a longer period of continuous ECG monitoring may be required. The Holter monitor records heart rate and rhythm for a period of 24–48 hours. After removal, the data are downloaded from the monitor and analysed for abnormal events (Figure 2.6).

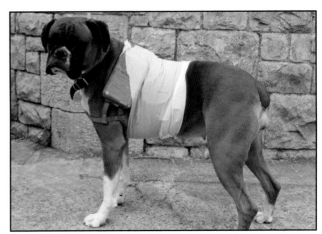

2.6 A Holter monitor attached to a Boxer with intermittent syncope. This dog is wearing an analogue monitor; these have been largely replaced by more compact digital units.

Placement

Adhesive electrodes are placed on the chest (the hair may need to be clipped to ensure good electrode contact) and attached to the monitor. The monitor is taped securely around the animal's body and a bandage applied for support and protection. It is important to ensure that the animal is not able to interfere with or damage the monitor. The owner should be advised to follow the normal routine with regard to exercise but should be reminded to avoid getting the monitor wet.

Telemetry

This is a method of continuous monitoring that can be recorded remotely. Telemetric devices are biosensors or electrical components that detect physiological parameters and convert them to a digital form, in a similar way that a pulse oximeter probe monitors oxygen saturation in capillary blood. The digital signal is then sent to a transmitting device via a cable connection or a wireless radiofrequency transmitter. The information is then received and recorded at a remote location. Some institutions prefer to use cardiac telemetry as an alternative to Holter monitoring for the diagnosis of rhythm abnormalities affecting hospitalized patients.

Echocardiography

This is a non-invasive method of imaging the heart and evaluating cardiac chamber size and myocardial function. Echocardiography also provides information regarding valve function and the appearance of surrounding great vessels (see Chapter 11 for further details).

Thoracic radiography

Thoracic radiographs are performed as part of the diagnostic assessment of patients with heart disease or heart failure, and complement echocardiography. Two radiographic views of the thorax (right lateral and dorsoventral) should be taken.

Blood pressure measurement

Heart disease can arise from systemic hypertension or be the cause of systemic hypertension, so measurement of arterial blood pressure is important in diagnosing cardiac disease and monitoring treatment. Blood pressure measurement must be performed using instrumentation validated in that species and for that size of patient.

Normal systolic blood pressure in dogs has been reported between 131 mmHg and 154 mmHg. In cats the range is 115–162 mmHg, although most studies describe a mean systolic blood pressure of <140 mmHg. Treatment of hypertension, in the absence of an underlying disease, is warranted and current recommendations are that the goal of treatment is to reduce systolic pressure to <150 mmHg. Arterial blood pressure measurement for diagnostic purposes is usually performed using an indirect (non-invasive) method; either the Doppler or oscillometric technique (Figure 2.7).

- The Doppler technique – this is described in the *BSAVA Manual of Practical Veterinary Nursing*.
- The oscillometric technique – a cuff is placed around a limb or tail where a palpable pulse

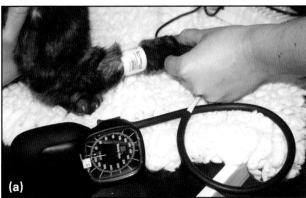

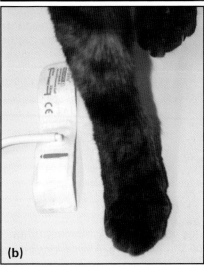

2.7

(a) Doppler measurement of blood pressure in a cat. **(b)** Cuff suitable for oscillometric measurement of blood pressure.

can be detected. The cuff is inflated to various pressures and at each cuff pressure the oscillations caused by the pulse are detected and read automatically.

Commonly, the sites of peripheral pulses on the fore- and hindlimbs of cats and dogs are used for indirect blood pressure measurement; the tail can also be used successfully in the cat. The cuff should fit the patient correctly, and not be placed too tightly or too loosely, otherwise inaccurate readings will be given. Oscillometric readings may be unreliable in cats and small dogs with tachycardia. Blood pressure readings should be carried out in a quiet environment and with the patient as still as possible. At least three measurements should be taken to see whether the readings are consistent. For blood pressure measurements to be valid, a cuff of the correct width must be applied. The correct cuff width is 40% of the circumference of the limb in question. The cuff should be firmly applied without causing vascular occlusion prior to inflation.

Fundoscopy

Retinal detachment can occur with systemic hypertension (see below for further details on the ophthalmic examination).

Nursing considerations

Patients with cardiovascular disease have special nursing requirements. The patient should be frequently reassessed as this will give valuable information about the animal's status and response to therapy.

- Information regarding circulation and peripheral perfusion can be gathered by making an assessment of pulse quality. Comparison should be made between pulses at different sites, for example, femoral and metatarsal pulses. A paradoxical pulse, where the pulse becomes weaker at inspiration and stronger at expiration, is sometimes evident if fluid has accumulated around the heart (pericardial effusion). Cardiac auscultation should also be carried out in conjunction with pulse assessment.
- Absence of a femoral pulse is a significant finding and may indicate the presence of aortic thromboembolism. With heart disease, the cardiac ventricles and atria can become enlarged, disrupting blood flow within the heart and making clot (thrombus) formation more likely. Part of the thrombus may then break loose and lodge (embolize). A common site for a thromboembolism is the point at which the aorta divides to become the femoral arteries. In animals with an aortic thromboembolism there will be no femoral pulse and the hindlimb(s) will feel cold.
- Animals with cardiac failure can develop pleural effusion so it is important to monitor respiration rates and respiratory effort, and instigate further nursing interventions as necessary.
- Continual or intermittent ECG and blood pressure monitoring may be required to assess a patient's response to medication.

- During hospitalization these patients may require emergency treatment and intravenous medication, thus venous access should be maintained.
- The veterinary nurse should consider seeking advice regarding administration of light sedation if a patient is stressed or overexcited, as hyperventilation can exacerbate pulmonary oedema.
- If fluid therapy is being administered to a patient with cardiovascular disease it is necessary to be aware of the possibility of fluid overload and pulmonary oedema.
- Exercise restriction may be necessary if the patient is active; however, most cardiovascular patients' exercise tolerance levels will be lower and therefore self-limiting. Patients with advanced cardiac disease should not be exercised.
- Any special instructions should be noted before handling drugs. For example, some cardiac drugs (glyceryl trinitrate) should be administered wearing gloves.
- Alterations in diet may be required: a low sodium prescription diet may be recommended for patients with cardiac disease as this may help to reduce the compensatory effects of heart failure on water retention. Weight loss may also be advised in the long term if the patient is overweight.

Pericardiocentesis

It is occasionally necessary to undertake drainage of a pericardial effusion as an urgent procedure.

- If the patient's clinical status allows, sedation may be administered.
- Ultrasonographic guidance (i.e. echocardiography) will be necessary.
- ECG monitoring during the procedure will detect any development of arrhythmia. Oxygen therapy should also be available if required.
- The patient is placed in left lateral recumbency on a comfortable surface and the hair clipped over the right chest wall from about the third to the seventh intercostal space. Drainage from the right side reduces the possibility of damage to the lungs and major vessels.
- The skin is prepared aseptically and aseptic technique is used throughout the procedure.
- Local anaesthetic is infiltrated under the skin and into the intercostal muscles.
- A small stab incision is made in the skin and an over-the-needle catheter of suitable diameter is introduced for pericardiocentesis and attached to a wide-bore extension set. A three-way tap is placed between the extension tubing and the collection syringe to allow the syringe to be emptied without disconnection.
- A large bowl or measuring jug should be readily available as significant quantities of fluid may be drained.

Therapeutics

Mild to moderate cardiac disease does not always merit therapeutic intervention. In cases demonstrating electrical dysfunction, medical (antidysrhythmic) therapy is selected on the basis of the type of rhythm disorder (Figure 2.8).

In cases of mild to moderate congestive heart disease, the compensatory mechanisms may be supporting circulatory function adequately so therapy is unrewarding. These patients require monitoring as the cardiac disease is likely to be progressive. In cases with severe congestive failure, the compensatory mechanisms that have increased cardiac filling pressure become life-threatening by increasing the work the heart has to do to maintain perfusion. Treatment is directed at reducing cardiac filling pressure, systemic arterial pressure and oedema, together with nursing interventions (Figure 2.9).

Indication	Therapeutic goal	Drug	Notes
Atrial fibrillation (AF)	Restoration of sinus rhythm	Amiodarone Sotalol Quinidine	Often unsuccessful and frequently reverts back to AF
	Reduce transfer of electrical impulses to ventricles	Digitalis glycosides: digoxin	Important interactions with other drugs, including cimetidine, metoclopramide, furosemide Narrow therapeutic window
		Beta-blockers: propanolol, atenolol	Usually used with digoxin at reduced dose rates
		Calcium channel blockers: diltiazem, verapamil	Usually used with digoxin at reduced dose rates
Third-degree heart block	Control ventricular rhythm	Drug therapy rarely useful	Surgical implantation of pacemaker indicated
Ventricular premature contractions/tachycardia	Reduce ventricular impulse generation	Oral agents: amiodarone, sotalol, mexilitine	Relatively slow onset of action but safer than traditional agents, e.g. procainamide
		Injectable: lidocaine	Used in hospitalized/anaesthetized patients

2.8 Medical therapy for cardiac dysrhythmia. Note: antidysrhythmic drugs carry a risk of inducing other rhythm disturbances and therefore use is reserved for cases in which quality of life is already under threat. Asymptomatic dysrhythmias may be best managed by regular monitoring.

Therapeutic goal	Drug	Notes
Reduce fluid retention	Furosemide	Most commonly used drug May cause hypokalaemia, avoid in renal insufficiency When using diuretics, care should be taken to monitor plasma potassium concentration; contraindicated in cases of renal insufficiency
	Hydrochlorothiazide	Causes hypokalaemia, avoid in renal insufficiency
	Amiloride	Weak potassium-sparing diuretic, can be co-administered with loop diuretics/thiazides Avoid in diabetes mellitus, hyperkalaemia
	Spironolactone	Potassium-sparing diuretic, can be co-administered with loop diuretics/thiazides Avoid in diabetes mellitus, hyperkalaemia
Improve tissue perfusion	Angiotensin converting enzyme (ACE) inhibitors: benazepril, enalapril, ramipril	Enalapril requires dose adjustment in renal insufficiency ACE inhibitors can induce hypotension
	Alpha-blockers: prazosin, carvedilol	Used as adjuncts to other therapies including, diuretics, ACE inhibitors, positive inotropes
	Hydralazine	Frequently used in conjunction with ACE inhibitors Can induce hypotension
Increase cardiac contractility	Digitalis glycosides: digoxin, digitoxin	Sensitive to interactions with other drugs including cimetidine, metoclopramide, furosemide Narrow therapeutic window Less commonly used than pimobendan
	Pimobendan	Contraindicated in hypertrophic cardiomyopathy
	Dobutamine	Intravenous use for short-term support
Reduce cardiac filling pressure	Glyceryl trinitrate ointment	Use in short-term management of oedema *Caution: wear gloves to apply*
Improve tissue oxygenation	Oxygen	Consider nasal prongs, oxygen tent
Increase lusitropy	Diltiazem	Indicated in hypertrophic cardiomyopathy; reduces cardiac contractility
Reduce blood pressure	ACE inhibitors: benazepril, enalapril, ramipril	Enalapril requires dose adjustment in renal insufficiency ACE inhibitors reduce proteinuria
	Amlodipine	Reduce dose in hepatic dysfunction
Normalize pro-coagulant state	Aspirin	Low dose therapy Risk of nephrotoxicity
	Dalteparin	Injectable agent; not fully validated

2.9 Treatment for congestive heart disease. In addition to drug treatment, other nursing actions, such as enforced rest and provision of a calm environment at a suitable temperature and humidity, should be provided for these patients.

Cardiac disease is a risk factor for the development of thromboembolism. The most likely explanation is sluggish blood flow in the atria caused by atrial dilatation as in mitral or tricuspid valve regurgitation in dogs or poor ventricular filling, e.g. in hypertrophic cardiomyopathy in cats. Patients at high risk may be suitable candidates for anticoagulant therapy (see Figure 2.9).

Nursing the patient with respiratory disease

Presenting complaints

Clinical signs may help to localize the problem (Figures 2.10 to 2.13), which in turn can direct appropriate diagnostic procedures.

Location	Clinical signs
Nose	Snorting (stertorous respiration), sneezing, nasal discharge, epistaxis, facial deformity
Throat/tonsils	Snorting, frequent swallowing, dysphagia, pain on swallowing, single hacking coughs
Larynx	Laboured breathing (stridorous respiration), marked exercise intolerance, cyanosis
Trachea	Cough, typically bouts of dry and non-productive coughing
Bronchi	Cough, dry and non-productive or moist and productive coughing
Bronchioles	Productive cough, lethargy
Alveoli	Lethargy, soft cough, audible moist sounds on auscultation
Pleura	Dry cough, exaggerated respiratory movements (hyperpnoea), shallow breathing (if painful)
Interstitial (structural) lung disease	Dry cough, weakness, fresh blood in sputum

2.10   Localization of respiratory disease by clinical signs.

Condition	Clinical signs	Cause	Comments
Congenital	Stertor Exercise intolerance	Typical component of brachycephalic obstructive syndrome	Often accompanied by soft palate hyperplasia and laryngeal collapse
Inflammatory (rhinitis)	Variable discharge Anorexia (especially cats)	Chronic viral infection (cats) Degenerative disease (dogs, hyperplastic rhinitis) Fungal or bacterial infection	Clinical signs resemble those seen with neoplasia
Neoplasia	Stertor Nasal discharge Epistaxis	Adenocarcinoma Lymphoma	May be managed by chemotherapy (lymphoma) or radiotherapy (carcinoma)

2.11   Diseases of the nasal passages.

Condition	Clinical signs	Cause	Comments
Congenital	Stertor Exercise intolerance	Typical component of brachycephalic obstructive syndrome	Often accompanied by stenotic nares and laryngeal collapse
Inflammatory	Pharyngitis Laryngitis Tracheitis	Typical features of an acute upper respiratory tract infection	Chronic cases are less common
Neoplasia	Stertor Stridor Cough Dyspnoea	Lymphoma Carcinoma	Lymphoma relatively common in cats Neoplasms at this site are generally rare in dogs
Degenerative	Dyspnoea Dysphagia Dysphonia Cough	Neuromuscular disorders (e.g. generalized neuropathy) Tracheal collapse	Canine laryngeal paralysis is sometimes associated with generalized neuromuscular disease See Chapter 8

2.12   Diseases of the pharynx, larynx and trachea.

Condition	Clinical signs	Cause	Comments
Inflammatory	Dyspnoea Cough Systemic illness	Bronchitis	Acute (with an upper respiratory tract infection) or chronic (e.g. due to irritation or allergy)
		Pneumonia	May be bacterial, viral, allergic or parasitic in origin
		Pleuritis/pyothrax	Typically bacterial, following penetration or haematogenous infection Coronavirus in cats
Neoplasia	Weight loss Cough Dyspnoea	Primary lung tumours	Relatively common in older dogs as a solitary mass Often large before clinical signs develop
		Metastatic (secondary) neoplasia	Multiple secondary masses (or diffuse disease) can be seen with primary malignancies elsewhere

2.13   Diseases of the lower airways, lungs and pleura.

Diagnostic procedures

The key techniques for investigating upper respiratory tract (URT) disease are radiography, advanced imaging and endoscopy (including thoracoscopy) (see Chapters 10 and 11).

Nasal biopsy

There are a number of techniques for collecting nasal biopsy samples, including:

- Nasal flush: saline is delivered by syringe into the nostril under pressure in an attempt to dislodge tissue (Figure 2.14), which is then collected at the back of the pharynx in a collecting device. A cuffed endotracheal tube must be used and the cuff must be properly inflated prior to the flush
- 'Grab' biopsy sample using forceps
- Nasal swabs and cultures
- Cytology brushing.

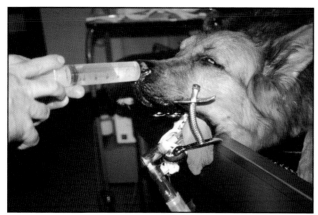

2.14 A patient positioned for a nasal flush biopsy.

Aspergillus serology

Serology for the detection of circulating antibodies to *Aspergillus* is one of the methods used in the diagnosis of nasal aspergillosis.

Tracheal lavage

Tracheal washing is generally carried out using a trans-tracheal technique as this can be undertaken in the conscious patient, although in an anaesthetized patient samples can be collected via an endotracheal tube.

- The patient should be restrained in a sitting position with the nose elevated.
- The ventral neck should be clipped and aseptically prepared.
- Local anaesthetic should be instilled at the site of entry over the cricothyroid ligament, which is located just above the cricoid cartilage.
- A 14- or 16-gauge over-the-needle catheter (18-gauge for a cat) should be introduced to the tracheal lumen. The stylet should be removed and either an endoscopy suction catheter or a through-the-needle jugular catheter introduced.
- The longer catheter, pre-filled with warm saline, should be advanced to the bronchial bifurcation; 3–5 ml of sterile saline should be gently instilled and aspirated immediately.

- The sample collected should be divided into an ethylene diamine tetra-acetic acid (EDTA) tube for cytology and a plain tube for bacteriology.

Bronchoalveolar lavage

Bronchoalveolar lavage (BAL) is a technique for collection of cytological samples from the pulmonary parenchyma and is routinely carried out under anaesthesia with the patient in sternal recumbency, but may be carried out in lateral recumbency with the affected side down at the clinician's discretion. Samples are collected via a suction catheter passed down the biopsy channel of an endoscope or by passing a suction catheter through the lumen of an endotracheal tube under endoscopic guidance.

Thoracic and pleural biopsy

Fine-needle aspirate samples of lung lobe or thoracic masses and pleural fluid may be obtained using ultrasonographic guidance. Blind percutaneous sampling is not advised as this may lead to pleural haemorrhage or pneumothorax. Patients should be monitored closely both during and following the procedure for deterioration in respiratory function. The thorax is clipped and prepared aseptically and the biopsy site infiltrated with local anaesthetic. Needle aspirate samples may submitted for cytological or microbiological analysis.

Thoracic drainage of pleural effusion

Drainage of effusions is both diagnostic (see Chapter 12) and therapeutic. Pleural effusions can be drained intermittently via thoracocentesis, or where effusions are likely to re-accumulate an indwelling thoracic drain can be placed. Thoracic drain placement can be performed under general anaesthesia, or sedation with additional local anaesthetic, depending on the status of the patient (see Chapter 8).

Blood gas analysis

Arterial blood samples are useful for evaluating respiratory function as they analyse the gaseous content of the blood. Equipment for in-house analysis of a patient's acid–base status is now more reasonably priced and therefore more widely available (see Chapters 6 and 7 for further details).

Faecal analysis for lungworm

Angiostrongylus vasorum and *Oslerus osleri* in the dog and *Aelurostrongylus abstrusus* in the cat shed larvae which are typically evident in faecal analysis. The larvae are also seen in tracheal or bronchial lavage samples.

Nursing considerations

Initial assessment

Triage should be completed when presented with a patient in respiratory distress. Sometimes the veterinary nurse will need to take action immediately if the patient is acutely dyspnoeic. Oxygen therapy should be administered if the patient is obviously unstable and an emergency management plan instigated. If the patient is stable a more thorough initial assessment can be carried out, including evaluation of respiratory noise and examination for evidence of trauma.

General care

- Venous access is vital in patients with compromised respiratory function; a peripheral intravenous catheter should be placed and maintained.
- Inhalation therapy. This technique allows administration of medication via an inhaler similar to that used by humans. A spacer device has a facemask at one end and an inhaler at the other.
  1. Hold the mouth closed and gently place the device over the nostrils, allowing breathing via the spacer.
  2. When breathing is calm and steady initiate the dose by pressing the inhaler. Allow 30 seconds of breathing to inhale the dose from within the spacer.

  A period of acclimatization to the technique may be necessary before this procedure will be tolerated. The animal should be allowed to get used to the presence of the spacer and inhaler initially from a distance, and then moving closer, the inhaler can be activated so that the patient becomes used to the noise associated with it. When the animal appears comfortable with the mask, place it over the nose with the mouth closed so that the patient gets used to breathing through it. The spacer should be added and the procedure repeated. Once the animal is comfortable with breathing through the mask and spacer, and used to the sound of the inhaler, the inhaler should be added and dosing initiated.
- When long-term oxygen therapy is administered either by mask or nasal catheter, it is beneficial to deliver the oxygen through a bubble humidifier to prevent damage to the respiratory tract from the drying effect of inhaled oxygen. A nebulizer can be used to humidify the respiratory system.
- Sudden changes in environmental temperature (either hot or cold) will often induce coughing. An air-conditioned or thermostatically controlled environment is ideal.
- Physical therapy (coupage) (see Chapter 4) may be beneficial in cases where pneumonia has developed.
- Use of a harness and lead instead of a collar is best if the patient has a compromised airway (especially tracheal disease). Exercise should be restricted but is often limited by what the patient can, or wants to, do.
- Patients should be kept as calm as possible. Handling should be minimized if the animal becomes stressed. Advice should be sought regarding sedation: light sedation in these cases will calm stressed, excitable or noisy dogs and thus improve respiratory function.
- Appropriate pain relief and comfortable bedding will help to encourage the animal to relax and it will be more inclined to take deeper, more effective breaths.
- Collecting blood samples from the jugular veins of cats with URT disease can cause distress. An alternative restraint technique to holding the head at the neck is to hold the muzzle from above, allowing the animal to mouth breathe if wished. If this still results in distress, samples should be collected from the cephalic vein.
- Nutrition is an important nursing consideration, especially in patients with upper respiratory disease. In cases where the nasal passages may be blocked, patients might need extra time and attention, and tempting with warm, stronger smelling food (see Chapter 3).
- Infection control protocols should be put into place to limit the spread of infection from diseases, especially potentially zoonotic conditions such as mycobacteriosis.
- When epistaxis occurs, especially after nasal biopsy procedures, the application of ice in a compress over the nose, with or without sedation, to limit haemorrhage should be considered.
- Patients with nasal discharge will require frequent face cleaning, and the use of barrier cream may prevent skin sores from developing.

Therapeutics

Mild to moderate rhinitis is typically self-limiting; if this is not the case, a diagnosis should be made. Chronic and severe rhinitis requires treatment directed at the inciting cause. Since diagnosis can be challenging, this is not always possible; at times these cases are managed by the speculative administration of antibiotic and anti-inflammatory therapies. Nebulization can also be helpful. Fungal rhinitis (typically aspergillosis in dogs) requires intensive, usually topical, therapy.

Medical management of cases presenting with non-nasal URT disease typically involves administration of appropriate pharmaceutical preparations (Figure 2.15). Drug delivery to airway tissues is incomplete when agents are administered by oral or injectable routes. More efficient drug delivery can be achieved with inhaled therapies. This permits the use of drugs with minimal absorption into the systemic circulation, reducing the risk of adverse systemic effects and allowing use of agents that would not achieve therapeutic levels by conventional drug delivery routes.

Drug	Effects	Further considerations
Corticosteroids: prednisolone, dexamethasone, beclometasone [a], budesonide [a], fluticasone [a]	Reduce inflammation Bronchodilation	Immunosuppression can promote the development of infectious disease Systemic consequences of inhaled therapy are minimal

2.15 Therapeutics used in chronic airway disease. [a] Inhalation therapy. (continues)

Drug	Effects	Further considerations
β-receptor agonists (non-selective): adrenaline (epinephrine), ephedrine, isoprenaline	Reduce inflammation Bronchodilation Reduce mucus viscosity Enhance ciliary activity	Can be used in acute emergency but systemic effects include tachycardia and hypertension
β-receptor agonists (selective): terbutaline, salbutamol [a]	Reduce inflammation Bronchodilation Reduce mucus viscosity Enhance ciliary activity	Systemic effects of orally administered agents include tachycardia and hypotension
Methylxanthines: theophylline, aminophylline, etamiphylline	Reduce inflammation Bronchodilation Reduce mucus viscosity Enhance ciliary activity	Long-acting theophylline preparation available Adverse effects include nausea, arrhythmias and restlessness
Anticholinergics: atropine, glycopyrrolate	Reduce sensitivity of irritant receptors Bronchodilation	Reduce mucus clearance Rarely used
Mucolytic: bromhexine	Reduce mucus viscosity	Reflex fluid secretion triggered by gastric irritation
Antitussives: codeine, butorphanol	Centrally acting cough suppression	Side-effects include respiratory depression, sedation and constipation
Antibiotics: ideally according to culture but empirically cephalosporins are often used	Treat acute or chronic bacterial bronchopneumonia	An underlying cause should be identified if possible (e.g. aspiration)

2.15 (continued) Therapeutics used in chronic airway disease. [a] Inhalation therapy.

Nursing the patient with gastrointestinal disease

Presenting complaints

Oesophageal disease (Figure 2.16) is frequently represented by regurgitation. It is diagnostically important to differentiate regurgitation from vomiting. The former is the production of ingested material from the oesophagus, the latter indicates that the food material arises from the stomach or beyond in some instances. Regurgitated food typically resembles the ingested product, with white frothy material mixed with it. Patients with oesophagitis are usually inappetent or anorexic and therefore simply regurgitate large volumes of thick frothy mucus. Regurgitation is not an active process and the material can be seen to exit with gravitational

Condition	Cause	Comments
Foreign body	Inappropriate ingestion	Usually requires endoscopic or (occasionally) surgical retrieval Rare in cats
Oesophagitis	Reflux during anaesthesia A complication of doxycycline therapy	Often painful Depressed Anorexia
Megaoesophagus	Congenital Acquired either as an isolated condition (idiopathic) or secondary to neuromuscular disease	Often present with a moist cough as the primary sign

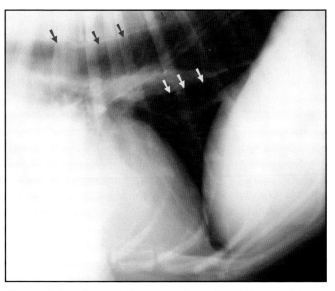

2.16 Oesophageal diseases. The lateral thoracic radiograph is of a standing conscious Great Dane with megaoesophagus. Dorsal and ventral borders of the dilated oesophagus are indicated by red and yellow arrows, respectively.

assistance, usually accompanied by a loud retching sound. Vomit can be variably digested if food material is present, depending on the duration of stomach dwell time. Sometimes there will be a lurid yellow bilious component to the fluid. Vomiting is an active process. Prior to vomition, patients exhibit abdominal heaving accompanied by premonitory respiratory efforts against a closed glottis; patients are also likely to drool immediately prior to vomition.

The cardinal signs of gastrointestinal disease are vomiting and diarrhoea. In simple terms, disease of any part of the intestine from the stomach to the colon, including the liver and pancreas can induce these signs, so they are of relatively little discriminatory value. Typically, upper gastrointestinal disease is accompanied by vomiting more than by diarrhoea and *vice versa*. Vomition of digested blood (haematemesis) is indicative of gastric ulceration. Passage of black tarry faeces (melaena) indicates upper gastrointestinal bleeding. Differential features of diarrhoea arising due to upper or lower gastrointestinal pathology are described elsewhere (see the *BSAVA Manual of Practical Veterinary Nursing*) but care should be taken in their application. The magnitude of the clinical signs is related to the severity of pathology rather than the underlying cause. A spectrum of signs can be seen ranging from mild, transient non-specific changes to severe life-threatening systemic consequences.

Hepatic disease can result in similar clinical signs to those of intestinal disease but generalized hepatic dysfunction can also cause jaundice, encephalopathy, oedema and coagulopathy. Pancreatic diseases include deficiencies of enzyme production and disorders of enzyme containment. Pancreatitis results from situations where the pancreas becomes inflamed (Figure 2.17); both cats and dogs can be affected by this condition. Clinical signs may include any of the following: anorexia, acute vomiting, cranial abdominal pain, pyrexia, diarrhoea and lethargy. Dogs are more likely than cats to show signs of abdominal pain and this often results in the dog assuming a posture referred to as the 'praying stance' (Figure 2.18). This is where the dog lowers itself on its front legs while the back legs stay upright in an attempt to relieve abdominal discomfort. Animals of any age can present with pancreatitis, although young animals are not so frequently affected.

Diagnostic procedures

Urinalysis

Routine urinalysis should be carried out, notably to aid diagnosis of dehydration and rule out protein-losing nephropathy as a cause of hypoproteinaemia (see the *BSAVA Manual of Practical Veterinary Nursing* for further information).

Imaging

Plain films are routinely taken. As endoscopy is now more widely used in practice for diagnostic investigation of stomach and small intestinal disease (see Chapter 10), the necessity to perform barium studies has been reduced (information on this technique

Causes	Comments
High-fat diet	Also seen following feeding after prolonged period of starvation
High circulating lipid concentration	Miniature Schnauzers can develop pancreatitis in association with idiopathic hypertriglyceridaemia
Pancreatic ischaemia	Seen following general anaesthesia (and hypotension)
Duodenal reflux	Stasis of duodenal fluid promotes reflux of activated enzymes
Pancreatic trauma or infiltrative disease	Disruption of pancreatic integrity allows enzymes access beyond pancreatic ducts
Pancreatic duct obstruction	Seen with parasitic infestation, tumours, pancreatic or biliary duct oedema, biliary calculus, surgical interference
Cushing's disease, steroid administration	Mechanism unknown
Diuretics	Furosemide and thiazide diuretics shown to induce pancreatitis
Chemotherapy	L-asparaginase in particular but also seen with others including vincristine, doxorubicin
Antibiotics: tetracycline, sulphonamides	Shown to induce pancreatitis
Hypercalcaemia	Mechanism unknown

2.17 Proven and suspected causes of pancreatitis.

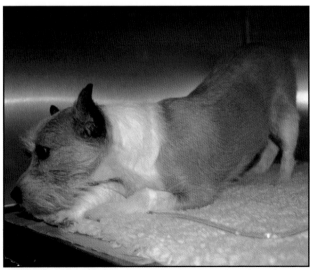

2.18 A dog with abdominal pain adopting the 'praying stance'.

can be located in the *BSAVA Manual of Practical Veterinary Nursing*). Portovenography (see Chapter 11) is used in some patients with liver dysfunction. Ultrasonography is particularly useful for evaluating intestinal wall thickness, gathering samples via fine-needle aspiration, obtaining needle core tissue biopsy (e.g. TruCut®) samples and assessment or drainage of abdominal fluid. Ultrasonography should be carried out in advance of endoscopy due to the accumulation of gas with endoscopic procedures. Endoscopic examination of the oesophagus, stomach, duodenum, colon and ileum is a key part of the investigation of these patients (see Chapter 10).

Biopsy

Liver biopsy

A liver biopsy may be indicated in order to establish a final diagnosis and prognosis where hepatic disease is suspected:

- To explain structural abnormalities or hepatomegaly of unknown cause
- To determine hepatic involvement in systemic disease
- To define the anatomical extent of neoplastic disease
- To explain abnormal hepatic function tests and/or response to treatment.

The method by which a liver biopsy is collected may be influenced by a number of things:

- Liver size and texture
- Size of specimen required
- Patient's suitability for anaesthesia
- Patient's coagulation status
- Available equipment.

Collection methods

The biopsy sample may be collected surgically or percutaneously (needle biopsy).

Laparotomy

Exploratory laparotomy allows examination of the entire gastrointestinal tract and the collection of multiple biopsy samples, larger than those obtained by endoscopy or other non-invasive methods. However, since there is significant morbidity associated with full-thickness biopsy of the small intestine, often endoscopic biopsy is recommended initially, with surgical biopsy performed if the results are unhelpful.

Patient care

The patient's coagulation status should be assessed regardless of which method of sample collection is selected. A complete coagulation profile includes activated clotting time (ACT), activated partial thromboplastin time (APTT), prothrombin time (PT), platelet count and buccal mucosal bleeding time (Figure 2.19). Von Willebrand factor should be measured in susceptible breeds in advance of liver biopsy.

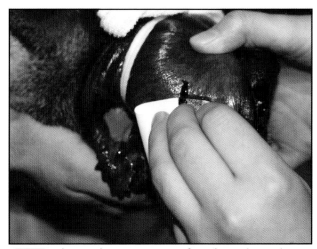

2.19 A veterinary nurse performing a buccal mucosal bleeding time test. Note the upper lip is everted by a bandage; filter paper is used to absorb excess blood without disturbing the primary clot.

Patients with liver disease and possible coagulopathies should be handled carefully and monitored for signs of spontaneous haemorrhage or bruising. The number of occasions that venepuncture is required should be minimized by collecting blood for all diagnostic analyses at one time. Food should be withheld from the patient prior to liver biopsy, even if the technique is to be performed with the patient conscious, as food in the stomach may inhibit visualization of abdominal structures during the ultrasound examination. The patient should be observed closely during the recovery period for signs of intra-abdominal haemorrhage.

Blood ammonia concentration

Ammonia is produced by intestinal bacteria and should be cleared by the liver as blood flows through the portal vessels. Increased plasma ammonia concentration is evidence of impaired hepatic function and/or the presence of a portosystemic shunt.

Liver tissue copper assay

Some breeds of dog are affected by inherited disorders that cause hepatic accumulation of copper, including the Bedlington Terrier, Dobermann and West Highland White Terrier. Copper analysis can be requested on formalin-fixed samples.

Canine pancreatic lipase immunoassay

Canine pancreatic lipase immunoassay (CPLI), also known as specific pancreatic lipase (SpecPL), is an immunological test for assessing serum levels of the lipase enzyme that is specifically produced by the (canine) pancreas. The specificity of the assay makes it a good diagnostic test for canine pancreatitis.

Nursing considerations

The advanced nursing considerations and therapeutics for gastrointestinal patients are outlined in Figures 2.20 and 2.21.

Condition	Cause	Nursing considerations	Comments
Nausea	Certain medications Vestibular disease Abdominal disease	Antinausea medication may be helpful	Nausea may be present without vomiting Salivation is an important clinical sign
Dysphagia	Oesophageal and pharyngeal disorders	Manipulate consistency of the diet Consider postural feeding	Aspiration pneumonia is an important complication Some patients may benefit from a gastrostomy tube
Acute pancreatitis	See Figure 2.17	Short-term withholding of oral intake (see Chapter 3)	Maintain hydration with fluid therapy Avoid exposure to food aroma, which may stimulate enzyme secretion
Abdominal distension	Many	Monitor carefully	Deep-chested dogs, in particular, are prone to aerophagia and gastric dilatation during hospitalization

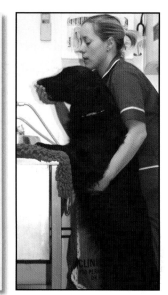

2.20 Nursing considerations for gastrointestinal disease. The photograph shows a dog with megaoesophagus being fed in an upright position by a veterinary nurse. Elevation of the head and thorax encourages passage of food into the stomach.

Condition	Treatment	Comments
Gastro-oesophageal ulceration	Gastroprotectants (sucralfate) Antacids (ranitidine, cimetidine, omeprazole)	Sucralfate suspension is preferred for oesophagitis Sucralfate may interfere with absorption of antacids and other drugs: check treatment intervals
Nausea and vomiting	Metoclopramide Maropitant Antihistamines	Should only be used if gastrointestinal obstruction or perforation have been ruled out Potentially may mask catastrophic disease
Dehydration/shock	Fluid therapy	Critical to address life-threatening secondary consequences of gastrointestinal disease Many acute cases are self-limiting and this is the prime treatment consideration
Inflammatory bowel disease	Exclusion diet therapy	Critical to emphasize the importance of the exclusion principle
	Corticosteroids: prednisolone	Polyuria/polydipsia/polyphagia. Risk of iatrogenic Cushing's disease, skin, coat and metabolic changes
	Corticosteroids: budesonide	Budesonide has limited systemic effects
	Other immunosuppressive agents: ciclosporin	Increased risk of certain malignancies Nausea, vomiting and diarrhoea seen Potentially nephrotoxic
	Other immunosuppressive agents: azathioprine	Avoid in cats Cytotoxic drug
	Other immunosuppressive agents: cyclophosphamide	Cytotoxic, myelosuppressive drug Risk of sterile haemorrhagic cystitis
Gastrointestinal lymphoma	Combination chemotherapy	See information on oncology (below)
Exocrine pancreatic insufficiency (EPI)	Exogenous enzymatic dietary supplements	Occasionally, patients may respond better to fresh chopped pancreas, although this is difficult to obtain
Hepatic disease	According to diagnosis	In severe insufficiency, treatment of encephalopathy with protein restriction, oral lactulose and antibiotics is useful (see Chapter 3)

2.21 Treatment for common gastrointestinal conditions.

Nursing the patient with neuromuscular disease

Presenting complaints

The presenting complaints of patients with neuro-muscular disorders are detailed in Figure 2.22.

Diagnostic procedures

In addition to routine haematology and biochemistry, specific tests are used to rule out systemic diseases (Figure 2.22).

Neurological examination

A detailed neurological examination is essential in the diagnosis and monitoring of patients with neuromuscular disorders, and is covered in detail in the *BSAVA Manual of Canine and Feline Neurology, 3rd edition.*

Serology

Serum samples are required in order to test for evidence of *Toxoplasma*, *Neospora*, canine distemper virus and feline coronovirus (FCoV), which causes feline infectious peritonitis (FIP).

Condition	Differential diagnoses	Comments
Focal brain and meningeal lesions	Neoplasia: glioma, pituitary tumour, solitary metastasis, choroid plexus tumour, meningioma	May be appropriate for intracranial surgery (see Chapter 8) or radiotherapy May present with a change in mental status and/or seizures and/or specific localizing signs (see Figure 2.23)
	Abscess	Rare
	Trauma	
Generalized brain and meningeal disease	Infectious: ■ Viral: feline infectious peritonitis (FIP) caused by feline coronavirus (FCoV), distemper, rabies ■ Bacterial: any ■ Protozoal: *Neospora*, *Toxoplasma* ■ Metazoal: *Toxocara*	Specific treatment indicated
	Inflammatory: granulomatous meningoencephalitis (GME), necrotizing encephalitis, steroid-responsive meningitis	May be responsive to corticosteroid therapy
	Vascular: transient ischaemic attack, infarction (failure of cardiac output)	Specific treatment not available Less common than in humans
	Developmental: hydrocephalus, lissencephaly	Specific medical and surgical treatments for hydrocephalus are described
	Nutritional: thiamine deficiency	Seen in cats, associated with a raw fish diet
	Toxic: heavy metal, lily poisoning, tetanus, organophosphate, other	Other clinical signs also usually apparent
	Metabolic: hypoglycaemia, portosystemic shunt, hepatic failure, renal failure, hypocalcaemia	Specific treatment indicated
Focal (solitary) spinal lesions	Intervertebral disc disease Vertebral/paravertebral neoplasia Fibrocartilaginous embolism (FCE) Discospondylitis Trauma	See Chapter 8
Diffuse spinal disease	Degenerative myelopathy	Typically seen in old German Shepherd Dogs and other large breeds Non-painful, progressive signs of weakness and ataxia Other diffuse diseases are rare except with diffuse brain disease
Focal peripheral neuropathy	Compression Trauma	May cause motor or sensory deficits Marked and rapid muscular atrophy can be a prominent feature
Polyneuropathy	Secondary to metabolic disease (e.g. hypoglycaemia, hypothyroidism) Protozoal, e.g. toxoplasmosis Immune-mediated (secondary to neoplasia elsewhere) Specific heritable conditions	Diagnosis and specific management is required

2.22 Presenting complaints of the central nervous and neuromuscular systems. (continues) ▶

Condition	Differential diagnoses	Comments
Neuromuscular junctional disorders	Myasthenia gravis (MG)	Most common example Immune-mediated in many cases May be generalized (causing weakness) or localized (commonly as megaoesophagus)
Muscular disease	Inherited degenerative (e.g. muscular dystrophy)	Breed-specific diseases are well recognized, e.g. in the Labrador Retriever
	Acquired degenerative	Associated with systemic diseases such as Cushing's disease and hypothyroidism
	Inflammatory (myositis)	Can be generalized (polymyositis) but also localized, especially masticatory myositis Muscle pain can be difficult to distinguish from generalized bone or joint pain

2.22 (continued) Presenting complaints of the central nervous and neuromuscular systems.

Imaging

Plain radiographs usually are insufficient without further investigations such as myelography, magnetic resonance imaging (MRI) (especially of the brain and spinal cord) and computed tomography (CT) (especially for bone lesions of the skull and vertebrae). Further details can be found in Chapter 11.

Cerebrospinal fluid collection and analysis

A sample of cerebrospinal fluid (CSF) can give useful diagnostic information about certain CNS conditions that may alter the CSF, such as infectious or inflammatory brain or spinal cord disease. Samples of CSF are collected from the subarachnoid space at the cisterna magna or lumbar cistern (see the *BSAVA Textbook of Veterinary Nursing, 4th edition* for more information). If myelography is to be performed, contrast material is injected via a spinal needle after CSF sample collection.

General considerations

If the proper technique is followed, the procedure for collecting a CSF sample is safe and simple; however, this is an invasive diagnostic procedure and there are a number of factors to consider:

- All less invasive tests should have been performed and interpreted first
- The patient must be stable enough for a general anaesthetic
- Complications may include subarachnoid bleeding, spinal cord trauma, respiratory arrest or death from brain herniation (especially with raised intracranial pressure)
- In cases where meningitis is a differential diagnosis, the CSF must be analysed prior to myelography as the introduction of contrast material may increase meningeal irritation
- Recent head trauma and skull or vertebral fractures are contraindications to the procedure.

CSF analysis

- At least 1 ml of fluid is ideal for routine analysis. It may be possible to obtain up to 2 ml from a cisternal puncture site in a large dog, but a lumbar puncture will yield smaller volumes.
- Routine analysis includes a number of tests: cell counts, determination of protein concentration and cytology. If <1 ml of CSF is collected not all of these tests can be performed.
- The physical appearance of the CSF should be noted: a normal sample is perfectly clear and colourless. A red tinge is indicative of haemorrhage and may clear after centrifugation if the haemorrhage occurred during the tap. Discoloration that remains may be due to earlier haemorrhage into the CSF. Turbidity or cloudiness is caused by an increased number of cells, either an increase in white blood cells or of protein content.
- CSF should be analysed as soon as possible after collection, ideally within 30–60 minutes as the cells begin to degenerate after this time and this may affect cell counts. If samples are to be sent to external laboratories a concentrating technique such as Cytospin should be used, where CSF is centrifuged and a slide prepared from the sediment prior to submission. Refrigeration of CSF samples will slow cellular degeneration.
- CSF can be analysed in-house but results may be unreliable unless these tests are carried out frequently. Either cytological examination after slide preparation and staining with a rapid cytological stain or red or white cell counts using a haemocytometer can be performed.

Electromyography

Electromyography (EMG) is a diagnostic procedure which is useful in differentiating primary muscle disorders from muscle weakness caused by neurological disorders, and to localize peripheral nerve disease or damage. Fine needle electrodes are placed through the skin into the muscle to sample electrical activity at the needle's tip. EMG needle electrodes are insulated except for the tip in order to reduce the possibility of interference from other muscles. Normal muscle is electrically silent at rest (except in the endplate region); as the needle electrodes are introduced some electrical activity will be seen, this is known as insertion potentials. Once the inserted needle is motionless the presence and extent of abnormal muscle can be examined, as denervated muscle fibres will exhibit spontaneous electrical activity.

Abnormal EMG findings will often necessitate further investigation, such as nerve conduction studies and muscle or nerve biopsy. It is possible that there may be both nerve and muscle disorders present.

Preparation of patient and environment

EMG should be carried out under general anaesthesia or heavy sedation; the animal will need to be motionless during the procedure, as movement will cause artefacts. The placement of needle electrodes in the muscle will also cause some discomfort to the patient. It may be necessary to switch off other electrical equipment (notably fluorescent lighting and heat pads) in the vicinity of the EMG machine in order to minimize additional electrical interference.

Interpretation

Electrical activity detected by the electrodes is displayed on a monitor as a wave form and may also be displayed audibly through speakers. The presence, size and shape of the wave form will give information about the ability of the muscle to respond to nervous stimulation. Several electrodes may need to be placed in order to obtain an accurate study. Correct interpretation is dependent on the operator being able to distinguish between normal and abnormal findings.

Normal and abnormal findings

Normal findings:

- **Insertion potentials: when a needle electrode is inserted into or moved within a normal muscle, electrical activity is stimulated and this appears on the monitor as a wave form. Although the presence of an insertion potential is a normal finding, some disorders may cause either a prolonged or reduced insertion potential.**

Abnormal findings:
A recording of prolonged spontaneous activity indicates peripheral nerve or muscular problems. Approximately 5–10 days after a peripheral motor nerve lesion occurs, denervated muscle fibres exhibit spontaneous activity and these are recorded in one of two forms:

- **Fibrillation potentials, which appear as biphasic wave forms**
- **Positive sharp waves, which appear as monophasic wave forms.**

Nerve conduction velocity

This test is carried out with similar apparatus to that required for EMG, and is used to evaluate the function of peripheral nerves where a peripheral neuropathy is suspected.

Nerve and muscle biopsy

Biopsy aids diagnosis of suspected peripheral nerve disorders or muscle disease. Biopsy sample collection is a relatively minor procedure carried out under general anaesthetic. Accurate interpretation is carried out in specialist laboratories and each will have specific instructions regarding collection and processing of samples; guidance should be sought from the laboratory regarding the preferred protocol prior to sample collection. Commonly, fresh (frozen) and fixed muscle specimens are required. If immediate freezing is not possible, the fresh sample should be wrapped in a saline-moistened swab and shipped to the laboratory on ice as quickly as possible.

Edrophonium response test

This is a test which may give a presumptive diagnosis of myasthenia gravis (MG). A short-acting anticholinergic drug, edrophonium chloride, is administered intravenously and a dramatic improvement in muscle strength and the animal's ability to move unaided will be seen if the test is positive. Not all responses are dramatic and the test can prove inconclusive. An intravenous catheter should be placed in order to administer the drug and atropine sulphate must be readily available in case of an adverse reaction.

Acetylcholine receptor antibody titre

Acquired MG is an autoimmune disease of neuromuscular transmission; it can be either focal or generalized. Animals affected by focal MG usually present with megaoesophagus as the weakness affects the oesophageal, pharyngeal and facial muscles. In generalized MG there is also weakness in the skeletal muscles. A serum sample is collected and analysed for the presence of acetylcholine receptor antibodies (AchRAb). A positive sample indicates acquired MG.

Type 2M muscle fibre antibody assay

Masticatory muscle myopathies can be diagnosed by analysis of the serum from affected animals for the presence of autoantibodies against type 2M muscle fibres.

Nursing considerations
Neurological assessment

Veterinary nurses caring for neurological patients will not usually be required to carry out a full neurological assessment of hospitalized patients, but these animals will need daily assessment as part of the care plan in order that progress can be monitored. It is important that this assessment is carried out methodically and that the information gathered is noted and interpreted correctly.

Observations

In addition to observing the patient's mental status and for signs of aberrant behaviour, the animal's posture, gait and postural reactions should also be evaluated.

Posture

- Head tilt (Figure 2.23) usually indicates vestibular dysfunction.
- Head turn is when the head is held level but the nose is turned to the right or left. Torticollis is abnormal curvature of the neck and may be demonstrated by animals with cervical lesions. Animals with forebrain lesions may tend to turn the head and circle in one direction.
- Recumbent animals may exhibit abnormally rigid limbs (Figure 2.24). Decerebrate rigidity produces extension of all four limbs and sometimes dorsiflexion of the head and neck. This posture is usually caused by a brainstem lesion and affected patients may have decreased consciousness.
- Decerebellate rigidity occurs with acute cerebellar lesions and is characterized by thoracic limb extension, dorsiflexion of the head and neck and normal mentation.
- The Schiff–Sherrington posture is where there is extension of the thoracic limbs with paralysis of the pelvic limbs, and is associated with a thoracic or lumbar spinal lesion.

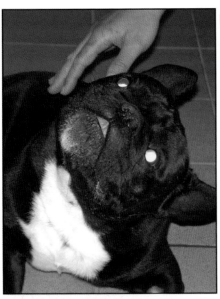

2.23 A French Bulldog demonstrating marked head tilt due to vestibular syndrome.

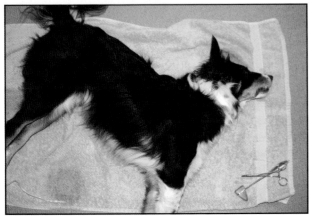

2.24 A dog adopting an opisthotonic posture due to immune-mediated meningitis. This dog is conscious though minimally responsive; the dog was ambulatory only 12 hours earlier.

Gait

The ability to stand and move requires intact motor and proprioceptive systems, so the animal's ability to make coordinated movements should be assessed. Gait should be evaluated on a non-slip surface and the patient should be observed from side, front and rear. Abnormal gait may be due to an abnormality in coordination (ataxia) or reduced strength of voluntary movement (paresis) or a combination of both.

Postural reactions

Assessing postural reactions discriminates between orthopaedic and neurological disorders. The normal animal has an awareness of the precise position and movements of its body (sensory function). Proprioceptors in joints, tendons and muscles, and also in the inner ear, are sensitive to these movements and send information to the cerebral cortex where it is consciously perceived.

- *Proprioceptive positioning*: With the patient standing squarely on all four limbs and supported if necessary, the paw is turned over so that the dorsal surface is in contact with the ground; if normal proprioception is present the foot should immediately be returned to its normal position.
- *Placing response*: This test is more practical for smaller animals that can be held or those that resent having the feet touched during proprioceptive positioning. As the patient is moved towards the edge of a table and the paw comes into contact with it, the normal animal places the limb forward and rests the paw on the table surface. The thoracic and pelvic limbs are tested and both sides compared. Often the patient will need to be blinded to the fact that the table or other surface is approaching.
- *Hopping reaction*: This test may highlight subtle weakness or ataxia. The patient is held so that all of its weight is supported by one limb and then as the animal is moved laterally, it should hop on that limb to maintain its centre of gravity. Each limb is tested individually and compared; an equal response should be seen on both sides in the normal dog.
- *Hemiwalking and wheelbarrowing*: During the hemiwalking test the animal's limbs on one side of the body are held up and the animal is moved laterally; this allows the animal's speed and coordination at correcting itself to be assessed. Wheelbarrowing tests the thoracic limbs; the animal is forced to move forward whilst its pelvic limbs are held off the ground.

Spinal reflex assessment

Spinal reflexes are assessed to evaluate whether the type of disorder is lower motor neuron (LMN) or upper motor neuron (UMN). This also allows more specific localization of spinal lesions. LMN disease results in paresis or flaccid paralysis with a loss of normal reflexes. UMN disease also result in paresis or paralysis but muscle tone is retained and typically increased.

There are a number of reflexes that are assessed in both thoracic and pelvic limbs as part of the neurological examination:

- Thoracic limb:
  - Triceps (involves spinal segments C7–C8, T1–T2)
  - Extensor carpi radialis (involves spinal segments C7, T1–T2)
  - Biceps brachii (involves spinal segments C6–C8)
  - Pedal withdrawal (involves spinal segments C6–T2).
- Pelvic limb:
  - Patellar (involves spinal segments L4–L6)
  - Cranial tibial (involves spinal segments L6–L7)
  - Gastrocnemius (involves spinal segments L7–S1)
  - Pedal withdrawal (involves spinal segments L4–S2).
- Perineum:
  - Stimulation of the perineum with haemostatic forceps should result in contraction of the anal sphincter and flexion of the tail. This tests the tail reflexes and highlights lesions in the spinal cord below S1.

The veterinary nurse is unlikely to check all spinal reflexes on a daily basis for each hospitalized patient but should be aware of the presence of the pedal withdrawal reflex and not confuse it with the patient's ability to perceive pain (deep pain perception).

Sensory evaluation

The purpose of testing pain perception is to detect and map out areas of sensory loss. The use of analgesic and sedative drugs prior to performing this test may alter results. If superficial pain responses are absent then deep pain perception can be tested. Haemostatic forceps can be used to compress the digits or tail, the degree of compression can be increased until a response is elicited. Withdrawal of the limb indicates only an intact reflex arc. A behavioural response such as turning the head or vocalization indicates conscious pain perception. All four limbs, the tail and the perineal region should be assessed. The presence or absence of deep pain perception is important in assessing the prognosis for recovery in patients with severe spinal cord injury.

Bladder function assessment

Animals that have spinal cord injury or disease may be unable to urinate voluntarily or effectively, and will be at risk of damage to the bladder wall as a result of over-distension and of developing a urinary tract infection (UTI). Bladder function is generally assessed by the presence or absence of muscular tone in the urethral sphincter muscle. In the non-ambulatory patient difficulty in expressing the bladder and spurting of urine may suggest an UMN lesion to the bladder. An easily expressed and a flaccid bladder implies a LMN lesion. LMN deficits generally carry a more guarded

prognosis. Bladder function is not easily assessed at a single examination. The size of the patient's bladder should be assessed at regular intervals throughout the day and this should be documented.

Seizures

Prolonged seizure activity (status epilepticus) will cause neurological damage. As a result of a prolonged seizure the patient may also become hyperthermic and suffer respiratory distress. These patients should be treated as emergency cases:

- The airway should be checked to see if it is patent
- Temperature, pulse and respiration rates should be evaluated
- Peripheral venous access should be obtained
- The clinician should be consulted regarding emergency treatment
- Hyperthermic patients should be cooled
- Blood samples should be obtained to determine glucose levels
- The patient should be placed in a quiet, darkened area for nursing.

Head trauma

The main nursing consideration with patients suffering from head trauma is the management of intracranial pressure. A rise in intracranial pressure can cause secondary brain damage, which can be life-threatening. Jugular occlusion, exaggerated respiratory movements and distress should be avoided.

Tetanus

Nursing involves care in a quiet, dark environment (cotton wool ear plugs may reduce reaction to noise) and nutritional support via feeding tubes until the animal is able to prehend and swallow. Urinary retention may require bladder catheterization. Full recovery may take weeks.

Myasthenia gravis

Patients may require assistance to walk outside and should only be taken a short distance. Myasthenic animals may also develop megaoesophagus, requiring postural feeding and treatment of aspiration pneumonia. Nursing these patients can be a very time-consuming and challenging process.

Peripheral nerve disorders

Animals with facial paralysis will require corneal lubrication in order to prevent corneal damage. Peripheral vestibular signs and Horner's syndrome, or drooping of the upper eyelid, may also be evident. Patients with facial nerve deficits may require assistance with feeding, and the mouth and face may need regular bathing to remove accumulated food from the buccal pouch and within the mouth.

Therapeutics

The treatment for patients with neuromuscular disorders is given in Figure 2.25.

CNS disorder	Treatment	Further considerations
Seizures	Phenobarbital	First line therapy. Can be given intravenously in status epilepticus or cluster seizures
	Potassium bromide	Used primarily in synergy with phenobarbital in refractory cases. Slow onset of action (weeks)
	Gabapentin	Used as sole therapy in refractory cases. Expensive treatment; data for its use are relatively sparse
	Propofol	Intravenous treatment for status epilepticus. Requires constant monitoring
	Diazepam	Used intravenously in status epilepticus and per rectum in preictal phase. Efficacy variable. Risk of hepatic failure in cats
	Midazolam	Used intravenously (infusion) as adjunct to phenobarbital in status epilepticus or cluster seizures
Protozoal encephalitis	Clindamycin	Clindamycin can induce transient vomiting
Thiamine deficiency	Vitamin B1	Complete resolution possible if diagnosed early
Bacterial meningitis	Bactericidal antibiotics	As indicated by bacteriology results
Granulomatous meningomyeloencephalitis	Prednisolone	Variably responsive to therapy, can relapse after apparent complete remission
	Cytarabine	Cytotoxic drug
Hydrocephalus	Surgical management	Stent placement can relieve fluid build up
Brain tumour	Radiotherapy	
Necrotizing encephalitis	Supportive care	
Lissencephaly	Supportive care	
Toxic disease	Supportive care	
Viral disease	Supportive care	
Lymphoma	Chemotherapy	
Steroid-responsive meningitis	Prednisolone	Can relapse but typically maintain complete remission
Meningioma	Surgical management	See Chapter 8
	Radiotherapy	
Intervertebral disc disease	Prednisolone	Conservative management can ameliorate mild to moderate clinical signs but subsequent progressive disease is possible or probable
	Surgical management	See Chapter 8
Discospondylitis	Bactericidal antibiotics	As indicated by bacteriology results
Fibrocartilaginous embolism (FCE)	Supportive care	Complete remission possible. Variable degrees of recovery seen
Paravertebral tumour	Supportive care	Specific neoplastic diagnoses may be amenable to chemotherapy
Degenerative myelopathy	Supportive care	Progressive disease ultimately results in loss of hindlimb/toilet function
Trauma	Anti-inflammatory therapy	As indicated by severity of presenting signs. Oedema can induce compressive damage

2.25 Treatment for central nervous system (CNS) disorders.

Nursing the patient with musculoskeletal disease

Diseases of the musculoskeletal system are detailed in Figure 2.26.

Diagnostic procedures

Arthrocentesis

This is often performed under anaesthesia at the same time as radiographic studies are carried out, but it is possible to collect synovial fluid samples from multiple joints under sedation. Even if only one joint is clinically affected, samples should be collected from other joints if polyarthritis is suspected.

- Hair over the joint should be clipped and the skin prepared aseptically.
- A sterile 21–23 gauge needle attached to a syringe is then inserted into the joint space. Generally, needles of 25 mm length are suitable for most joints but a longer spinal needle may be required for the hip joint.

	Condition	Cause	Treatment
Immature animals	Osteochondrosis	Multifactorial disease affecting articular cartilage	Management of pain, diet and exercise Surgical intervention in selected cases
	Panosteitis	Unknown cause affecting fast-growing immature large-breed dogs	Analgesia Self-limiting
	Rickets	Vitamin D deficiency	Note: rare where commercial pet foods used
	Dwarfism	Thyroid or growth hormone abnormalities	Note: rare
Mature animals	Neoplasia	Osteosarcoma	In cats, often cured by removal (amputation) In dogs, typically has metastasized at the time of diagnosis and requires adjunctive therapy
	Hypertrophic pulmonary osteopathy	Secondary to intrathoracic masses (mechanism unknown)	Improves after treatment of underlying cause
	Osteomalacia	Dietary Also associated with severe chronic renal disease, gastrointestinal disease and hyperparathyroidism	Managed by treatment of underlying cause Note: dietary form rare where commercial pet foods used
	Arthritis	Degenerative joint disease due to congenital malformations Immune-mediated polyarthritis	Treatment of underlying cause Management of bodyweight and exercise Analgesia, especially non-steroidal anti-inflammatory drugs (NSAIDs)

2.26 Medical disorders of the musculoskeletal system.

- Once the tip of the needle is in the joint, gentle suction is applied and synovial fluid removed. Negative pressure on the syringe should be released prior to removal of the needle.
- Only a few drops of synovial fluid are required for cytological examination, and smears on microscope slides should be prepared straight away. Larger samples can be placed into an EDTA tube for further cytological analysis and culture.

Biopsy

Synovial membrane biopsy

This can be useful for diagnosing joint infection and synovial neoplasia. Samples are usually obtained via arthroscopy or arthrotomy where a specific site can be selected. The tissue samples for histopathology should be pinned at either end on to cardboard before being placed in formalin to prevent them from curling up at the edges.

Bone biopsy

Closed biopsy techniques include the use of a Michel trephine or a wide-bore Jamshidi needle to obtain biopsy samples. A trephine may be better for sampling dense bone lesions but it needs to be sharp with an undamaged surface to be effective. Needles manufactured specifically for bone marrow biopsy are often not strong enough to sample bone and therefore retrieve fragmented samples; a 14-gauge Jamshidi needle collects better bone biopsy samples. Bone sampling devices are shown in Figure 2.27. After collection the 'plug' of bone should be placed in formalin as soon as possible so that it does not dehydrate.

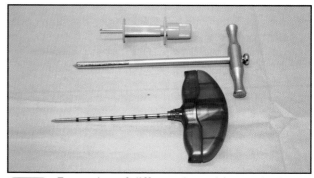

2.27 Examples of different bone biopsy devices. Top: Bone marrow needle. Middle: Michel trephine. Bottom: Jamshidi needle.

Imaging

In addition to standard views, arthrography, spinal survey films, CT and scintigraphy may be useful (see Chapter 11).

Antinuclear antibody and rheumatoid factor assays

These serology tests are indicated when non-infectious, immune-mediated arthritis is suspected. This form of inflammatory joint disease occurs as a result of immune complex deposition within the synovium, leading to a sterile synovitis. Immune-mediated arthritis is often an idiopathic syndrome but can be a feature of systemic lupus erythematosus (SLE). An antinuclear antibody (ANA) titre is required to rule out SLE. Rheumatoid arthritis is another form of immune-mediated polyarthritis; it is characterized by progressive joint destruction. Serology to analyse rheumatoid factor (RF) in addition to a synovial membrane biopsy will confirm the diagnosis.

Serology can also be performed to rule out the presence of infection from the tick-borne spirochaete *Borrelia burgdorferi*, which causes a multi-systemic inflammatory disease known as Lyme disease. In dogs this disease often causes an inflammatory arthritis and lameness. A positive test result would demonstrates elevated levels of antibodies to *Borrelia burgdorferi* but must be interpreted in the light of clinical signs.

Nursing considerations

Pain management

Disease and interventions that involve bone are painful and consequently assessment of pain in these patients is essential. Some breeds are known to be more stoical than others and may not vocalize even if in pain or discomfort. Orthopaedic pain will limit mobilization but this should not be used as a method of exercise restriction: a comfortable animal will be more responsive to rehabilitation techniques such as physiotherapy (see Chapter 4).

Therapeutics

NSAIDs are frequently prescribed for control of chronic orthopaedic pain; this should be noted on the patient's hospital record as it is important that steroid treatment is not used concurrently. Oral NSAIDs should not be administered on an empty stomach or if the animal is vomiting or has diarrhoea. A gastroprotectant drug may also be prescribed in conjunction with this treatment to reduce the likelihood of gastric ulceration.

Diet and physiotherapy

For information on diet and physiotherapy see Chapters 3 and 4, respectively.

Nursing the patient with urogenital disease

Presenting complaints

Kidney disease is defined as chronic or acute. Chronic renal failure is considerably more common than acute renal failure. Due to the production of large volumes of poorly concentrated urine, these patients are susceptible to ascending UTIs and may also develop cystitis. Clinical signs arise due to failure of water conservation and failure to eliminate metabolic toxins. The diseased kidney tubules are usually irreversibly damaged and therefore therapy is directed at supporting the function of whatever viable renal tissue remains.

Acute renal failure is more sudden in onset. There is often a toxin- or drug-induced aetiology (Figure 2.28). Other causes include infection and hydronephrosis due to obstruction of the ureters or urethra. Rather than overproduction of urine, these patients may produce little or no urine (oliguric or anuric renal failure). These cases are considerably more challenging to manage and require aggressive supportive therapy with very close monitoring of all renal functions.

Aetiology	Comments
Non-steroidal anti-inflammatory drugs (NSAIDs): aspirin, ibuprofen, phenylbutazone	All NSAIDs can induce renal failure: fluid deficits should be corrected before these drugs are used
Hypercalcaemia	Secondary to malignancy or vitamin D toxicosis
Haemoglobin (or myoglobin)	Associated with intravascular haemolysis or muscle breakdown (rhabdomyolysis)
Aminoglycoside antibiotics: gentamicin, amikacin, streptomycin	Systemic use is contraindicated in patients with renal compromise
Sulphonamide antibiotics	Can induce sulphonamide crystal formation in dehydrated patients
Iodinated contrast media	Fluid deficits should be corrected before use
Chemotherapy: cisplatin, carboplatin, doxorubicin	Cisplatin use requires intensive diuresis. All chemotherapy can induce nephrotoxicity
Lily poisoning	Ingestion of the leaves or flowers of lilies is fatal to cats
Ethylene glycol	Constituent of antifreeze
Snake/insect envenomation	Snakebite antiserum can also induce renal failure

2.28   Aetiology of acute renal failure.

Diagnostic procedures

Urinalysis

Urinalysis, including bacterial culture, is an essential first step in these cases. See Chapter 12 and the *BSAVA Manual of Practical Veterinary Nursing* for more information.

Imaging

Diagnostic imaging is a key method of diagnosis in these cases and is covered in Chapter 11 and in the *BSAVA Manual of Practical Veterinary Nursing*.

Urine protein:creatinine ratio

This test is useful as an indication of glomerular disease. When there is an excess of protein in the urine and no evidence of urinary tract disease, it is likely that the protein is leaking through the glomerular filters within the kidney. The higher the urine protein:creatinine ratio, the more severe the glomerular disease. The test is performed on a plain sample, preferably collected by cystocentesis.

Water deprivation test

This test is occasionally used as an indicator of the patient's ability to concentrate urine as part of the evaluation of polyuria. Urine specific gravity (SG), packed cell volume (PCV) and total protein (TP) are measured at the start of the test, the bladder is then emptied, and food and water are withheld. Urine SG, PCV and TP are checked every 4 hours during the test and at the end of the test. The test must not continue for more than 24 hours and must be stopped when the urine concentrates or if the animal shows signs of dehydration, i.e. 5% of bodyweight is lost. The water deprivation test should only be performed when other causes of polyuria have been ruled out.

Prostatic wash

This test is used for further investigation of suspected prostatic disease. The patient is placed in lateral recumbency, the prepuce is cleaned and water-soluble lubricant is applied to the catheter tip to facilitate its insertion into the urethra. The bladder is drained and a urine sample collected. A gloved assistant, with the use of lubricant, then places a digit via the rectum over the prostate and feels for the urinary catheter. The catheter is pulled out until the tip is palpable within the prostatic urethra. The assistant increases pressure to massage the prostate in order to release cells. A 10 ml syringe of saline is connected to the urinary catheter and the saline expelled into the prostatic area. The sample is then collected via the syringe and split into two pots: one plain and one with formalin at 2 drops/ml. The first sample pot is submitted for bacteriology and the second sample pot for cytology.

Serum progesterone and oestrogen levels

The assessment of progesterone levels may be used to approximate ovulation in the bitch and to monitor dioestrus. Oestrogen determination may also be a useful diagnostic test for the presence of functional ovarian tissue remnants after ovariohysterectomy.

Vaginal examination

The patient may require sedation for visual examination using a speculum and light source. Vaginoscopy can be useful for evaluating stages of the oestrus cycle and identifying anatomical abnormalities. Microbiology swabs can be taken for culture and sensitivity testing, a smear may also be prepared for cytological examination.

Urolith analysis

Uroliths or calculi are stones that form in the urinary tract. There are a number of reasons for urolith formation. It is important to send the entire stone away for analysis to a specialist laboratory to establish its composition (it may be made up of layers of different types of crystal). Dietary changes may help in preventing further urolith formation once analysis has been carried out.

Nursing considerations

Acute renal failure

Patients that are known to have pre-existing renal disease or a major systemic disease are at risk of developing acute renal failure and consequently must be monitored closely. Administration of nephrotoxic drugs or prolonged anaesthesia may be sufficient to precipitate acute renal failure. At-risk patients should have urine output monitored and be observed for signs of dehydration. Patients in acute renal failure often develop a subnormal body temperature and are weak, pale and lethargic. Supportive nursing includes:

- Correction of dehydration and fluid imbalance with fluid therapy
- Monitoring of vital signs (temperature, pulse, respiration and blood pressure measurement) and the correction of hypothermia
- Monitoring of bodyweight daily
- Urinalysis, including urine SG and proteinuria tests, and urine output
- Correction of electrolyte imbalance (hyperkalaemia or metabolic acidosis)
- Blood sampling for monitoring of blood urea nitrogen and serum creatinine
- Close monitoring for signs of volume overload (e.g. regular recording of respiratory rate, repeated thoracic auscultation).

Idiopathic feline lower urinary tract disease

Idiopathic feline lower urinary tract disease (FLUTD) is a condition that affects both tomcats and queens but the risk of urinary obstruction is greatest in tomcats. It is thought that one of the contributory factors to this condition is stress or anxiety. A change in the cat's environment or circumstances (e.g. not being allowed outside to urinate, as happens with hospitalized cats) may induce feline idiopathic cystitis, which can in turn lead to urethral obstruction, due to the formation of a urethral plug, and then bladder distension. Feline patients should be monitored to ensure urine output is adequate and that they are not developing signs of cystitis (dysuria, haematuria or inappropriate urination). In order to reduce the possibility of this condition occurring, methods to reduce stress in hospitalized cats should be used, including:

- Separate wards for feline patients
- Ensuring a peaceful environment
- Using pheromones
- Client questionnaires to find out about the cat's normal behaviour
- Using the same cat litter as is used at home; litter trays should be changed as soon as they have been used
- Providing a bed or box for the cat to hide within
- Providing water fountains and moist food to increase water intake
- Feeding the same diet as is given at home if possible; a change in diet may induce stress.
- Spending time with the cat: grooming and hand feeding may reduce stress
- Using techniques requiring minimal restraint for handling.

If the cat's lower urinary tract does become obstructed, the urethral obstruction will need to be relieved and an indwelling urinary catheter placed. The metabolic state of the cat will need to be assessed and corrected prior to anaesthesia, so cystocentesis may be necessary in the short term. In addition, there is a risk of potassium changes with urinary obstruction both during (hyperkalaemia) and after (hypokalaemia) removal of the obstruction.

Therapeutics

The treatment for patients with urogenital disorders is given in Figure 2.29.

Condition	Cause	Treatment
Urinary tract infection (UTI)	Typically bacterial	Antibacterial therapy according to culture and sensitivity Persistent cases should be investigated for underlying causes: urolithiasis, diabetes mellitus, Cushing's disease
Urolithiasis	Metabolic abnormalities Dietary abnormalities Chronic UTI	May require surgical intervention Stone analysis is essential to direct treatment
Chronic renal disease	Often not apparent at the time of presentation In some breeds, inheritable conditions are important	Dietary management (see Chapter 3) Angiotensin-converting enzyme (ACE) inhibitors Monitor for UTI and hypertension
Acute renal failure	See Figure 2.28	Supportive care Closely monitored fluid therapy Furosemide, mannitol or dobutamine if required to maintain urine production
Urinary incontinence	Various congenital and acquired conditions, notably urethral sphincter mechanism incompetence	Medical (phenylpropanolamine, oestrogens) or surgical
Neoplasia	Various types Transitional cell carcinoma is the most common bladder tumour	Gonadal and uterine tumours are generally managed surgically Transitional cell carcinomas are best managed by non-steroidal anti-inflammatory drugs (NSAIDs) and chemotherapy
Oestrogen-induced aplastic anaemia and thrombocytopenia	Oestrogen-secreting tumours of the gonads	Supportive care Surgical removal of the neoplasm In some instances, bone marrow suppression is irreversible
Pyometra	Cystic degeneration in the endometrium accompanied by bacterial infection	Ovariohysterectomy is the treatment of choice. In selected cases, medical therapy consists of supportive care, antibacterial therapy and use of prostaglandins or progesterone-antagonists Bitches managed in this way should be subsequently bred from or neutered to prevent recurrence

2.29 Treatment for urogenital disorders.

Nursing the patient with disorders of the haemopoietic system

Presenting complaints

Anaemia is the most common primary disorder affecting blood cells. There are many different causes of anaemia; efforts should be made to classify the type of anaemia as this helps to define a specific diagnosis, treatment and prognosis (Figure 2.30). White blood cells primarily serve to indicate the presence of other pathological processes by the nature of their response to disease. Cytopenias arise in conjunction with bone marrow disease, including acute leukaemia.

Platelet disorders (see Chapter 12) result in spontaneous bleeding or failure of coagulation. Spontaneous haemorrhages are frequently noted in the skin or mucous membranes and are described by whether they are small, pinpoint-sized petechial haemorrhages or large ecchymotic haemorrhages.

Type	Cause	Treatment	Prognosis
Regenerative anaemia			
Haemorrhage	Trauma Clotting or bleeding disorders	Supportive care Control of haemorrhage Management of underlying cause	Excellent if haemorrhage controlled
Immune-mediated haemolytic anaemia	Often idiopathic	Immunosuppressive: Prednisolone Azathioprine Ciclosporin Cyclophosphamide Antithrombotic: Aspirin Dalteparin	Variable, often recurrent Occasionally non-regenerative if immune response is to precursors

2.30 Causes and treatment of anaemia. (continues) ▶

Type	Cause	Treatment	Prognosis
Infectious	*Haemoplasma* feline infectious anaemia	Doxycycline	Not all strains appear pathogenic Doxycycline is associated with oesophageal stricture
Toxic	Zinc (dogs) Onions (dogs) Paracetamol (cats)	Specific therapy where available, e.g. acetylcysteine	Generally poor
Non-regenerative anaemia			
Red cell dysmaturity disorders	Several breed-specific diseases described	Supportive care	Poor since no specific treatment is available
Bone marrow toxicity	Oestrogen-induced aplastic anaemia/thrombocytopenia	Removal of oestrogen source (e.g. gonadal tumour) Supportive care	Guarded, some cases are irreversible
Neoplasia	Bone marrow infiltration with, for example, lymphoma	Chemotherapy	Guarded, although remission may be possible
Chronic disease	Various chronic diseases cause non-specific bone marrow suppression	Supportive care	Depends on underlying cause
Iron deficiency	Rare except due to severe parasitism	Supportive care Parasiticides	Good unless advanced at presentation
Chronic renal failure	Erythropoietin deficiency	Supportive care Exogenous erythropoietin	Poor due to irreversible underlying cause
Polycythaemia			
Polycythaemia vera	Bone marrow neoplasia (red cell progenitors)	Chemotherapy Repeated phlebotomy	Good with ongoing treatment
Polycythaemia of other cause	Cardiorespiratory disease Renal tumours	Management of underlying disease	Variable
Leucocytosis			
Leukaemia	Bone marrow neoplasia (white cell progenitors)	Chemotherapy	Variable, poor for acute leukaemia
Reactive leucocytosis	Systemic inflammation/infection	Management of underlying cause	Variable
Leucopenia			
Primary leucopenia	Bone marrow toxicity, e.g. oestrogen, trimethoprim, chloramphenicol	Supportive care	May be irreversible
	Bone marrow failure (neoplastic infiltration or myelofibrosis)	Supportive care Chemotherapy	Poor
Secondary leucopenia	Acute severe inflammation	Management of underlying cause	Generally poor
	Immune-mediated neutrophil destruction		Rare

2.30 (continued) Causes and treatment of anaemia.

Diagnostic procedures

Haematology profile

Detailed haematology, including assessment of a smear for morphological characteristics and platelet numbers, is essential. In cases of anaemia, reticulocyte counts are also indicated (see Chapter 12).

Coagulation studies

Coagulation studies may be performed in-house using an analyser or sent to an external laboratory. Any sample collected for a coagulation study must be placed in sodium citrate anticoagulant. A coagulation study typically includes the following tests:

- *Activated clotting time*: This test assesses the intrinsic and common coagulation pathway; whole blood is placed in pre-warmed (37°C) tubes containing Fuller's earth. Normally clot formation occurs in 2 minutes
- *Prothrombin time*: This test assesses the extrinsic and common coagulation pathways
- *Activated partial thromboplastin time*: This is a more accurate test than ACT for assessing the intrinsic and common coagulation pathways.

Buccal mucosal bleeding time

Buccal mucosal bleeding time (BMBT) (see Figure 2.19) is a simple test that can performed in-house.

1. Expose the buccal mucosa by folding back the top lip and securing it with a bandage.
2. Using either a spring-loaded device or a surgical blade make a small incision.
3. As the cut bleeds, dab the blood using filter paper adjacent to the incision every 5–10 seconds. Take care not to dislodge any clot.

Normal bleeding time in dogs is <3.5 minutes. Bleeding time assesses platelet function in particular, rather than clotting factors, although it is useful to identify dogs that are severely affected by von Willebrand's disease (vWD).

von Willebrand factor

von Willebrand factor (vWF) is required for normal platelet function so a deficiency leads to prolonged bleeding time. The most accurate diagnosis is made by assessing the concentration of vWF in the blood. A blood sample in sodium citrate anticoagulant is required for this test. Specialist laboratories are able to carry out this analysis.

Biopsy and aspiration

Bone marrow

Core biopsy samples of bone marrow are taken for histological examination and bone marrow aspirates for cytological examination. These procedures can be performed under a general anaesthetic or sedation and local anaesthetic.

Bone marrow samples may be taken from the iliac crest, proximal humerus or proximal femur. The chosen site should be prepared and draped aseptically. Sterile gloves should be worn by the person collecting the samples. A Jamshidi bone marrow needle is used to collect core biopsy samples. With this device, a stylet within the needle aids insertion through the bone cortex. The stylet is removed as the needle is advanced into the marrow cavity and after removal from the bone, a probe is used to remove the core sample, which is placed in formal saline.

Alternatively, a Klima biopsy needle can be used. It is advanced into the bone cortex and when in place, the stylet is removed and a sterile 10 ml syringe containing 0.5 ml of 3% EDTA or sodium citrate is attached to the needle. The anticoagulant in the syringe will help to prevent the marrow from clotting before smears are made. Once aspirated, a drop of the bone marrow is placed at the top end of a number of glass slides, which should be propped at an angle to allow blood to run to the bottom of the slide leaving the marrow particles remaining. The smear is created by placing a clean microscope slide on top of the sample at right angles and then drawing the sample out along the slide. The smears are then air-dried and stained before cytological examination.

Lymph node

Fine-needle aspiration is a relatively non-invasive technique for gathering a sample for cytological examination. The primary haemopoietic indication is lymphadenopathy to distinguish inflammatory from neoplastic causes. Surgical excision of a lymph node can be carried out with the tissue sent for histological examination.

Virology

Testing for feline immunodeficiency virus (FIV) and feline leukaemia virus (FeLV) is commonly performed using in-house test kits, but blood samples can be sent for more specific testing by virus isolation at an external laboratory.

Antibody tests

Tests for immune-mediated haemolytic anaemia can be carried out in-house, such as the direct agglutination test. For this test, a drop of whole blood (EDTA anticoagulant) is mixed with a drop of normal saline on a slide and if agglutination occurs this indicates the presence of antibody-coated erythrocytes. However, this test is prone to error and a Coombs' test carried out by an external laboratory is preferred. In specific cases, assessment of antiplatelet antibodies and antinuclear antibodies can be performed at specialist laboratories, although the results can be difficult to interpret.

Iron metabolism evaluation

When anaemia is being investigated, an evaluation of the animal's iron metabolism may be helpful in distinguishing the cause. A serum sample can be sent to specialist laboratories for evaluation of serum iron and total iron binding capacity.

Polymerase chain reaction

Polymerase chain reaction (PCR) is a sensitive test for tick-borne diseases, FeLV, FIV and haemoplasmosis and is offered by specialist laboratories.

Faecal analysis

Faecal examination is used to investigate anaemia that may be due to gastrointestinal blood loss, in particular for evidence of parasites (worm eggs) and faecal occult blood.

Fibrin degradation products

This test assays the concentration of fibrin degradation products (FDPs) in the blood, which can be elevated in some clotting disorders, notably disseminated intravascular coagulation (DIC).

Nursing considerations

Coagulopathies and bleeding disorders

Where these conditions are suspected the patient must be handled gently to avoid further bleeding and bruising. Other considerations include:

- Interviewing the owners about the possibility of exposure to anticoagulant rodenticides
- Collecting all blood samples required at one time, using the smallest gauge needle possible, to reduce the necessity for venepuncture
- A person proficient in sampling technique should collect samples and place catheters
- Applying a compressive bandage following venepuncture or intravenous catheter removal
- Providing adequate padded bedding in the kennel
- Ensuring that should the patient be anaesthetized it is not injured during movement and has a smooth recovery.

Immunosuppressed patients

Patients suffering from disease that suppresses the immune system or those being treated with immunosuppressive drugs are at risk of nosocomial infection. These patients, therefore, must be highlighted as 'at risk of infection' and barrier nursed accordingly.

Therapeutics

The objectives of therapy for anaemic patients are to restore circulating oxygen-carrying capacity and to manage the underlying cause of the disease (see Figure 2.30). It is not always possible to identify an underlying cause and this may be reflected by the relatively poor prognosis with certain forms of anaemia. Restoration of oxygen-carrying capacity requires either the transfer of whole blood (or packed red cells) or administration of a blood substitute (see Chapter 6).

Immune-mediated anaemia is managed by the administration of immunosuppressive therapy. A frequent manifestation of haemolytic anaemia is concurrent vasculitis, which results in the development of thromboembolic disease; for this reason antithrombotic therapy is also indicated. Coagulopathy due to thrombocytopenia can be managed by the administration of fresh whole blood (platelets do not survive in stored blood). Increased thrombotic tendency is managed by administration of antithrombotic agents (see Figure 2.30).

In vWD, patients with a partial lack of vWF can respond to the administration of desmopressin. This is of clinical use in cases of prolonged bleeding in which the available vWF is at risk of being consumed, or in cases of elective surgery, when mild to moderate haemorrhage is anticipated. Haemorrhage due to coumarin toxicity is ameliorated by administration of Vitamin K. This treatment needs to be given as long as the toxic product remains functional, which can be up to 3 months.

Nursing the patient with skin disease

Presenting complaints

A significant problem when attempting to identify cutaneous disease by the physical presenting signs is the fact that most cutaneous diseases are represented by the same set of changes. It is relatively unusual to see primary cutaneous lesions as cutaneous pathogens promptly proliferate in the altered ambient conditions, resulting in inflammation, pruritus and often self-excoriation. For this reason, the diagnostic pathway for cutaneous disease frequently follows the same track, as one cannot afford to exclude potential differential diagnoses on clinical signs alone. A glossary of frequently encountered dermatopathological features can be found in Figure 2.31 and a typical diagnostic flow chart is given in Figure 2.32. Frequently patients are presented due to the development of a skin mass; common skin tumours of the dog and cat are presented in Figure 2.33.

Feature	Description
Primary lesions	
Macule	Skin spot with altered pigmentation, no change in skin thickness
Patch	Area of altered pigmentation of ≥2 cm in diameter
Papule	Raised area <1 cm in diameter, often circular
Plaque	Raised area >1 cm in diameter, often irregularly shaped
Pustule	Raised lesion containing pus Rarely noted intact
Vesicle	Blister, <1 cm in diameter Rarely found intact
Bulla	Large blister, >1 cm in diameter Rarely intact
Nodule	Mass >1 cm in diameter Causes include tumour, cyst or inflammatory process
Wheal	Well demarcated raised red lesion Colour dispersed by direct pressure but promptly returns Often short-lived
Secondary lesions	
Scale	Colourless flakes of skin still partially attached
Epidermal collarette	Circular scaling lesion, often with thin red rim
Comedo	Plugged hair follicle, usually appears dark, with hair absent
Lichenification	Thickening of the skin
Erosion	Superficial lesion, graze
Ulcer	Full-thickness skin lesion, will heal by scar formation

2.31 Frequently encountered dermatopathological features.

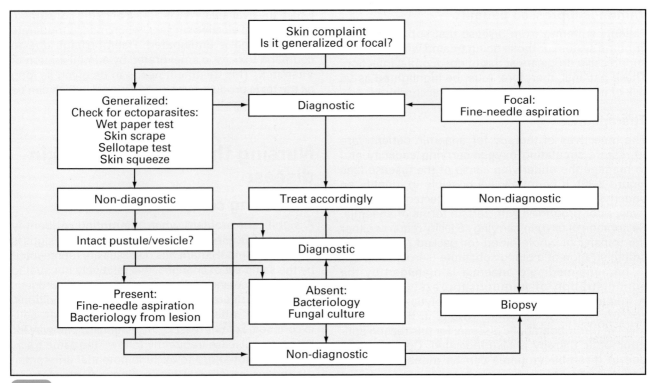

2.32   Diagnostic flow chart for investigation of skin disease.

Frequency	Type	Benign (B)/ malignant (M)	Clinical features	Species
Very common	Sebaceous hyperplasia [a]	B	Typically hairless, lobulated and exophytic. Usually non-invasive but minimal invasive growth can be seen, particularly with malignant variants	Dog and cat
	Sebaceous adenoma [a]	B		
	Sebaceous carcinoma [a]	M		
Less common	Basal cell tumour	B	Rounded intradermal or subcutaneous mass Often alopecic	Cat
	Trichoepithelioma and pilomatricoma	B	Tumours of hair follicle origin contain keratin or calcified debris	Dog
	Squamous cell carcinoma	M	Associated with UV light exposure. Often ulcerated	Dog and cat
	Cutaneous histiocytoma	B	Can spontaneously regress. Typically affects young dogs	Dog
Uncommon	Plasmacytoma	B	Usually solitary and benign. Can be multiple	Dog
	Melanocytoma	B	Pigmented. Usually slow growing and amenable to excision	Dog
	Malignant melanoma	M	Pigmented. Usually progressive and fatal. May ulcerate	Dog and cat
Rare	Papilloma	B	Viral origin, can be multiple	Dog
	Sweat (apocrine) gland carcinoma [b]	M	Frequently in axillary or inguinal sites	Dog and cat
	Multicentric squamous cell carcinoma *in situ*	M	Purative association with viral infection. Non-metastatic	Cat

2.33   Skin tumours in the dog and cat. [a] Specialized modified sebaceous glands can undergo the same changes as unmodified glands. These specialized glands include meibomian glands, arising on the inner aspect of the eyelid (tumours uncommon in dogs, exceptionally rare in other species), and hepatoid glands, primarily in the perineal region (these are only present in dogs). [b] Specialized modified apocrine glands can undergo the same changes as unmodified glands. These glands can be found in the perianal region (tumours rare in cats and dogs) and in the apocrine glands of the anal sacs (tumours uncommon in dogs, very rare in cats).

Immune-mediated skin disease is common but it can be challenging to identify correctly. It is important to note that many patients can be affected by more than one cutaneous disorder at a time. Simple diagnostics should be performed and potential confounding conditions eliminated before entering into more complex procedures or lengthy treatment trials.

Systemic disease can manifest primarily as a skin complaint. The most notable examples include the endocrinopathies, hypothyroidism and Cushing's disease. When an underlying systemic disease is suspected, the diagnostic plan should be changed accordingly. Histological changes are sometimes characteristic of specific underlying systemic disorders.

The diagnostic pathway (see Figure 2.32) may culminate in the acquisition of a biopsy sample. In the event that this indicates a probable immune-mediated disease this is likely to be food-related, atopic (inhaled allergens) or a contact allergy. A food allergy does not necessarily present in the company of gastrointestinal signs. Diagnosis is made by resolution of clinical signs in response to feeding an exclusion diet, food that comprises basic foodstuffs that have not previously been encountered by the patient's immune system. Strictly speaking, re-challenge with the offending food is also required but few clinicians or owners decide to actively induce relapse of clinical signs if a resolution is achieved. The most sensitive and specific test for atopic skin disease is the intradermal skin test. This involves the direct intradermal administration of refined allergen and measurement of the magnitude of any resulting inflammatory response. Serological tests for canine atopy are also available, although the reliability of these tests remains controversial.

Diagnostic procedures

The common laboratory tests (e.g. skin scraping, coat brushing and fungal culture) are described in the *BSAVA Manual of Practical Veterinary Nursing*.

Skin biopsy

For nodular disease an excisional biopsy technique is preferred. For generalized skin disease, the biopsy should obtain specimens that are representative of the underlying pathology. This sometimes means that areas of the greatest abnormality should be avoided as these are likely only to yield evidence of secondary changes. Primary lesions (see Figure 2.31) should be identified and sampled if possible. Limited skin preparation is carried out prior to fine-needle aspiration and biopsy of skin lesions. It is important that the skin surface is not disrupted by rough handling. Punch biopsy devices are useful for obtaining skin biopsy samples but the rotational shearing action involved can disrupt fragile dermatopathological changes, so this technique should be avoided for junctional areas between normal skin and vesicular or pustular lesions; excisional biopsy is indicated instead. Similarly, normal aseptic skin preparation techniques can disrupt pathological changes so care must be taken in getting the patient ready for the biopsy procedure. Opinions differ as to how best to prepare the patient and therefore the best recommendation would be to discuss this with the veterinary surgeon and analysing laboratory first. Skin biopsy samples, whether collected by punch biopsy or excisional methods, should be handled carefully to avoid damage and placed in formalin immediately to prevent deterioration.

Intradermal skin tests

Intradermal skin tests could be used as part of an investigation for an atopic animal. It is a process where selected allergens are injected intradermally; if sensitized mast cells are present in the animal's skin, a red wheal will develop at the site showing a positive allergic reaction.

Blood tests

Blood tests for allergies are less specific than the intradermal test.

Hormone assays

Endocrine diseases, such as hypothyroidism and Cushing's disease, cause hormone imbalances that result in bilateral flank alopecia or coat thinning.

Exclusion diet

Food allergies and food intolerances often display dermatological clinical signs. An exclusion diet can be used to try and identify the food product responsible. The animal should be fed exclusively on a new diet that it has not experienced before for 6 weeks; if the skin is better after this time a food allergy must be suspected but cannot be confirmed until the old diet is reintroduced to see what effect that has on the skin. The animal should then go back on the exclusion diet and the original foods should be reintroduced one by one in an attempt to find the ingredient that caused the allergy.

Nursing considerations

It is not common for patients to be hospitalized for treatment of skin conditions alone, but patients hospitalized for management of other systemic diseases might exhibit physical changes to the skin or coat that may require treatment.

Barrier nursing

Patients with zoonotic skin disease (e.g. dermatophytosis, sarcoptic mange) should be barrier nursed in order to protect staff and other patients from the disease. These conditions, although not serious in humans, will produce irritation and itching and usually require symptomatic treatment. Actions to prevent further spread, including reverse zoonosis, should be used.

Therapeutics

A number of different systemic drugs may be prescribed. Corticosteroids are likely to induce an increase in thirst, appetite and urination. In the long term, liver and adrenal function may be affected. Staff and owners must wear gloves when applying topical corticosteroid preparations.

Ectoparasitic disease is managed by appropriate parasiticidal treatment. Consideration should be given to the entire lifecycle of the organism in question or the complaint is bound to relapse. Superficial pyoderma and malassezia dermatitis can be managed by the topical administration of antibacterial and antifungal shampoo. Many patients require regular administration of such products as the persistent changes that result from the underlying dermatological disease perpetually promote the development of these commensal cutaneous organisms.

Many cutaneous disorders are essentially inflammatory diseases that require management with anti-inflammatory therapy. Prednisolone is the drug of choice in many cases. Since this therapy is typically longstanding, the hazards associated with chronic corticosteroid administration are seen in this group of patients perhaps more than any other. These include polydipsia, polyuria, polyphagia, body condition change, metabolic derangements, exercise intolerance and susceptibility to infection (including cutaneous infection). Other immunomodulatory drugs are employed in conjunction with prednisolone, primarily for their steroid-sparing effects; these include azathioprine, ciclosporin, omega-3 fatty acid sources such as evening primrose oil, and antihistamines. Immunomodulation by controlled allergen exposure can also be used and has been extremely successful in the management of atopy in some cases.

'Vaccines' are composed using the results of intradermal skin testing (or serological testing), and the controlled administration of these vaccines at increasing doses is intended to induce a level of immune system tolerance of the offending allergens. In the majority of cases this achieves partial control of the underlying disease process but continued low dose or periodic anti-inflammatory therapy may still be required.

Nursing the patient with ophthalmic disease

For information on the common presenting conditions of the eye, see the *BSAVA Manual of Small Animal Ophthalmology, 2nd edition*.

Diagnostic procedures

Ophthalmic examination

A systematic approach should be used when conducting an eye examination. Following a routine ensures that no signs are overlooked. The examination should be carried out in a quiet room, capable of being darkened; a noisy environment will distract the patient and cause ocular movement. Both eyes should be examined even if the problem is only apparent in one eye. Full details of the ophthalmic examination can be found in the *BSAVA Manual of Small Animal Ophthalmology, 2nd edition*.

Patient restraint

Ocular examination is best performed with minimal restraint, supporting the patient's head under the chin with one hand and placing the other hand behind its head to prevent sudden movement backwards. Small dogs and cats should be placed on a non-slip table surface. Patients with ophthalmic conditions may be 'head shy' and sedation might occasionally be necessary to allow full examination; however, this will alter the appearance of the eyelids and eye shape. Scruffing of the patient should be avoided as eyelid conformation in animals with loose skin will be altered; there is also the risk of globe proptosis in brachycephalic breeds. Restriction around the patient's neck will also falsely elevate intraocular pressure readings.

Schirmer tear test

The Schirmer tear test (Figure 2.34) indicates whether there is normal tear production. The Schirmer test strips are longitudinal lengths of filter paper. By placing these between the eyelid and cornea it is possible to assess the tear production over a 1-minute interval. There must be adequate contact between the corneal surface and the filter paper strip for the results to be interpreted. A reading of 15 mm or more equates to normal tear production.

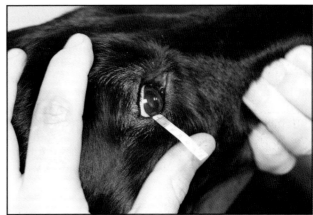

2.34 Performing the Schirmer tear test in a dog. (© D Gould)

Fluorescein stain

Fluorescein stain (Figure 2.35) is used to diagnose corneal ulceration. Fluorescein is a water-soluble stain that, when applied to the surface of the eye, adheres to any ulcerated areas; these stained areas will then fluoresce green under blue light.

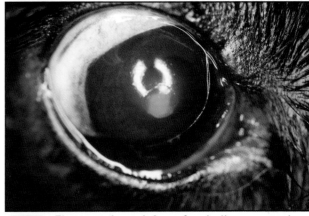

2.35 Fluorescein staining of a shallow corneal ulcer. (© D Gould)

Tonometry

A tonometer is a device that measures intraocular pressure; increased pressure indicates glaucoma, which could cause blindness and pain. A topical local anaesthetic, such as proxymetacaine, should be applied to the eye prior to this test being performed. There are various types of tonometry, including indentation tonometry and applanation tonometry.

Types of tonometry

Indentation tonometry: **determines intraocular pressure by indenting the cornea. The Schiøtz tonometer is the most common indentation tonometer (Figure 2.36).**

Applanation tonometry: **determines intraocular pressure by flattening the cornea. The Tonopen tonometer is the most common applanation tonometer.**

Normal measurements depend on the method of tonometry used:

Type of tonometer	Normal intraocular pressure for dogs (mmHg)	Normal intraocular pressure for cats (mmHg)
Schiøtz	17–26	12–26
Tonopen	12–20	14–25

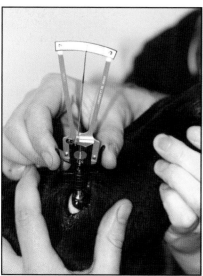

2.36 Using the Schiøtz tonometer to measure intraocular pressure. (© D Gould)

Culture and cytology

Where corneal or conjunctival disease is present it may be necessary to carry out culture and sensitivity to determine antimicrobial therapy. Contamination of the swab by touching the eyelids should be avoided. The swab should be placed in the appropriate transport medium. Cytology samples can be collected from the conjunctiva with a cytology brush or spatula and applied directly to a microscope slide for cytological examination after staining.

Gonioscopy

This is the examination of the iridocorneal angle, also known as the drainage angle. The technique is used mainly to screen dogs for evidence of goniodysgenesis, an abnormal narrowing of the drainage angle, which can lead to glaucoma. Some breeds of dog are known to suffer from inherited primary glaucoma such as the Basset Hound and Flat-coated Retriever. A goniolens is placed on the topically anaesthetized cornea, which allows the refraction to be altered in order for the drainage angle to be assessed.

Ophthalmic ultrasonography

This may be carried out in the conscious patient after application of local anaesthetic eye drops and gives information about the structures within the eye (e.g. retinal detachment and intraocular neoplasia). The transducer is placed directly on the cornea and specific ophthalmic ultrasound gel or a gel pad is used.

Magnetic resonance imaging and computed tomography

MRI and CT (see Chapter 11) may be used to examine the eye, orbit and optic nerves for the presence of foreign bodies, infection or neoplasia.

Electroretinography

This is an objective method of evaluating retinal function by recording the electrical response of the retina to a flashing light stimulus. Retinal function should be evaluated prior to surgical removal of cataracts.

Nursing considerations

Patients with corneal ulceration or intraocular disease or those recovering from surgery may have a 'fragile eye'. It is important with these patients to minimize the occurrence of raised intraocular pressure and possible damage to the eye. This can be achieved by:

- Not allowing excitable patients to bark excessively
- Sedating hyperactive patients as required
- Using a harness during exercise to avoid pressure around the neck
- Not using drugs that may induce vomiting, e.g. morphine
- Minimizing handling and not scruffing the animal
- Regular assessment and administration of pain relief
- Taking care not to struggle with the patient to apply the medication
- Preventing patient interference through the use of collars or paw bandages. It should be checked that the animal is not using cephalic intravenous catheters to rub the eye
- Following medication regimes precisely and correctly updating the hospitalization sheet for each day's treatment in the light of changes to medication following an ophthalmic examination
- Providing guidance to blind patients to avoid collision with obstacles when being exercised and showing patience as these animals are slow
- Avoiding the use of the ipsilateral jugular vein for blood sampling.

Observations of the hospitalized patient

- The presence and characteristics of the ocular discharge should be noted. Relevant comments should be made on the hospitalization sheet. If any ocular discharge develops it should be brought to the clinician's notice, especially if the side of the face appears wet as this may indicate rupture of the globe. The eyelids may require gentle cleaning with gauze swabs and sterile saline. The same swab should not be used for cleaning both eyes, and care must be taken not to touch the surface of the eye itself with swabs. It should be ensured that no pressure is exerted on the eye during cleaning.
- The patient should be observed from a distance. The eye(s) should be checked to see whether they are open or shut. It should be ensured that the patient has received adequate pain relief either topically or systemically. The eye may have been protected either by the application of a soft bandage contact lens or the eyelids may have been partially sutured together. If the eyelids have been partially sutured together (temporary partial tarsorrhaphy) the eye will appear half closed; this should not be confused with eye pain. The contact lens has a blue pattern on it to help identify whether it is in the eye or not. With both techniques the eye should be comfortable. The clinician should be asked for advice if the animal appears to be in discomfort or there is excessive discharge.
- The patient's vision should be assessed.

Medicating the eye

- **Always medicate a clean eye (take care when cleaning especially if the eye is fragile).**
- **Only apply one drop of medication, any more will spill out of the eye.**
- **Leave at least 5 minutes between different medications and always apply drops before ointment.**
- **Avoid touching the corneal surface with the tip of the bottle or tube.**
- **Some medication should be stored in the refrigerator; this method of storage will also reduce the likelihood of medication stinging as it is applied.**
- **Ensure that the medication is clearly labelled with dosage instructions and with which eye is to be medicated.**

Nursing the patient with endocrine disease

Information on presenting complaints, diagnostic procedures and therapeutics is detailed in Figure 2.37.

Disorder	Cause	Specific blood tests	Other diagnostic tests	Treatment	Comments
Diabetes insipidus (DI)	Central/hypothalamic: failure of the hypothalamic–pituitary axis to produce antidiuretic hormone (ADH) in response to increasing plasma tonicity. May be congenital or due to acquired brain disease Renal/nephrogenic: failure of the kidney tubules to express receptors for ADH. May be primary (rare and congenital) or be mimicked by other causes of failure of tubular function	None A definitive diagnosis of true DI requires exclusion of other potential causes of hyposthenuria	Urine specific gravity (SG) Water deprivation test Modified water deprivation test Urine SG consistently in the hyposthenuric range (<1.012) In complete DI, the ability to concentrate urine is not altered on water deprivation Partial central DI states exist in which urinary concentrating ability is seen on water deprivation but the urine SG will be unlikely to exceed 1.015–1.020	Central DI is managed by administration of the synthetic ADH desmopressin (DDAVP), provided as eye drops. Primary nephrogenic DI can be treated to a degree by salt and water restriction Thiazide diuretics can also induce a reduction in urine production in DI True DI is not dangerous so long as the patient has adequate access to fresh drinking water: for this reason, not treating these patients at all is a valid approach to treatment	Check for other diseases Important to recognize that increased urinary concentration in response to DDAVP does not prove the presence of central DI
Panhypo-pituitarism	Congenital pituitary dysfunction affecting growth hormone (GH) and thyroid-stimulating hormone (TSH) production	Thyroxine (T4) TSH		GH supplementation However, a canine GH formulation has not been produced and there are significant problems associated with the use of human, bovine or porcine GH products GH does not work in conditions of hypothyroidism, so T4 supplements are also indicated	The primary presenting complaint in these cases is failure to grow properly, resulting in a form of dwarfism, and retention of the puppy coat The life expectancy for these cases is always limited

2.37   Tests for endocrine disease in the dog and cat. (continues) ▶

Disorder	Cause	Specific blood tests	Other diagnostic tests	Treatment	Comments
Acromegaly/ hypersomato- tropism	A condition of adult patients which results from GH excess The excessive hormone is produced by a pituitary tumour. These can be large macroadenomas, or small microadenomas. Macroadenomas can respond to radiotherapy	Insulin-like growth factor-1 (IGF-1) Blood glucose Lower limit of acromegalic range uncertain for IGF-1 assay	Magnetic resonance imaging (MRI) of the pituitary gland Computed tomography (CT) of the pituitary gland	The only available therapy is pituitary radiation There is evidence that pituitary irradiation reduces insulin resistance but makes little impact on the progressive clinical signs of organ hyperplasia Diabetic patients undergoing radiotherapy should be monitored as the alteration in exogenous insulin requirement is unpredictable	Bone growth leads to characteristic changes of facial structure, with a prominent forehead and gaps developing between incisor teeth, and characteristically oversized paws. Soft tissue hyperplasia can lead to cardiac or renal complications Increasingly recognized in cats with a primary presenting sign of insulin-resistant diabetes mellitus (DM)
Hypothyroid- ism	Most commonly due to progressive immune-mediated destruction of the thyroid gland Under these circumstances, the drive to produce T4 increases, resulting in a measurable excess of TSH	Diagnosis of hypothyroidism is best made by concurrent evaluation of multiple test results Low T4 in the presence of elevated TSH Early or subclinical cases are recognized but can be very hard to differentiate from cases of sick euthyroid syndrome, in which T4 levels are also decreased as a physiological response to concurrent disease	Free T4 by dialysis Serum thyroglobulin antibody TSH stimulation test Thyrotropin-releasing hormone (TRH) stimulation test Trial T4 therapy is used as a diagnostic test in some instances. Under these circumstances a significant improvement in patient activity levels within 4 weeks of implementing therapy would be expected; failure to improve must prompt re-evaluation of the diagnosis	Administration of synthetic levothyroxine There is debate about whether the dose is best calculated on the basis of bodyweight or metabolic rate, for which body surface area (BSA) serves as a proxy indicator	Hypothyroidism is relatively common in dogs but rare in cats Stimulation tests do not definitively rule out sick euthyroid syndrome
Hyperthyroid- ism	Cats: due to thyroid gland hyperplasia and thyroid adenomas in almost equal proportions Dogs: rare, may occur in association with a small proportion of thyroid carcinomas	T4 Renal parameters	Systemic blood pressure (BP) Retest borderline cases after 3 months A palpable enlarged thyroid gland (goitre) is frequently found in the ventral neck of affected cats	Thyroidectomy Medical therapy Radioiodine	Surgical therapy should be preceded by medical therapy for approximately 2 weeks to stabilize haemodynamic parameters
Hyperpara- thyroidism	Secondary to systemic disease (dietary or chronic renal failure) Primary due to parathyroid neoplasia Also humoral hypercalcaemia of malignancy due to parathyroid hormone-related peptide (PTHrP) that mimics the effects of parathyroid hormone (PTH). Commonly associated malignancies are lymphoma and anal sac carcinoma	PTH PTHrP Ionized calcium phosphate	Cervical ultrasonography Search for malignancy elsewhere (lymphoma, anal sac)	Primary cases: removal of parathyroid tumour Humoral calcaemia of malignancy: treatment of underlying cause (surgical excision and/or chemotherapy)	Total calcium concentration is a less specific indicator of hypercalcaemia than ionized calcium Some cases become hypocalcaemic postoperatively and require intensive management
Addison's disease	Adrenal cortex failure (cause usually unknown)	Na$^+$/K$^+$/Cl$^-$ Renal parameters Adrenocorticotrophic hormone (ACTH) stimulation Aldosterone assay	Electrocardiography if acutely affected	Initial stabilization Oral therapy can be implemented once clinical signs of vomiting and weakness have resolved: fludrocortisone and prednisolone. Most cases do not require chronic prednisolone administration, although occasional low-dose therapy is recommended when periods of stress are anticipated	Despite the fact that clinical signs relate almost entirely to inadequate aldosterone, failure to respond to ACTH is characteristic finding An uncommon disease in dogs and very rare in cats

2.37 (continued) Tests for endocrine disease in the dog and cat. (continues) ▶

Disorder	Cause	Specific blood tests	Other diagnostic tests	Treatment	Comments
Cushing's disease	Excessive glucocorticoid production, predominantly cortisol, arises with ACTH-secreting tumours of the pituitary gland or glucocorticoid-secreting tumours of the adrenal glands	Alkaline phosphatase (ALP) ACTH stimulation test Low-dose dexamethasone suppression test (LDDST) High-dose dexamethasone suppression test (HDDST) coagulation screen	Urine analysis Urine cortisol Urine protein:creatinine ratio MRI of pituitary gland Ultrasonography of adrenal glands BP	Cushing's disease does not consistently affect patient quality of life adversely Since treatment and monitoring can be expensive, and is not without some risk of complications, some patients may be best managed conservatively Surgical therapy (adrenalectomy or hypophysectomy) occasional used Medical therapy: ■ Trilostane is an authorized veterinary product and therefore should be used in all cases unless there is a compelling reason not to such as failure to control the disease or drug-induced toxicity. Trilostane successfully manages Cushing's disease in approximately 70% of cases ■ Mitotane: cytotoxic and therefore care must be taken when handling this drug. Mitotane successfully manages Cushing's disease in approximately 80% of cases; overdose can also induce Addisonian crises	Elevated cortisol level seen with intercurrent disease or stress can complicate diagnosis During and after therapy, regular ongoing monitoring of cortisol levels after ACTH stimulation testing is required
Phaeochromo-cytoma	Tumours of the adrenal medulla which secrete adrenaline and noradrenaline Rare	Coagulation screen	BP Urine protein:creatinine ratio Ultrasonography of adrenal glands	Surgical Substantial perioperative risks due to hypertension and coagulopathy Cases without metastases can be cured by successful surgery	Definitive diagnosis can only be made on histopathology Dramatic changes in BP are particularly indicative
Insulinoma	Insulin-secreting tumours of the pancreas Uncommon in dogs and very rare in cats	Blood glucose Serum insulin Fructosamine	Ultrasonography of liver and duodenum Exploratory laparotomy	Insulinoma can be cured by surgical intervention but frequently relapses are noted, sometimes years after initial surgical intervention Partial pancreatectomy carries a 10% mortality rate due primarily to induction of pancreatitis. Patients who are not candidates for surgery such as those with metastatic disease can be managed medically	Numerous diagnostic manipulations of glucose and insulin ratios in use but none is categorically definitive of insulinoma
Diabetes mellitus	Loss of functional islet tissue of the pancreas (type 1 diabetes) associated with chronic pancreatitis or immune-mediated destruction Tissue resistance to insulin (type 2 diabetes), often associated with obesity, Cushing's disease or acromegaly	Blood glucose Glucose curve Blood gas analysis $Na^+/K^+/Cl^-$	Urine glucose Urine culture Urine ketones	See text	Hyperglycaemia and glucosuria also seen with stress

2.37   (continued) Tests for endocrine disease in the dog and cat.

Nursing considerations

Veterinary nurses are most commonly closely involved with the care of patients with diabetes mellitus (DM) and this disease is covered in-depth in this section.

Diabetes mellitus

In DM, glucose fails to enter cells in adequate quantities, resulting in excessive glucose delivery to the kidneys and osmotic diuresis. When glucose persists in the plasma filtrate above a level that the kidneys' resorptive capabilities can deal with, this results in glucosuria. The glucose in the urine draws fluid with it, forcing increased water loss. These patients are typically polyuric and polydipsic as a result. They are also frequently polyphagic and show exercise intolerance, weakness and lethargy. Glucosuria also promotes the development of bacterial UTIs; clinical signs of cystitis may be what prompts initial veterinary presentation. In severe disease, advanced ketoacidosis can develop. This is a metabolic crisis state with a rapidly progressive combination of acidosis and hypovolaemia. Patients typically present with anorexia, vomiting, listlessness and rapid, shallow breathing. In severe cases these patients can be comatose. Some people have the ability to smell ketones on the patient's breath; others do not. The characteristic smell is described as similar to that of 'pear drops'.

Protocol

A protocol should be adopted for the daily management of all diabetic patients within the hospital environment so that consistent care is given.

- Daily (morning) urine sample. The urine SG should be checked for the presence of glucose, ketones, blood and protein.
- Daily (morning) blood samples for blood glucose levels and as requested by the clinician. The smallest gauge needle and volume of blood possible should be used. Jugular samples and careful venepuncture should be used. If a jugular sample is not possible then an insulin syringe and the cephalic vein should be used, although this vein should be preserved for intravenous catheterization wherever possible. A small quantity of blood can be obtained from the pinna using commercially available blood spot devices (Figure 2.38). Notably in cats, this can avoid stress-induced hyperglycaemia and reduce the risk of jugular thrombosis.

Feeding and exercise
Dogs

- Accurately measured amounts of the correct type of food should be fed.
- No titbits should be allowed.
- Feeding should occur at specified times.
- Plenty of water should be offered, especially to large-breed dogs overnight.
- Frequent opportunities to urinate should be offered. Exercise should be approximately the same each day.

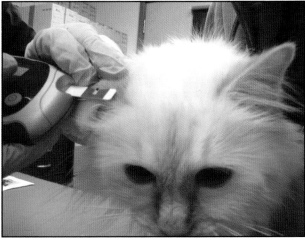

2.38   Ear prick blood collection for monitoring blood glucose levels in a cat.

Cats

Feeding and exercise in cats are less directly controlled under normal circumstances. Feeding a diet high in complex carbohydrates can make a significant impact on disease control (see Chapter 3). Ensuring adequate access to clean litter or the outdoors for toilet purposes will limit the development of urinary retention-related illness.

Insulin administration

For information on the considerations for the storage and administration of insulin see the *BSAVA Manual of Practical Veterinary Nursing*.

Hypoglycaemia

The patient should be observed for the clinical signs of hypoglycaemia. The following action should be taken if clinical signs of hypoglycaemia occur:

- Assistance should be called for
- A blood sample should be collected to determine the blood glucose level
- The animal should be fed immediately (if conscious) or glucose syrup be rubbed on its gums (if safe to do so)
- If unable to feed, 10 ml of 20–50% dextrose solution should be drawn up for intravenous administration. The relevant clinician should be checked with before administration (dextrose solution can be irritant; therefore, it may need to be diluted further in small dogs).

For further details see the *BSAVA Manual of Practical Veterinary Nursing*.

Glucose curves

During stabilization, blood samples may be taken regularly throughout the course of the day to produce a glucose curve, which will give an indication of the patient's glycaemic stability. Important information can be gained as to when the insulin is taking effect, by how much the insulin is taking effect and the duration of the insulin effect. The aim of the glucose curve is to keep the blood glucose levels below that of the renal threshold

(10 mmol/l in dogs and 14 mmol/l in cats) and above that which would cause hypoglycaemia or a Somogyi overswing (below 5 mmol/l). Blood glucose levels should be checked every 2 hours initially, reducing to 4 hourly as stabilization is being achieved. Examples of glucose curves are given in Figures 2.39 to 2.41.

It is not always practical to carry out a glucose curve in the hospitalized cat as stress may induce hyperglycaemia and invalidate results. Cats may also be reluctant to eat specialized prescription diets or eat at all in the hospital environment and this can create stabilization problems.

Glycaemic control can also be evaluated by measuring the plasma protein fructosamine. Fructosamine is a combination of a plasma protein bound with glucose. Persistently high levels of glucose will increase

fructosamine and because proteins last up to 2 weeks in the blood, measuring fructosamine can give an indication of blood glucose levels over this time. This test is particularly useful in cats where stress hyperglycaemia is common.

Urinary tract infections

UTIs are often seen in patients with DM. Glucosuria combined with a low urine SG is an ideal environment for bacteria to breed and grow. The presence of an UTI can cause insulin resistance, and a urine sample collected in a sterile manner, e.g. by cystocentesis, should be periodically cultured to check for this. A diabetic patient that is difficult to stabilize or one that has become unstable should also have this test performed.

Unstable diabetic patients

Dogs and cats may become unstable or be difficult to stabilize for many reasons including:

- Incorrect storage, handling, dosing and administration of insulin
- Infection (commonly UTI)
- Obesity
- Transient diabetes
- Ineffective insulin type.

Incorrect storage, handling, dosing and administration of insulin

It is common that patients become unstable at home due to human error. Owners should be questioned about the storage and handling of insulin, and asked

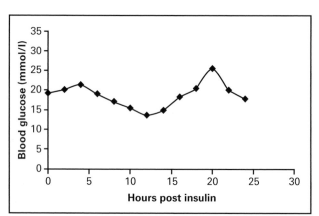

2.39 Blood glucose curve showing persistent hyperglycaemia due to inadequate insulin or insulin resistance.

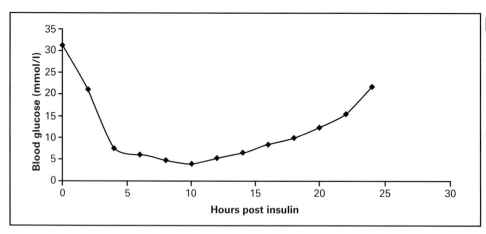

2.40 Blood glucose curve showing a rapid decrease in blood glucose levels, causing hypoglycaemia, due to an insulin overdose.

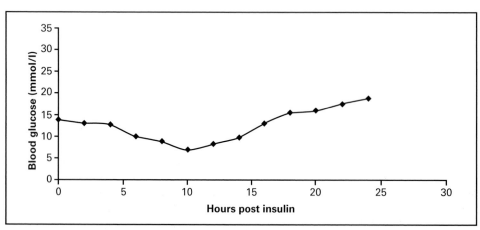

2.41 Blood glucose curve showing good stabilization.

to demonstrate how it is prepared and administered. A patient that has been receiving insulin for some time may have developed an absorption problem if it has been injected into the same area each time. Simply moving injection sites may be all that is required.

Infection
See information on UTIs (above).

Obesity
This can cause insulin resistance as well as difficulty in insulin absorption. Diabetes can sometimes be reversed following a safe weight loss programme.

Transient diabetes
Diabetes can sometimes be transient, particularly in animals with pancreatitis. Patients should be monitored carefully and should be investigated in cases of sudden episodes of hypoglycaemia.

Ineffective insulin type
Cats and dogs may be more responsive to certain types of insulin. As well as the different duration of action, how the patient responds to insulin may be determined by whether it is a bovine or porcine insulin.

Anaesthetic considerations
Diabetic animals that are to be anaesthetized will need reduced levels of insulin on the morning of the procedure as they will have had food withheld (see Chapter 7).

Diabetic ketoacidosis
Prolonged insulin deficiency will cause ketoacidosis. Animals may arrive in a collapsed or comatose state and these will need emergency treatment. Soluble insulin is given intravenously in these animals, as absorption from subcutaneous administration will be too slow. Ketoacidotic patients will exhale ketones; these have a characteristically sweet odour but this can only be detected by some people. Acid–base status and electrolyte levels will often be severely abnormal and the patient dehydrated. This should be addressed promptly through supplemented intravenous fluids as indicated. While patients presenting in ketoacidosis require urgent efforts to correct hyperglycaemia, hypovolaemia and electrolyte disturbances, rapid correction can lead to terminal consequences. It is recommended that glucose, fluid and electrolyte disturbances are corrected over a period of approximately 48 hours. Rapid correction of hyperglycaemia or hypovolaemia can lead to cerebral oedema. Short-acting soluble insulin preparations are available, which are given intravenously or intramuscularly. Another important consideration is the impact of correction of hyperglycaemia on potassium concentrations. Ketoacidotic patients often have low plasma potassium concentrations at presentation. Glucose uptake into cells is always accompanied by potassium uptake, so plasma potassium concentrations will fall with insulin therapy. Hypokalaemia can induce fatal arrhythmias; therefore, potassium concentration must be monitored very closely. Intensive nursing is needed with these patients. Measuring vital signs, urine output, blood pressure and repeated blood analysis is essential.

Nursing the patient with cancer
The treatment of cancer in veterinary patients is a challenging issue for many reasons, all of which are pertinent to the veterinary nursing team.

- A diagnosis of cancer carries a stigma that is sometimes disproportionate. In reality, when the prognosis for many cancers is measured against other disease types which may be invariably fatal (e.g. kidney or heart failure), the expected lifespan is similar.
- Cancer therapy carries the risk of inducing unwanted side-effects which, when they occur, can be significant. However, the frequency and severity of these events are in reality considerably less than many clients (and veterinary surgeons) expect.
- The non-surgical therapies employed in veterinary oncology do pose a tangible personnel health hazard in themselves and so appropriate precautions must be taken to safeguard the welfare of staff and clients as well as the patient.

The experienced veterinary nurse should be able to play a relatively central role in the management of veterinary cancer cases. Undoubtedly, owners of animals undergoing chemotherapy will benefit from the opportunity to discuss matters with a well informed and sympathetic individual. These cases, by the nature of the disease and the treatment, can change regularly. Achieving the right balance between risk taken in terms of the therapy administered and the patient's quality of life is a very dynamic and very personal thing. Knowledgeable support is invaluable. The practice of oncology is as much (if not more) about education and counselling of owners to help them make the right choices for their pet as it is about administering the right therapy in the right way.

Definitions

Cancer is defined by the acquisition of living tissues of biological features that enable them to grow without adherence to usual constraints. In order to grow, cancer cells must be able to:

- **Undergo cell division (mitosis), thus multiplying in number**
- **Be resistant to antigrowth signals from surrounding cells**
- **Be able to resist internal suicide messages (apoptosis)**
- **Be resistant to immune system protection against tumour growth**
- **Be able to spread to distant sites and grow (metastasis)**
- **Be able to develop a blood supply**
- **Be resistant to death from 'old age'.** ▶

Cancer typically arises as a 'lump' and this lump will have a certain potential for growth and for spread to distant sites. Cancer can arise in any living cell in the body and tend to be defined by the perceived cell of origin, as identified by histopathology.

Cancer patients can present with any degree of illness from none at all aside from the presence of a mass, through to the most severe cases of cachexia, respiratory distress or coma. Each case must be addressed on its own merits but there are principles of the approach to cancer patients that can be applied widely.

Approach to the cancer patient

The information required when presented with a cancer patient is:

- What is the tissue diagnosis?
- Is it low- or high-grade?
- Is it solitary or has it spread?
- Are there any signs of intercurrent disease?
- How infiltrative is the primary tumour?

Tissue diagnosis

A diagnosis is made by biopsy; however, there are instances when this is impractical or too hazardous, such as bone tumours that have undergone pathological fracture or intracranial masses. The simplest technique is fine-needle aspiration. Not all tumours can be diagnosed by fine-needle aspiration and there are some modifications of technique that can influence the likelihood of a useful result. If fine-needle aspiration proves non-diagnostic or is not considered appropriate, an incisional biopsy can be performed. This can take the form of a surgical biopsy, or a spring-loaded device can be used, which saves time and allows the biopsy to be performed through a tiny incision. On occasion it is considered appropriate to perform an excisional biopsy; for example, in a case such as a fracture through a bone tumour when other imperatives dictate that the lesion needs to be removed in its entirety anyway, or it may be in the hope that the biopsy might prove curative. In all circumstances, laboratory evaluation is required to define the nature of the mass.

Tumour grade

If a tissue specimen is obtained then histopathological evaluation can yield further information about tumour grade; this gives a more reliable indication of the likelihood of local relapse or spread. Tumour grading is a measure of biological activity (aggressiveness) that is applicable to certain tumour types, such as canine mast cell tumours (see below).

Metastasis

Different cancers spread by different routes. The presence of metastases has a significant impact on prognosis in many cases. All cancer patients must have a rigorous lymph node evaluation performed as part of their initial clinical examination. Any enlarged lymph nodes should undergo analysis by fine-needle aspiration or biopsy. For tumours that are known to metastasize to the lungs (Figure 2.42) or within the abdomen, pulmonary radiography or abdominal ultrasonography should form part of the diagnostic workup. All high-grade tumours have the potential to spread. With lower grade tumours the propensity to spread is more tumour-specific.

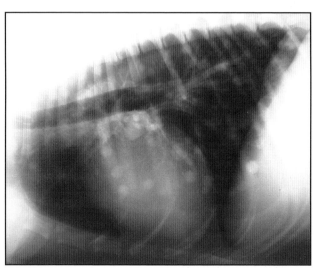

2.42 Lateral thoracic radiograph of a dog with pulmonary metastases from a malignant oral tumour.

Intercurrent disease

The purpose of evaluation of a cancer patient is to attempt to generate a complete picture of that patient's health status so that rational plans for therapy can be presented. It is critical that consideration is given to the possibility that patients may also be suffering other systemic illnesses, either as a consequence of the cancer or as an unrelated problem. Decisions about proceeding with cancer therapy are based not only on the potential impact of therapy on the tumour, but also the impact of therapy on the patient. Intercurrent disease states can shorten life expectancy, diminishing the value of cancer therapy, and may affect the patient's tolerance of cancer therapy.

Infiltrative disease

The most successful sole cancer therapy is surgery. It is critical that the surgery performed is appropriate and will not be curative if parts of the tumour are left behind. Prior to the advent of advanced MRI in veterinary oncology, surgical margins were defined by arbitrary assessments of the invasion of tumours based upon their histological type and grade. Such an approach is still employed but the addition of information from appropriate MRI studies can provide a much more specific assessment of the extent of tumour growth in an individual patient. The benefits of this are that appropriate surgery can be more readily performed and that surgery can be cancelled if it is evident from preoperative imaging studies that the desired outcome will not be achieved.

Common cancer presentations

Common cancer presentations include canine and feline lymphoma, canine cutaneous mast cell tumour and canine spindle cell sarcoma. Other notable presentations include canine mammary tumour, canine osteosarcoma, feline oral squamous cell carcinoma and feline injection site sarcoma.

Lymphoma

This is a cancer of the lymphocyte lineage of white blood cells and is the most common systemic malignancy in cats and dogs. The typical presentation in dogs is a generalized lymphadenopathy; in cats the alimentary form is most common and these patients typically present with reduced appetite, vomiting and an abdominal mass. A diagnosis can often be made with a fine-needle aspirate alone; sometimes a whole lymph node is required for histological evaluation. There are different sub-types of lymphoma, some of which carry different prognoses and may warrant a different therapeutic approach. Further tests, such as incisional biopsy and flow cytometry, may be performed by specialist veterinary oncologists to define the lymphoma sub-type. Lymphoma in dogs and cats is managed by the administration of systemic chemotherapy. Drugs used as first line therapy in dogs include vincristine, cyclophosphamide, prednisolone, doxorubicin and L-asparaginase; in cats they are vincristine, cyclophosphamide and prednisolone.

Canine cutaneous mast cell tumour

These are common in dogs. There is great variation in the degree of malignancy of these tumours and to aid prediction of biological behaviour a histological grading scheme is applied, which separates them into three groups: low-, intermediate-, and high-grade. A diagnosis can be made with a fine-needle aspirate but a tissue biopsy sample is required to provide a tumour grade. Low-grade tumours are minimally invasive and rarely metastatic, so local surgery is usually curative. Intermediate-grade tumours are moderately invasive and spread in about 15% of cases. High-grade tumours are highly invasive and metastasize in most cases. Systemic chemotherapy is administered to cases with proven metastasis. Radiotherapy is used in the management of incompletely resected primary tumours.

Canine spindle cell sarcoma

These are a form of soft tissue sarcoma that tend to be relatively benign in behaviour with moderate invasiveness and a low incidence of metastasis. Often a fine-needle aspirate fails to yield a diagnostic specimen so a tissue biopsy sample is required. Surgery often fails to achieve complete excision of these masses due to their moderately invasive growth; under these circumstances radiotherapy can be used postoperatively.

Canine mammary tumours

These are extremely common amongst entire bitches but routine ovariohysterectomy results in a significant reduction in the incidence of mammary tumours. Canine mammary tumours are benign in approximately 50% of cases. Small tumours are nearly always benign and the larger the tumour becomes, the more sinister becomes its behaviour. A fine-needle aspirate is rarely diagnostic so a tissue biopsy sample is required. In most cases, in which a discrete mass is present, excisional biopsy is appropriate. For cases with evidence of lymph node metastasis, chemotherapy has been used but the benefits are inconsistently seen.

Canine osteosarcoma

Primary bone tumours in dogs are almost invariably osteosarcoma. A presumptive diagnosis on the basis of radiography is often considered adequate to justify amputation as bone biopsy is notorious for yielding non-diagnostic information, the anatomical and radiographic presentation is highly predictable and most of the alternative diagnoses are also managed by amputation. Cases that do not meet the expected presentation should undergo a more complete evaluation prior to surgery. Thoracic radiography is mandatory as a very high proportion of osteosarcoma cases undergo metastasis. Ideal therapy is a combination of amputation and chemotherapy. However, because of emotional, cultural and social attitudes to amputation, not all owners will consent to it. Additionally, concurrent orthopaedic disease of other limbs may limit its application.

Feline oral squamous cell carcinoma

Older cats presented with a reduced appetite and focal or unilateral gingival redness and swelling should be considered to be potential cases of oral squamous cell carcinoma (Figure 2.43). This condition is very hard to treat; chemotherapy offers no benefit and radiotherapy offers such a modest benefit to most cases that it is rarely worth pursuing. Surgery can be curative but only if performed at the earliest possible stage. It is therefore critical that practitioners are aware of this potential diagnosis so that biopsy samples are taken early in the course of disease whilst surgery might still be applicable.

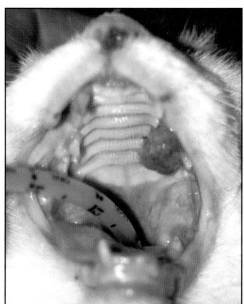

2.43 Oral squamous cell carcinoma in a cat.

Feline injection site sarcoma

Injection site sarcoma is still an unusual condition but the fact that it is triggered by the administration of veterinary products, mostly vaccines, that are given to otherwise healthy patients makes this a potentially controversial subject. Injection site sarcomas arise primarily between the scapulae. Any swelling noted in this site should be considered a potential injection site sarcoma. These tumours do not metastasize in most cases but they are highly invasive. Surgery can be curative but if the normal tissue planes have been disturbed prior to definitive surgery, the chance of a curative outcome diminishes dramatically. All potential cases of injection site sarcoma should be assessed by minimally invasive biopsy techniques (fine-needle aspiration, core or incisional biopsy), and if a diagnosis is made advice should be sought from a veterinary oncologist before further action is taken.

Chemotherapy

Chemotherapy carries risks of inducing two principal side-effects: gastrointestinal toxicity and myelosuppression. All owners of patients embarking on a course of chemotherapy must be informed of the potential risks and how to manage them should they arise. In addition, cytotoxic drugs pose certain risks to the individuals involved in their preparation and administration, and to those who are caring for the patients receiving them.

Effects of chemotherapy

Mild gastrointestinal signs are seen in up to 50% of cases but are typically short-lived and considered acceptable if a significant benefit is also being seen. Patients can also exhibit more severe consequences from prolonged anorexia, more frequently seen in cats, through to severe haemorrhagic gastroenteritis. These patients should be managed in the same way that a patient would be managed with the same clinical signs but with a different aetiology. Gastrointestinal signs typically develop within 24–72 hours of treatment administration.

Myelosuppression arises from a direct cytotoxic effect on haemopoietic precursors. Myelosuppression happens after every single chemotherapy administration. However, most animals have an adequate compensatory reserve capacity in the cell populations so the temporary cytotoxic effect has no overall effect on function. The cell populations preferentially affected are neutrophils, platelets and red blood cells in that order. Neutrophil numbers can change very acutely and need to be checked regularly. Platelet and red blood cell numbers are more stable and tend to only change with more chronic chemotherapy administration. Myelosuppresion typically affects patients 7–10 days after treatment administration. The typical presentation is neutropenic sepsis; in this instance cases are profoundly depressed and pyrexic. Prompt broad-spectrum antibiotic therapy is required. A useful guideline is not to administer chemotherapy to patients with neutrophil numbers $<3.0 \times 10^9$/l or platelet numbers $<100 \times 10^9$/l.

In the event that an adverse reaction develops, it must be recorded and consideration must be given to either a withdrawal of therapy or a subsequent dose reduction.

Safety

Chemotherapy drugs are cytotoxic. This means that they kill living cells and they do not have to be ingested or injected in order to do this. Different drugs carry different degrees of risk, which should be identified and actions taken to diminish them. Principal routes of inadvertent exposure include contact with skin or mucous membranes (spillage or splashing), inhalation (pressurized vial) and ingestion (food and drink in chemotherapy preparation area). This is contrary to the popular misconception that accidental exposure usually occurs through inadvertent needlestick injuries.

Acute exposure effects

Light headedness, nausea, ocular and cutaneous irritation have been reported.

Chronic exposure effects

Undoubtedly, the most important risk of occupational exposure arises through chronic low-level contact. Objective quantifiable data are lacking for obvious ethical reasons. The principal concerns are that these drugs are mutagenic and carcinogenic and this is certainly borne out by animal studies. Of less doubt is the fact that these drugs can be teratogenic; concerns prevail about the incidence of birth defects, miscarriage and low birth weight among workers suffering chronic occupational exposure.

Legal responsibilities

Employers have a legal duty to protect employees and the public from any consequences of their work, including exposure to cytotoxic drugs (Health and Safety at Work etc. Act 1974 and Management of Health and Safety at Work Regulations 1999). It is the employers' legal obligation to have a health and safety policy and to consult with their employees and safety representatives on the risks identified within the workplace and the measures needed to prevent or control these risks. Cytotoxic drugs are considered as hazardous as defined by the Control of Substances Hazardous to Health Regulations 2002 (COSHH). Carcinogenic substances are subject to Appendix 1 of the COSHH Approved Code of Practice (ACoP), which provides additional guidance. Under COSHH, employers have a legal duty to assess the risks from handling cytotoxic drugs for employees and anyone else affected by this type of work, and to take suitable precautions to protect their health.

Employers need to ensure that employees handling cytotoxic drugs are given suitable and sufficient information, instruction and training. Employees also have a duty to take care of their own health and safety at work and those around them who may be affected by their actions.

Prevention or control of exposure

Ideally totally enclosed systems should be used for the preparation of cytotoxic substances (Figure 2.44). In circumstances where this is not possible or practical, substances should be handled in areas with adequate ventilation, with low human traffic levels and where eating, drinking and smoking are prohibited. All staff who may be involved in handling and administration of

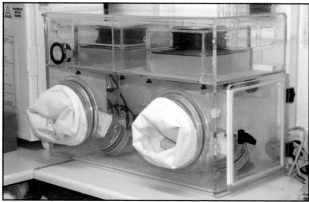

2.44 Glove box isolator used for the preparation of drugs required for chemotherapy.

cytotoxic substances should be appropriately trained. If risk of exposure cannot be adequately prevented or controlled by the means stated above, protective clothing should be provided for all staff who may be at risk of exposure. This should include some or all of the following:

- Protective gloves
- Respiratory protective equipment
- Goggles
- Protective gown or apron.

While latex gloves will protect the wearer from accidental splashes, natural rubber is not impermeable to some chemotherapy agents. In addition, latex gloves tend not to be a snug fit and therefore they reduce dexterity. Nitrile rubber gloves are recommended for handling chemotherapy agents. There is no protective glove that will be completely chemical proof for extended periods. Glove type is irrelevant if chemical exposure arises by contact via the cuff.

If chemotherapy drugs cannot be prepared in a safety cabinet or pharmaceutical isolator, suitable respiratory protective equipment should be provided and used (see COSHH Regulations, above). Surgical facemasks do not protect against the inhalation of aerosols. Gowns and aprons can help protect against accidental spillage. Liquid can seep through cloth gowns and so these are less protective than some operators assume. Conversely, impermeable materials lead to discomfort with prolonged wear and this must also be a consideration when constructing a protocol for use.

Administration

Chemotherapy drugs should ideally be prepared in a closed system (see above) so that they can be administered to the patient without risk of accidental spillage or leakage. Oral chemotherapy must not be handled without gloves. Under no circumstances should chemotherapy tablets be divided; if smaller doses are required then a pharmacist must be employed to formulate the appropriate product. Intravenous chemotherapy should always be administered via an intravenous cannula. The consequences of perivascular injection range from loss of local skin and soft tissues in less severe cases, for example, following vincristine extravasation, to severe, extensive, protracted necrotic changes usually necessitating amputation as would be the case following extravasation of doxorubicin.

Administration should be carried out in an area away from disturbances and away from food or drink items. A chemotherapy 'spill kit' (Figure 2.45) should be considered a mandatory requirement before handling cytotoxic liquids.

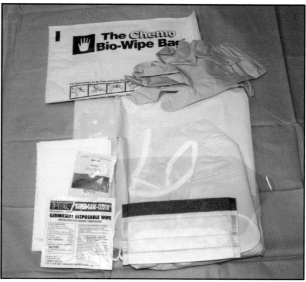

2.45 Items found in a chemotherapy 'spill kit'. Note the aerosol-proof facemask with eye protection. Other items include a water-impervious long-sleeved gown, nitrile rubber gloves and a self-sealing cytotoxic waste and absorbent wipe bag.

Any inpatient who has received chemotherapy in the preceding 72 hours should be handled as if its excreta remain cytotoxic; appropriate signage to indicate the animal's cytotoxic status is mandatory.

Cytotoxic waste

Staff must be aware that urine and faeces from patients receiving chemotherapy can contain active metabolites or unchanged chemotherapy drugs and suitable protective equipment should be worn and handling measures taken. Soiled bedding should be disposed of promptly and double-bagged in the appropriate waste bags. Separate containers for cytotoxic waste, including chemotherapy preparation and administration consumables should be available and clearly labelled. Syringes and sharps contaminated by chemotherapy should be disposed of as cytotoxic sharps. Waste should not be allowed to accumulate. It is a requirement in law that veterinary practices hold a document, written or ratified by the practice principal, outlining procedures with respect to inpatient care, including details of where patients should urinate, handling and storage of cytotoxic substances and measures taken to protect staff, patients and owners. These constitute the local rules that govern an individual practice (see above). As a general rule, urine that is potentially toxic should be copiously diluted. Faeces should be collected as usual but double-bagged and disposed of as hazardous waste.

Advice for owners

Studies have not been performed to define the range of duration of cytotoxic metabolite excretion in domestic animals. Owners of all patients receiving chemotherapy must be advised to treat urine, faeces and vomit from their pet as though it were contaminated by cytotoxic drugs for the duration of a chemotherapy protocol. Faeces should be recovered, wherever they were deposited, and disposed of down the toilet. Urination can be permitted in the local environment; owners must carry a bottle of water with them at all times when exercising their dog, with which to dilute any urine passed, thus sanitizing the area.

Radiotherapy

Radiation therapy represents one of the three principal therapeutic modalities in the arsenal of the veterinary oncologist for use against cancer. Radiation can be in different forms, with X-ray radiation being the form most commonly used. A beam of radiation carries energy from the radiation source to the target, where all or part of that energy is deposited. Other forms of radiation energy used therapeutically include electron beams, alpha particles and neutron beams. The various types of radiation differ in depth of penetration before depositing their energy and in how much energy a radiation beam has to deposit. Radiotherapy cannot be applied without the oversight of a specially qualified Radiation Protection Advisor (RPA).

Effects of radiation

Radiation therapy harms cancer by exploiting differential sensitivities between the normal healthy tissue and the cancer cells. In essence, the cancer cells are less able to tolerate a certain dose of radiation and so can be killed more easily than the surrounding normal cells. When radiation deposits its energy in a target tissue, it precipitates a series of chemical reactions that result in damage to critical cellular machinery, particularly DNA. Healthy tissues can identify and correct that damage much of the time. Cancer cells can too but not so effectively. This explains the differential sensitivity of normal and neoplastic cells to radiation.

Comparative oncology

In human oncology, certain cancers are considered curable with radiation therapy, for example, early Hodgkin's lymphoma. If they are not curable, certain cancers can be managed as well by radiation as they can by surgery, for example, certain forms of prostate cancer in men and cervical cancer in women. Achieving this outcome requires intensive radiation treatment with exquisitely high degrees of accuracy and complexity of administration. Whilst it may be a valid goal of veterinary radiotherapy to emulate the outcomes achieved in human oncology, there are issues of tolerability of side-effects, access to facilities, financial cost and practical difficulties that limit the success of veterinary radiotherapy.

General indications

Different body tissues have different sensitivities to radiation therapy; this can be a significant limiting factor in the application of radiotherapy in certain anatomical locations. For instance, the spinal cord, lungs and gastrointestinal tract have a low tolerance of radiation; a full course of treatment could cause fatal consequences if these organs were in the target site. Other tissues, such as skin, the brain, the oral mucosa, bone and muscle have a relatively good tolerance of radiation. A decision to undertake radiotherapy is therefore determined not only by tumour type but also by anatomical considerations.

Tumours that are particularly suited to management with radiotherapy are presented in Figure 2.46. Without doubt, radiation therapy plays a vital role in the management of veterinary cancer. Perhaps the strongest indication for radiotherapy is as part of a multimodality treatment plan. Surgery, chemotherapy and radiation therapy all have strengths and weaknesses in the management of cancer; by combining these treatments, when appropriate, far superior outcomes can be seen.

Location	Tumour type
Oral	Squamous cell carcinoma, melanoma, fibrosarcoma, lymphoma
Nasal	Adenocarcinoma, carcinoma, lymphoma, sarcoma
Brain	Meningioma, glioma, ependymoma, granulomatous meningoencephalitis (GME) (non-neoplastic application)
Distal limb	Mast cell tumour, haemangiopericytoma, spindle cell sarcoma, sweat gland tumour

2.46 Tumours amenable to management by radiotherapy.

Radioiodine therapy

Hyperthyroidism can be managed by the administration of radioactive iodine. This radionuclide emits gamma rays, which constitute a radiation hazard to personnel, and therefore these patients must only be handled minimally during the period of confinement. Isolation of these patients can be prolonged (8 weeks) and therefore preliminary investigations are undertaken to rule out the possibility of chronic illness that might develop into a life-threatening problem during that time. Nursing care of isolated patients is minimized, although disposable environmental enrichments are permitted.

Future developments

There is no doubt that radiotherapy will become increasingly important in the management of veterinary cancer. Access to facilities for the administration of radiation therapy is improving around the world and, with this, veterinary oncologists' experiences and expectations are burgeoning. With improved technology, the accuracy of targeting of radiation will improve and this will diminish the risk of side-effects. In the future there will become a greater reliance upon the veterinary oncologist to perform radiation therapy, predominantly in the context of the multidisciplinary team of veterinary professionals. This team will attend to all aspects of the care of the oncology patient, drawing on proficiencies in surgery, radiology, medicine, nutrition and most importantly, nursing care.

Conclusion

Advanced medical nursing is a skill that encompasses all aspects of veterinary nursing. Patients must be nursed in the context of the whole patient and its environment, not just as an isolated medical problem. The advanced medical veterinary nurse makes regular observations, some conscious, some subconscious, and continually compares these observations with an expectation of what is normal for the patient in question. This allows early recognition of abnormalities and implementation of appropriate measures to prevent progression of clinical signs and to assist in diagnosis.

Acknowledgements

The authors would like to thank the following people for use of images within this Chapter:

Dr Sebastien Behr; Dr Clive Elwood; Rachel Garrod; Dr David Gould; Theresa McCann; and Dr Paul Wotton.

References and further reading

Chandler EA, Gaskell CJ and Gaskell RM (1993) *Feline Medicine and Therapeutics, 2nd edn.* Blackwell Publishing, Oxford
Day M, Mackin A and Littlewood J (2000) *BSAVA Manual of Canine and Feline Haematology and Transfusion Medicine.* BSAVA Publications, Gloucester
Dobson J and Lascelles D (2003) *BSAVA Manual of Canine and Feline Oncology, 2nd edn.* BSAVA Publications, Gloucester
Elliott J and Grauer G (2007) *BSAVA Manual of Canine and Feline Nephrology and Urology, 2nd edn.* BSAVA Publications, Gloucester
Foster A and Foil C (2003) *BSAVA Manual of Small Animal Dermatology, 2nd edn.* BSAVA Publications, Gloucester
Gorman NT (1998) *Canine Medicine and Therapeutics, 4th edn.* Blackwell Publishing, Oxford
Hall E, Simpson J and Williams D (2005) *BSAVA Manual of Canine and Feline Gastroenterology, 2nd edn.* BSAVA Publications, Gloucester
King L and Boag A (2007) *BSAVA Manual of Canine and Feline Emergency and Critical Care, 2nd edn.* BSAVA Publications, Gloucester
Luis Fuentes V and Swift S (1998) *BSAVA Manual of Small Animal Cardiorespiratory Medicine and Surgery.* BSAVA Publications, Cheltenham
Mooney C and Peterson M (2004) *BSAVA Manual of Canine and Feline Endocrinology, 3rd edn.* BSAVA Publications, Gloucester
Mullineaux E and Jones M (2007) *BSAVA Manual of Practical Veterinary Nursing.* BSAVA Publications, Gloucester
Petersen-Jones S and Crispin S (2002) *BSAVA Manual of Small Animal Ophthalmology, 2nd edn.* BSAVA Publications, Gloucester
Platt S and Olby N (2004) *BSAVA Manual of Canine and Feline Neurology, 3rd edn.* BSAVA Publications, Gloucester
Ramsey I and Tennant B (2001) *BSAVA Manual of Canine and Feline Infectious Diseases.* BSAVA Publications, Gloucester
Villiers E and Blackwood L (2005) *BSAVA Manual of Canine and Feline Clinical Pathology, 2nd edn.* BSAVA Publications, Gloucester

3

Clinical nutrition

Rachel Lumbis and Daniel L. Chan

This chapter is designed to give information on:

- The role and limitations of nutrition in modulating various diseases in dogs and cats
- Creating and applying a nutritional plan for hospitalized patients
- Selecting methods of assisted feeding (feeding tubes, parenteral nutrition and drug therapy)

Introduction

Small animal veterinary nutrition initially focused on the essential nutrients and minimal requirements needed to meet the basic biological needs of animals. It was later recognized that health and vitality could be further improved by modifying nutrient levels to the lifestage, lifestyle and breed of an individual animal (see *BSAVA Manual of Practical Animal Care* and *BSAVA Manual of Practical Veterinary Nursing*). In addition, the metabolic changes associated with certain disease states could be corrected or controlled by adjusting levels of key nutrients. Complete nutrition is essential for maintaining good health and plays an important role in modulating many common diseases in animals. Clinical nutrition entails understanding basic nutritional principles and the application of nutrition in optimizing health and well being.

An increasing number of therapeutic foods are now available for various medical disorders, from diabetes mellitus to canine cognitive dysfunction. Previously, clinical nutrition was considered adjunctive therapy to common diseases but in recent years it has emerged as a foundation of treatment in certain instances. Ongoing research is contributing to the understanding of clinical nutrition and its critical role in animal health and disease, and in the future modulation of certain diseases may primarily involve nutritional rather than pharmacological therapy.

As veterinary nurses play an instrumental role in educating pet owners about nutrition and in implementing the majority of nutritional support therapies to hospitalized animals, it is vital that they are aware of the current issues surrounding nutrition of both healthy and clinically affected companion animals. Various diseases require at least some modification of the dietary plan, and having an appreciation of these requirements is vitally important. Additionally, having a greater understanding of special techniques and protocols for providing nutritional support of hospitalized and critically ill animals is becoming essential for veterinary nurses. With these goals in mind, this chapter aims to prepare veterinary nurses for their pivotal role in ensuring good nutrition of companion animals.

Diets for dogs and cats with specific conditions

Hepatic disease

The diet should aim to achieve these objectives:

- **Maintain optimal bodyweight**
- **Support protein synthesis**
- **Decrease protein catabolism**
- **Slow disease progression**
- **Improve clinical signs, e.g. reduce hepatic encephalopathy**
- **Support liver regeneration**
- **Encourage food intake (many patients with liver disease have a reduced appetite).**

The complexity and variety of disorders involving the liver make it impossible to describe an 'ideal diet'. Depending on the exact pathology involved, certain modifications to the diet may be helpful; however, not all patients with hepatic disease may benefit from dietary modification. For example, for cats with hepatic lipidosis, the most important management strategy is ensuring adequate food intake, and the composition of the diet itself is less important. As cats with hepatic lipidosis are typically managed with feeding tubes, the use of energy-dense, high-fat diets makes it easier to deliver the required amount of calories. Some of the most common modifications for patients with liver disease include:

- Moderate protein restriction
- High-fat, energy-dense source of non-protein calories
- High carbohydrate intake
- Control of copper intake.

Moderate protein restriction

Excess dietary protein leads to an abundance of protein byproducts, which are converted to ammonia by bacterial action in the gut. The ammonia is normally absorbed into the bloodstream, converted to urea by the liver and excreted in the kidneys. In cases of liver failure or portosystemic shunts (i.e. severe hepatic dysfunction) this conversion may be incomplete, leading to accumulation of ammonia, which is believed to be responsible for many signs of encephalopathy. Providing high biological value protein sources minimizes the production of protein byproducts and maximizes protein uptake and assimilation. This allows for the overall content of protein to be reduced without compromising absolute protein requirements. However, most patients diagnosed with liver disease do not have this advanced form of liver dysfunction and protein restriction is not required. What dictates whether a patient would benefit from dietary protein restriction is the presence of clinical signs compatible with hepatic encephalopathy (e.g. head-pressing, depression, vocalization, seizures).

It was previously thought that proteins rich in certain types of amino acids (branched-chain amino acids) would be beneficial to animals with severe liver dysfunction. Many diets formulated for patients with liver disease have been designed with a purported optimal ratio of branched-chain to aromatic amino acids. Unfortunately, the determination of this 'optimal ratio' has not been made, and there is insufficient evidence to support such an approach for effectively controlling signs of encephalopathy.

High-fat, energy-dense source of non-protein calories

Fat increases the caloric density and palatability of food, provides essential fatty acids and enhances absorption of fat-soluble vitamins. In patients where protein restriction is required (e.g. in hepatic encephalopathy) fat may be added to increase caloric density. However, in certain types of liver disease there may be an impaired ability to digest and absorb fat, due to reduced bile salt synthesis and bile stasis; therefore, increasing the fat content of the diet is not desirable. Patients with chronic diarrhoea and/or steatorrhoea should be evaluated for impaired fat assimilation, which would preclude feeding high-fat diets.

High carbohydrate intake

As discussed above, with severe liver dysfunction there may be a need to reduce dietary protein significantly. However, this may lead to breakdown (catabolism) of lean muscle, which leads to greater formation of nitrogenous waste and thus ammonia formation. In this situation, there may be a benefit from shifting energy metabolism to carbohydrate sources instead of protein. Liver disease may also lead to glycogen depletion which may be ameliorated by provision of simple carbohydrates.

Furthermore, addition of specific fermentable sugars (lactulose solution) to the diet of patients with hepatic encephalopathy has been shown to reduce clinical signs. Fermentation of the lactulose is believed to achieve this by acidification of colonic contents, resulting in trapping of ammonia in the lumen and restricting bacterial growth, and by producing a laxative effect.

Control of copper intake

In certain conditions (e.g. copper hepatopathy) the uptake of specific micronutrients, such as copper, becomes significantly altered and can lead to pathological consequences. Copper restriction is recommended in breeds suffering from hepatic copper storage disease, e.g. Bedlington Terrier, Cocker Spaniel, Dobermann. In cases where dogs refuse specially formulated prescription diets, a homemade diet formulated by a board-certified veterinary nutritionist may be used.

Renal disease

> ## The diet should aim to achieve these objectives:
>
> - **Ameliorate clinical signs of uraemia if present**
> - **Slow down disease progression – this is best achieved if dietary management is started during early renal insufficiency and not delayed until the animal is uraemic and in overt renal failure.**

The diets recommended for cats and dogs with renal disease will depend on the nature and degree of renal compromise and include:

- Restricted levels of high biological value protein
- Increased levels of non-protein calories
- Reduced phosphorus intake
- Increased levels of water-soluble vitamins
- Additional management strategies.

Restricted levels of high biological value protein

Decreased protein intake may help to reduce signs of uraemia; the inclusion of protein sources of high biological value may decrease production of nitrogenous waste products that have to be eliminated by the kidneys. Animals with severe proteinuria resulting from glomerular disease may also benefit from protein restriction. It is important to realize that the presence of azotaemia alone is not sufficient to recommend a diet with reduced protein content. There are many mechanisms of azotaemia and not all are amenable to dietary modification. The decision to reduce protein is mostly based on whether the azotaemia is believed to be resulting in adverse clinical signs such as anorexia and vomiting.

Increased levels of non-protein calories

Many animals with advanced renal disease are already in a catabolic state and further protein restriction can worsen their condition. Supplying calories from carbohydrate or fats may aid in minimizing catabolism of body protein and improve caloric density of the diet.

Reduced phosphorus intake

Minimizing hyperphosphataemia is an important goal for patients with advanced renal disease. A reduction in dietary phosphorus may also slow the progression of some forms of renal disease and reduce the risk of renal secondary hyperparathyroidism – a complication of chronic renal failure characterized by increased endogenous levels of parathyroid hormone (PTH). Renal secondary hyperparathyroidism is seen frequently in dogs and occasionally in cats. With progressive renal disease, serum hyperphosphataemia develops as the glomerular filtration rate decreases. Hyperphosphataemia leads to a lower serum calcium concentration and PTH concentrations progressively increase, leading to the clinical manifestations of renal secondary hyperparathyroidism. As a result of accelerated resorption of cancellous bone of the maxilla and mandible, bones become softened and pliable ('rubber jaw' syndrome), and the jaw is unable to close completely. Renal secondary hyperparathyroidism is diagnosed by laboratory abnormalities consistent with renal insufficiency accompanied by an increase in serum PTH.

Increased levels of water-soluble vitamins

Animals with significant renal disease may have significant increased urinary loss of water-soluble vitamins and therefore may have higher requirements for them. Overt manifestation of deficiency is rare, but supplementation of these vitamins in diets is thought to be beneficial.

Additional management strategies

Depending on the type and severity of renal pathology, additional management strategies may need to be addressed; however, these may be independent of the diet used to manage the disease process. Increasing water intake has been recommended for some patients with renal disease but this is likely to be inadequate to meet water requirements in some polyuric patients. Potassium supplements may also be required for some, though not all, patients with renal disease, and can be added to the food directly by the owner. In the stable patient, dietary supplementation with potassium is preferred to parenteral supplementation because it is more convenient and is safer.

Cardiac disease

The diet should aim to achieve these objectives:

- **Reduce sodium and water retention**
- **Alleviate clinical signs such as pulmonary congestion and peripheral oedema**
- **Decrease workload of the heart**
- **Maintain lean body mass and restore the animal to normal bodyweight.**

Depending on the type and severity of cardiac dysfunction, diets designed for dogs and cats with heart disease may have the following properties:

- Increased energy density and high digestibility
- Avoidance of dietary sodium excess
- Additional B vitamins and magnesium
- Optimized potassium intake.

Increased energy density and high digestibility

Cardiac failure elicits a chronic inflammatory state that increases overall energy demands and promotes various other metabolic changes, such as altered substrate metabolism and oxidative stress. At the same time, many animals with cardiac disease will have a reduction in appetite. This leads to lean body wasting, which is sometimes referred to as cardiac cachexia. Inclusion of certain fatty acids such as omega-3 may be beneficial with certain types of cardiomyopathies by modulating the inflammatory response as well as increasing the caloric density of the diet. Omega-3 fatty acids are a subset of polyunsaturated fatty acids which play an important role in reducing inflammation and may even reduce the rates of certain tachyarrhymias. Some research has also demonstrated that omega-3 fatty acids may enhance appetite in certain patient populations.

Avoidance of dietary sodium excess

In heart failure, sodium, chloride and water are retained by the body following activation of the aldosterone–angiotensin cascade. This may lead to oedema, ascites, pulmonary congestion and coughing. These deleterious effects are exacerbated by consuming diets with a high salt content, which is typical of many maintenance diets. Most treats are also very high in sodium and should be avoided in patients with congestive heart failure. Feeding a diet that is restricted in sodium (less than minimum requirements) is not usually necessary, and in fact may accentuate activation of the aldosterone–angiotensin system. A gradual reduction in sodium levels (or avoidance of sodium excess) in the diet, especially if the animal has been fed a diet high in sodium, is preferred over actual sodium restriction. Furthermore, restricting sodium reduces palatability of the diet, which is undesirable. Appreciating the difference between avoidance of sodium excesses and sodium restriction is an important point in the dietary management of patients with cardiac disease.

Additional B vitamins and magnesium

The use of diuretic agents increases the requirements for water-soluble vitamins and therefore supplementation may be necessary, although deficiencies leading to clinical manifestations are uncommon. Additionally, diuretics also increase the requirement for magnesium. If hypomagnesaemia develops, this could lead to an increased risk of cardiac arrhythmias. The risk for the development of cardiac arrhythmias due to hypomagnesaemia may be ameliorated with diets enriched in magnesium.

Optimized potassium intake

Body potassium may also be depleted by the use of diuretics, notably furosemide. For this reason, diets designed for patients with cardiac disease are fortified with potassium to compensate for increased requirements. In animals with a tendency towards potassium depletion, the use of potassium-sparing diuretics, such as spironolactone, may be preferrable. Animals concurrently receiving angiotensin-converting enzyme (ACE) inhibitors usually do not need potassium-supplemented diets.

Pancreatitis

Acute pancreatitis is the sudden onset of inflammation of the pancreatic acinar tissue. Pancreatitis occurs as a consequence of intracellular pancreatic acinar enzyme activation and resultant autodigestion of the pancreas. Acute pancreatitis is an important differential diagnosis for dogs with vomiting and abdominal pain. Pancreatitis is less commonly diagnosed in cats because of difficulties in diagnosis. Pancreatitis in dogs is very distinct from that in cats, and nutritional management of the disorder is also very different. Because there is much less known about the pathophysiology of pancreatitis in cats, there are very few dietary recommendations available. One important distinction is that withholding food from cats with pancreatitis appears to be unnecessary and may even increase the risk of developing hepatic lipidosis, although this has not been demonstrated.

Chronic pancreatitis is less commonly recognized in companion animals than in humans, and dietary modification may be required. Histopathological examination of tissues from dogs and cats with chronic pancreatitis often shows irreversible fibrotic changes. Both chronic and recurrent pancreatitis may result in acquired exocrine pancreatic insufficiency (EPI) in which animals have a reduced capacity to digest and assimilate fat and fat-soluble vitamins (see below).

Discontinuation of food and water (*nil per os*) is recommended as initial therapy for acute pancreatitis in dogs. Avoidance of oral feeding is recommended because feeding contributes to abdominal discomfort and vomiting. Stimulation of pancreatic secretion was once thought to be another reason for the need to avoid feeding, but this does not appear to be the case. After vomiting and abdominal discomfort have resolved or lessened in severity, food and water can be introduced gradually over several days. Normal feeding methods can be reintroduced after several days provided there is resolution of clinical signs – unless the original diet was thought to have contributed to the problem (e.g. high-fat diet triggering pancreatitis). If clinical signs have not resolved after 3 days of *nil per os*, patients should receive either enteral or parenteral nutritional support. In most cases, some form of enteral nutrition is appropriate; however, in more severe cases parenteral nutrition may be necessary to meet the patient's energy, protein, electrolyte and vitamin requirements (Figure 3.1).

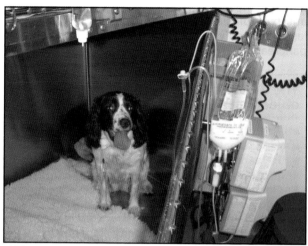

3.1 Some dogs with pancreatitis are subject to severe vomiting, which necessitates feeding via the parenteral route.

Enteral feeding may be accomplished via naso-oesophageal, oesophagostomy, gastrostomy or jejunostomy feeding tubes (see later), depending on the severity of clinical signs and the need for surgical exploration (e.g. pancreatic abscess). With the exception of naso-oesophageal tubes, all other tubes require general anaesthesia for placement. Once placed, these feeding tubes can be used to deliver specific diets.

Diets for acute pancreatitis should aim to achieve these objectives:

- **Meet nutritional requirements without exacerbating pancreatitis**
- **Be easily digestible and minimally reliant on pancreatic enzymes for digestion.**

Diets for **dogs** with pancreatitis may involve the following:

- Reduced levels of fat
- High digestibility.

Reduced levels of fat

Fat digestion is very reliant on pancreatic enzymes; therefore, patients with pancreatitis may benefit from low-fat diets. Fat also delays gastric emptying, which may increase the tendency for vomiting. As cats with pancreatitis do not tend to vomit (<30% of cats with pancreatitis are reported to have vomiting as a clinical sign) and the disease process tends not to be related to fat in the diet, fat restriction is not necessary for cats. In fact, cats diagnosed with pancreatitis are often fed high-energy dense diets that have high fat levels.

components, allowing the osmolarity of the solution to be tolerated in a large peripheral vein, such as the lateral saphenous vein in dogs or the femoral vein in cats. Because PPN only provides a portion of the patient's requirements, it is intended for short-term use only in a non-debilitated patient with average nutritional requirements. For example, an animal with acute vomiting and diarrhoea may only need nutritional support for 3 days and therefore PPN would be sufficient, but an animal with chronic malabsorptive diarrhoea resulting in severe malnutrition should receive TPN for nutritional support. Other considerations for choosing one form of PN over the other include: whether the patient can have a central line placed (central lines are contraindicated in patients with severe coagulopathy); and cost.

Equipment and solutions

Regardless of the exact form of PN, intravenous nutrition requires catheters that are placed specifically for nutrition using strict aseptic technique. Multi-lumen cathethers (in which up to three different solutions can be administered via separate ports) are often recommended for PN because they can remain in place for longer periods of time than normal jugular catheters, and they provide other ports for blood sampling and administration of additional fluids and intravenous medications (Figure 3.10). The expertise required for placing these catheters is another limiting factor. Suitable materials for these catheters include silicone and polyurethane.

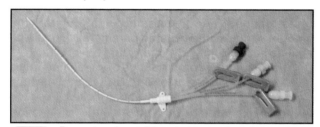

3.10 Parenteral nutrition is best administered via dedicated catheters designed for long-term use. A triple-lumen central catheter such as this is commonly used.

Most PN solutions are composed of a carbohydrate source (e.g. 5% or 50% dextrose), a protein source (e.g. 8.5% or 11% amino acids), and a fat source (e.g. 20% lipids) (Figure 3.11). Vitamins and trace metals can also be added. Calculations for formulating PPN and TPN diets are shown in Figures 3.12 and 3.13.

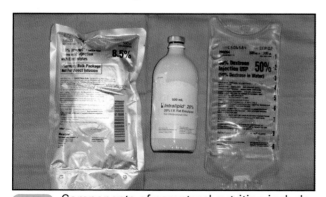

3.11 Components of parenteral nutrition include (left to right) an amino acid source, a lipid source and a carbohydrate source.

---

1. **Calculate resting energy requirement (RER)**

   RER = 70 x (current bodyweight in kg) $^{0.75}$
   or for animals 2–30 kg, RER = (30 x current bodyweight in kg) + 70

   RER = _____ kcal/day

2. **Calculate the partial energy requirement (PER)**

   Plan to supply 70% of the animal's RER with PPN:
   PER = RER x 0.70 = _____ kcal/day

3. **Proportion of nutrient requirements according to bodyweight:**
   (*NB For animals ≤ 3kg, the formulation will exceed maintenance fluid requirements*)

   Cats and dogs 3–5 kg:
   PER x 0.20 = _____ kcal/day carbohydrate
   PER x 0.20 = _____ kcal/day protein
   PER x 0.60 = _____ kcal/day lipid

   Cats and dogs 6–10 kg:
   PER x 0.25 = _____ kcal/day carbohydrate
   PER x 0.25 = _____ kcal/day protein
   PER x 0.50 = _____ kcal/day lipid

   Dogs 11–30 kg:
   PER x 0.33 = _____ kcal/day carbohydrate
   PER x 0.33 = _____ kcal/day protein
   PER x 0.33 = _____ kcal/day lipid

   Dogs >30 kg:
   PER X 0.50 = _____ kcal/day carbohydrate
   PER x 0.25 = _____ kcal/day protein
   PER x 0.25 = _____ kcal/day lipid

4. **Volumes of nutrient solutions required:**

   Carbohydrate
   5% dextrose solution = 0.17 kcal/ml
   _____ kcal carbohydrate required/day ÷ 0.17 kcal/ml
   = _____ ml/day dextrose

   Protein
   8.5% amino acid solution = 0.34 kcal/ml
   _____ kcal protein required/day ÷ 0.34 kcal/ml
   = _____ ml/day amino acids

   Lipid
   20% lipid solution = 2 kcal/ml
   _____ kcal lipid required/day ÷ 2 kcal/ml
   = _____ ml/day lipid

   = _____ total ml of PPN to be administered over 24 hours

3.12 How to calculate partial parenteral nutrition (PPN) requirements.

1. Calculate resting energy requirement (RER)

RER = 70 x (current bodyweight in kg) $^{0.75}$
or for animals 2–30 kg, RER = (30 x current bodyweight in kg) + 70

RER = _____ cal/day

2. Protein requirements

	Dogs (g/100 kcal)	Cats (g/100 kcal)
Standard	4	6
Reduced (hepatic/renal disease)	2–3	3–4
Increased (excessive protein losses)	6	6

(RER ÷ 100) x _____ g/100 kcal = _____ g protein required/day
protein req

3. Volume of nutrient solutions required

Protein
8.5% amino acid solution = 0.085 g protein/ml

_____ g protein required/day ÷ 0.085 g/ml = _____ ml/day of amino acids

Non-protein calories
The calories supplied by protein (e.g. 4 kcal/g) are subtracted from the RER to calculate the total non-protein calories needed:

_____ g protein req/day x 4 kcal/g = _____ kcal provided by protein

RER – kcal provided by protein = _____ total non-protein kcal/day required

Non-protein calories are usually provided as a 50:50 mixture of lipid and dextrose

20% lipid solution = 2 kcal/ml
To supply 50% of non-protein calories
_____ lipid kcal required ÷ 2 kcal/ml = _____ ml of lipid

50% of dextrose solution = 1.7 kcal/ml
To supply 50% of non-protein calories
_____ dextrose kcal required ÷ 1.7 kcal/ml = _____ ml of dextrose

4. Total daily requirements
_____ ml of 8.5% amino acid solution
_____ ml of 20% lipid
_____ ml of 50% dextrose

_____ total ml of TPN solution to be administered over 24 hours

3.13 How to calculate total parenteral nutrition (TPN) requirements.

TPN and PPN solutions must be mixed and handled aseptically (Figure 3.14a). This requires special training and equipment, e.g. a special PN compounder (Figure 3.14b). For these reasons, PN is not feasible in most practices, though using TPN compounding services at some human hospitals may be an alternative. When compounding PN diets, components with the highest osmolarity are added first to specially made fluid bags intended for PN (Figure 3.14c). These special bags limit the oxidation of components, preserving the quality of the product. Typically, amino acid solutions are the first component to be added, followed by dextrose and finally lipids. Other fluids can be added to adjust the osmolarity of the solution.

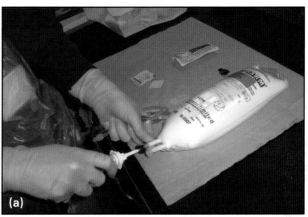

(a)

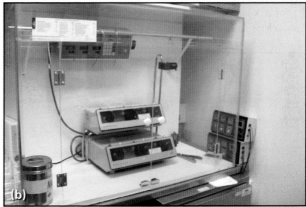

(b)

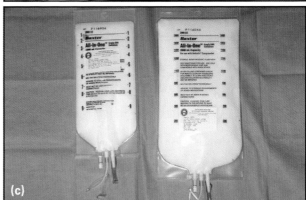

(c)

3.14 Parenteral nutrition requires absolute attention to aseptic technique. **(a)** Bags and infusion lines must be handled with sterile gloves. **(b)** Solutions are ideally mixed in a specially made total parenteral nutrition compounder, which mixes precise amounts of the components in a closed sytem, thereby maintaining absolute sterility of the solution. **(c)** The solutions are held in specially made bags.

Alternatively, commercial ready-to-use preparations of glucose and amino acids are available for peripheral use but these only provide approximately up to 70% of the total required calories (when administered at maintenance fluid rate) and should only be used for short-term or interim nutritional support. A product that could be used in practice is Vamin® 9 Glucose (Fresenius Kabi) which is a 5.9% amino acid and 10% dextrose solution. A worksheet for calculating infusion rates using Vamin® 9 Glucose is shown in Figure 3.15. Advantages of such solutions are that they are already mixed and require no specialized equipment other than fluid infusion pumps to be used. However, the major disadvantage is that they cannot be individualized to the patient's needs as the components are fixed in proportion.

Administration and nursing considerations

Due to the high osmolarity of the TPN solution (usually 1100–1500 mOsm/l), it must be administered through a central venous (jugular) catheter. Administering a solution with very high osmolarity increases the risk of thrombophlebitis. PPN is formulated to have a lower osmolarity (<1100 mOsmo/l) so can be administered through a peripheral catheter.

This parenteral nutrition solution has a relatively low osmolality and thus can be administered via a peripheral catheter. Strict asepsis should be adhered to when delivering the solution. The solution contains **20 mmol/l potassium chloride,** thus adjustments to supplementation rates may be necessary.

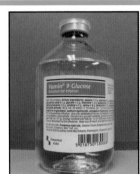

1. **Calculate resting energy requirement (RER)**

RER = 70 x (current bodyweight in kg) $^{0.75}$
or for animals 2–30 kg, RER = (30 x current bodyweight in kg) + 70

RER = _____ kcal/day

2. **Calculate protein requirement**

	Dogs (g/100 kcal)	Cats (g/100 kcal)
Standard	4	6
Reduced (hepatic/renal disease)	2–3	3–4
Increased (excessive protein losses)	6	6

(RER ÷ 100) x _____ g/100 kcal = _____ g protein required/day
protein req

3. **Calculate rate of Vamin® 9 Glucose required**

Vamin® 9 Glucose is a 5.9% amino acid solution (9% nitrogen) and thus has 0.059 g protein/ml.

PPN rate required = _____ g protein/day ÷ 0.059 g prot/ml ÷ 24 hours = _____ ml/h of PPN

> ⚠️ **WARNING**
> **Make sure this rate of infusion is acceptable for this patient.**

4. **Calculate proportion of RER provided at this rate**

Vamin® 9 Glucose contains 0.65 kcal/ml of energy.

Energy provided by PPN = 0.65 kcal/ml x _____ ml/h of PPN x 24 hours = _____ kcal/day

Proportion of energy from PPN = _____ PPN energy ÷ _____ RER x 100 = _____ %

5. **Calculate rate of glucose infusion at calculated PPN rate:**

Vamin® 9 Glucose is a 10% glucose solution, i.e. 100 mg/ml

Glucose infusion rate = _____ ml/h PPN ÷ 60 min x 100 mg/ml ÷ kg bodyweight
= _____ mg/kg/min

> ⚠️ **WARNING**
> **Glucose infusion rate should not exceed 4 mg/kg/min, as this may cause hyperglycaemia. It may be necessary to decrease the infusion rate and recalculate.**

 3.15 How to calculate the infusion rate required for partial parenteral nutrition (PPN) using Vamin® 9 Glucose. PPN should ideally provide 40–70% of resting energy requirement (RER) and should not be continued beyond 5 days.

As with enteral nutrition, PN should be instituted gradually over 48–72 hours. With both TPN and PPN, the animal's catheter and lines must be handled aseptically to avoid complications. Other intravenous fluids should be adjusted accordingly for the amount of fluid being administered via PN to avoid volume overload. For example, if a dog requires 50 ml/h of fluids to meets its fluid requirements and is currently receiving 50 ml/h of crystalloids, the addition of PN being administered at 20 ml/h should prompt a reduction by the same volume of the crystalloid fluid.

Monitoring and reassessment

Monitoring parameters include:

- **Vital signs**
- **Bodyweight**
- **Serum electrolytes**
- **Gastrointestinal signs (e.g. vomiting, regurgitation, diarrhoea)**
- **Signs of volume overload or pulmonary aspiration**
- **Tube/catheter patency**
- **Appearance of tube/catheter exit site.**

Bodyweight should be monitored daily for patients receiving either enteral or parenteral nutritional support. The use of the RER as the patient's caloric requirement is merely a starting point. The number of calories provided may need to be increased to meet the patient's changing needs, typically by 25% if well tolerated. In patients unable to tolerate the prescribed amounts, the veterinary surgeon may consider reducing amounts of enteral feedings and supplementing the nutritional plan with PPN.

Complications of enteral nutrition

Possible complications of enteral nutrition include: mechanical difficulties, such as clogging of the tube or early tube removal: and metabolic complications, such as electrolyte disturbances, hyperglycaemia, volume overload and gastrointestinal signs (vomiting, diarrhoea, cramping, bloating). Patients being tube-fed may experience complications that require adjustments to the nutritional plan. Patients with vomiting may be managed with antiemetics; however, if they do not respond to antiemetic therapy, tube-feeding may need to be reduced or discontinued. Patients with delayed gastric emptying may regurgitate or vomit and could respond to prokinetic agents such as metoclopramide and erythromycin. Decreasing the amount of food per feeding, increasing the interval between feeds, or lowering the fat content may help in these situations. Animals receiving mostly liquid diets via tube-feeding may develop diarrhoea. This may require decreasing the amount of food being tube fed temporarily, or changing the composition of the diet.

Complications of parenteral nutrition

Possible complications of PN include: sepsis; mechanical complications of the catheter and lines; thrombophlebitis; and metabolic disturbances, such as hyperglycaemia and electrolyte shifts. The frequency of monitoring required for such complications depends on the severity of illness. In some patients, monitoring these parameters once daily is adequate, whilst in others monitoring every 4–6 hours may be necessary. Avoiding serious consequences of complications associated with PN requires early identification of problems and prompt action. Frequent monitoring of vital signs, catheter-exit sites and routine biochemistry panels may alert the veterinary surgeon to developing problems (Figure 3.16).

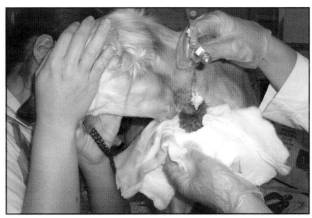

3.16 Intravenous catheters used for parenteral nutrition must be checked daily for any abnormal discharge. This catheter is suspected of having become infected and must be removed and submitted for bacteriological culture.

Transition

With continual reassessment, the veterinary surgeon can determine when to transfer the patient from assisted feeding to voluntary consumption of food. The discontinuation of nutritional support should only begin when the patient can consume approximately its RER without much coaxing. In patients receiving TPN, the progression from PN to enteral nutrition should occur over the course of at least 12–24 hours, depending on the patient's tolerance of enteral nutrition.

References and further reading

Abood SK, McLoughlin MA and Buffington CA (2006) Enteral nutrition. In: *Fluid, Electrolyte, and Acid-Base Disorders in Small Animal Practice, 3rd edn*, ed. SP DiBartola, pp. 601–620. Saunders Elsevier, St Louis

Buffington T, Holloway C and Abood A (2004) Clinical dietetics. In: *Manual of Veterinary Dietetics*, ed. T Buffington *et al.*, pp. 49 –141. Saunders Elsevier, St. Louis

Chan DL (2007) Nutritional support for the critically ill patient. In: *Small Animal Emergency and Critical Care for Veterinary Technicians, 2nd edn*, ed. AM Battaglia, pp. 85 –108. Saunders Elsevier, St Louis, MO

Freeman LM and Chan DL (2006) Total parenteral nutrition. In: *Fluid, Electrolyte, and Acid-Base Disorders in Small Animal Practice, 3rd edn*, ed. SP DiBartola, pp. 584–600. Saunders Elsevier, St Louis

Zoran DL (2005) Feeding tubes. In: *BSAVA Manual of Canine and Feline Gastroenterology, 2nd edn*, ed. EJ Hall *et al.*, pp. 288–296. BSAVA Publications, Gloucester

4

Physiotherapy and rehabilitation

Brian J. Sharp

This chapter is designed to give information on:

- The principles of physiotherapy with special reference to veterinary physiotherapy and the role of the veterinary nurse
- The indications for physiotherapy and the modalities used in the treatment of the canine and feline patient
- The principles of therapeutic exercise and hydrotherapy and their role within the rehabilitation process
- Incorporating physiotherapy into nursing care plans for patient groups commonly encountered in small animal practice

---

Introduction

Physiotherapy (or physical therapy) is involved with physical function, and physiotherapists regard movement and physical potential to be central to the health and well being of individuals. It is a 'hands-on' science-based healthcare profession concerned with the assessment, diagnosis and treatment of disease and disability through physical means. It is based upon the principles of medical science, and is generally held to be within the sphere of conventional (rather than alternative) medicine. Human physiotherapy is an internationally recognized discipline, and the positive benefits of physiotherapeutic intervention have been well documented.

Physiotherapy involves identifying and maximizing movement potential through health promotion, disease prevention, treatment and rehabilitation. A range of physical modalities are used to treat and prevent injuries, restore movement and function, and maximize physical potential by:

- Reducing pain
- Promoting the healing process
- Increasing and maintaining muscle strength and joint flexibility

- Promoting and restoring normal movement patterns
- Increasing cardiovascular fitness.

Rehabilitation is an integral component of physiotherapy, and is the process of helping an individual with an illness or injury to achieve the highest level of function, independence and quality of life as possible.

The modern practice of physiotherapy began in London in 1894, but it was as a result of the rehabilitation of large numbers of amputees from the World Wars of the early 20th century, and the care of patients suffering from diseases such as polio, that the development of medical physiotherapy was galvanized worldwide. In 1944 the Chartered Society of Physiotherapy (CSP) was formed in the UK. In 1977 professional autonomy for physiotherapists was instituted, and in 1978 physiotherapists were finally allowed to treat patients without prior medical referral. Today, physiotherapy is a graduate profession. Some physiotherapists have achieved consultant status within human healthcare and are often the first point of referral from primary (general practice) care into secondary (hospital) care.

Circular frictions

Circular frictions are performed into the muscle fibres, progressively increasing in depth.

Percussion techniques

Percussion (tapotement) is a series of techniques in which the hands strike the body. The hands usually work alternately and the wrists are kept flexible so that the movements are springy and invigorating. Some of these techniques are used in chest care of the postoperative or recumbent patient, in addition to their musculoskeletal use.

Hacking

This is performed with the ulnar border of the little finger, either alone or supplemented by other fingers. The operator's elbows are flexed to approximately 90 degrees, the wrists are held in extension and the fingers are relaxed. The striking movement is one of alternate pronation and supination. Hacking is a good technique for the back muscles and the thicker muscles of the hindquarters (Figure 4.8).

Clapping (coupage)

During clapping the operator's hands are cupped and the forearms pronated. The elbows are bent, and alternate flexion and extension of the wrists bring the hands sharply into contact with the patient's body, resulting in a deep toned clapping sound. This can be used over most muscular areas, but the pressure must be kept light over more bony areas such as the scapula. It is often used over the ribs to loosen secretions.

Beating

This is similar to clapping but is performed with a loosely clenched hand so that the dorsal aspect of the fingers and the base of the hand come into contact with the part being treated. Beating should be used only over large muscle groups.

Pounding

This is a movement similar to hacking but with a loosely clenched fist striking the part being treated with the ulnar border of the hand.

Shaking and vibration techniques

These techniques are commonly used in chest care of the postoperative or recumbent patient for loosening secretions, in addition to their role in musculoskeletal treatment.

Shaking

This is a rhythmic shaking of part of the body performed by holding the part with one or both hands and moving it from side-to-side, up and down, or in and out (Figure 4.9). This stimulates circulation, but care must be taken over bony areas.

Vibration

This is a fine form of tremor conveyed through the hands or fingertips for a few seconds. This technique relaxes the nervous system and is useful over joints and around bony prominences, as well as near healed scar tissue to reduce adhesions.

A summary of the major massage techniques and their specific benefits is given in Figure 4.10.

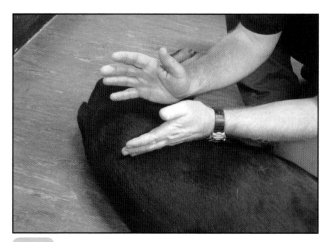

4.8 Hacking massage.

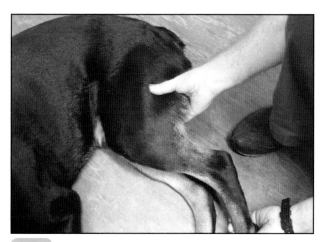

4.9 Shaking massage.

Massage technique	Major benefits	Other benefits
Stroking	Accustoms animal to touch Reduces tension and anxiety Lowers muscle tone	Useful to start and finish massage session Useful as a link between different techniques
Effleurage	Reduces swelling and oedema	Removes chemical byproducts of inflammation Maintains mobility of soft tissues Stretches muscle

4.10 Benefits of the various massage techniques. (continues) ▶

Massage technique	Major benefits	Other benefits
Kneading Picking-up Wringing	Increases circulation and lymphatic flow Mobilizes soft tissues	Removes chemical byproducts of inflammation Sensory stimulation and invigoration (fast technique) Relaxation and lowering of muscle tension (slow technique)
Skin rolling	Mobilizes skin and scar tissue	
Frictions	Break down adhesions	Local hyperaemia
Hacking Clapping Beating Pounding	Increases circulation Loosens chest secretions and stimulates coughing Sensory stimulation	
Shaking Vibration	Increases circulation Mobilizes soft tissues Loosens chest secretions and stimulates coughing	Sensory stimulation Reduces adhesions

4.10 Benefits of the various massage techniques.

Contraindications to massage

Massage should *not* be performed on an animal if any of the following apply:

- Acute inflammation
- Unstable fractures
- Infectious diseases
- Pyrexia (temperature over 40°C)
- Shock
- Infectious skin problems (e.g. ringworm)
- Open wounds
- Acute haematoma
- Neoplasia.

Massage should be undertaken with care in the following situations:

- Acute neurological conditions such as disc disease, where stimulation may be uncomfortable
- Arthritis, where pressure may be uncomfortable.

Passive movements and stretches

ROM is a term used to describe the full range that a joint (or muscle) may be moved through, and this can be affected by the joint structure as well as the type and integrity of the muscles and other soft tissues surrounding the joint. Tissues that limit ROM may be normal or pathological. Joints may develop arthritic changes; wounds and surgical procedures may result in adhesions and fibrosis between tissues; muscles may shorten because of spasm, contracture or hypertonicity. All of these may result in restriction of ROM.

The loss of ROM at a joint is a common consequence of injury or surgery. This loss may be only temporary, but it can become permanent if full ROM is not achieved within 2 weeks of surgery. Loss of range will inevitably limit an animal's functional abilities and create a background for subsequent muscle and joint problems in other body areas, due to compensatory postures and gaits.

To diminish the effects of disuse and immobilization and maintain ROM, joints and muscles must be moved through their available range on a regular basis, and this can be carried out by passive, active–assisted, or active means (see Therapeutic exercise below). It is generally appropriate to initiate passive movements as soon after injury as possible, provided there are no contraindications, but it is important that the movements are comfortable for the patient, and that tissues are not further injured by exceeding the limits of the damaged or repairing tissues. Passive ROM can be improved through the use of passive movements and stretches and, as the animal's condition improves, ROM exercises can be progressed through active–assisted and active modalities, depending on the amount of muscle activity the animal can produce.

As well as being important procedures for animals following surgery, after injury or with chronic conditions, passive movements and stretches can be used preventively to help maintain extensibility of muscle and other soft tissue, and to prevent further injury to joints, muscles, tendons and ligaments.

Passive movements

Passive movement is the movement of a joint by external forces. It is generally used when a patient is incapable of moving the joint on its own, or when active motion may be injurious to the patient (such as contracting a muscle soon after surgical repair of that muscle). The most common indications for passive movements in small animal practice are immediately after surgery and during recovery of patients with neurological conditions. In the latter case, if the patient does not regain functional neuromuscular control quickly, it is likely that some degree of contracture will occur, despite the best efforts of the therapist. It is important to understand that passive movements will not prevent muscle atrophy or increase (maintain) strength. It is equally important that passive movements are performed correctly if the full benefits are to be achieved (see Technique 4.1).

Effects of passive movements

- Increases blood circulation and lymphatic return.
- Prevents adhesions in articular capsules and joints. Maintains joint range.

- Improves articular nutrition by increasing synovial fluid production and diffusion.
- Prevents shortening and contracture of soft tissues such as ligaments, tendons and muscles. Maintains muscle length.
- Maintains mobility between different tissues.
- Reduces pain.
- Produces or maintains a pattern of movement.
- Aids relaxation of muscle.
- Stimulates mechanoreceptors in joints, muscles, skin and other soft tissues. Improves proprioceptive awareness.

Contraindications to passive movements

- Ligament, muscle or tendon repair where the repaired tissue is not yet able to withstand stress.
- Fractures.
- Haemarthrosis.
- Joint infection.
- Intravenous fluid catheters in the area being treated.
- If motion may result in further injury or instability.

Stretches

Stretches are often carried out in conjunction with passive movements to improve flexibility and help prevent muscle weakness that may occur as a result of tissue shortening. *Tightness* is a mild shortening of a muscle with no specific pathology, and is commonly found in muscles that cross two joints (such as biceps brachii and rectus femoris). Stretching exercises can normally restore range to tight muscles. *Contracture* is a significant shortening of the muscles and/or other soft tissues around a joint, causing a limitation in joint range; this is often due to scar tissue and adhesions between different tissues. Muscle hypertonicity due to upper motor neuron (UMN) lesions may also result in contracture.

There are several different types of stretching, but the most useful in small animal practice are static stretching and prolonged mechanical stretching.

Static stretching

This form of stretching (see Technique 4.2) utilizes a low-intensity stretch, which is generally more comfortable, less likely to induce tension in the muscles through stimulation of muscle spindles and Golgi tendon organs, and less likely to damage the tissues. Low forces applied over a period of time allow collagen fibres to realign.

Prolonged mechanical stretching

Prolonged mechanical stretching is similar to static stretching in that a low-intensity stretch is applied, but it is held much longer, for a minimum of 20 minutes up to several hours daily. It requires the use of splints (static or dynamic), which can also be used in a serial manner.

Effects of stretching

- Maintains or increases muscle length and flexibility; sarcomere numbers increase with slow, low-load passive stretches.

- Prevents loss of ROM caused by shortening and contracture of soft tissues such as ligaments, tendons and muscles.
- Prevents adhesions in articular capsules and joints and therefore maintains joint range.
- Maintains mobility between different tissues.
- Produces or maintains normal patterns of movement.
- Stimulates mechanoreceptors in joints, muscles, skin and other soft tissues and therefore improves proprioceptive awareness.
- Improves articular nutrition by increasing synovial fluid production and diffusion.
- Prevents injuries.

Contraindications to stretching

- Acute injury to a ligament, muscle or tendon, where the repair tissue has not yet reached a stage where it is able to withstand some stress.
- Be careful if the limb has been immobilized for a length of time.
- Take care when stretching areas close to recent fractures.
- Do not stretch joints when they are cold.

Hot and cold therapy

The use of heat and cold are simple and effective modalities used in the treatment and rehabilitation of animals. However, their successful use requires proper assessment of the problems encountered and the effects desired, which should be appropriate to the stage of the inflammatory process reached.

Heat

Heat (thermotherapy) has been used for centuries as a means of managing acute and chronic conditions. It can be applied to the body in many different ways.

Superficial heating

This includes the use of hot packs/wraps, baths/spas, hosing, heat pads, infrared lamps and warm air dryers. Damp forms of heating are preferable as these can penetrate to a depth of approximately 1–2 cm. Infrared lamps are *not recommended* for animal use due to the dangers of burning.

The superficial forms of heating are the simplest and most practical to carry out in small animal practice. They are particularly useful in subacute and chronic conditions, in situations where there is a reduced ROM due to stiffness or contracture, to relieve pain, and as a prequel to passive movements, stretches or exercise. However, as heat is carried away by the circulation, it will have effects on other organs, so care must be taken when using any form of heating.

Deep heating

This includes electrotherapy modalities such as therapeutic ultrasound, which must only be carried out by operators trained and competent in its use due to the potential dangers. Ultrasound waves can penetrate to a depth of 4 cm or more.

Application of heat

- Hot packs are generally applied to the area being treated for 15–30 minutes, but they may be left for longer as they will gradually cool.
- Commercial hot packs contain various substances to retain the heat. Sometimes a gel is used, which may be toxic. When using these packs the patient must be observed to ensure it does not bite the pack.
- It is generally recommended that hot packs are wrapped in a towel prior to application, but the number of layers will depend on the temperature of the pack. The therapist should always check the temperature on themselves before applying a hot pack, especially if it has been microwaved, as it will continue to build up more heat even when the microwaving has stopped. The temperature of the pack should not exceed 75°C.
- Spas or whirlpools have the same advantages as hot packs, but a larger surface area can be treated. There is also the benefit of greater hydrostatic pressure with increasing water depth, which will improve lymphatic and venous return. Water temperature should not exceed 35°C.

Effects of heat

- Reduces pain.
- Reduces blood pressure.
- Reduces muscle spasm and aids muscle relaxation.
- Increases local circulation (vasodilation) and metabolism.
- Increases capillary pressure and blood vessel permeability (which can promote oedema).
- Increases leucocyte migration into the heated area and accelerates tissue healing.
- Improves tissue elasticity.
- Increases nerve conduction velocity.

Contraindications to heat therapy

- Acute inflammation.
- Active or recent haemorrhage.
- Open wounds.
- Cardiac insufficiency.
- Impaired circulation in the area to be treated.
- Pyrexia.
- Malignancy.
- Poor body heat regulation.
- Decreased sensation, e.g. following a neurological event or under anaesthesia.
- Devitalized tissue, e.g. after radiotherapy.

Precautions for heat therapy

- **Take care when using electric heat pads.**
- **Be careful of overheating animals immersed in heated spas/whirlpools. Check rectal temperature regularly if in any doubt.**
- **Take care with sedated animals as they are unable to react to burning.** ▶

- **Take care with heavy hot packs on small bodies.**
- **Never allow a patient to lie on top of a hot pack, particularly if treating the trunk.**

Cold

Cold (cryotherapy) penetrates deeper and lasts longer than heat because of the decreased circulation. It is most effective when used immediately after trauma (accidents or surgery) during the acute phase of inflammation to provide analgesia, reduce inflammation, control bleeding and reduce muscle spasm.

Application of cold therapy

- The simplest method of cold application is to wrap a freezer bag containing crushed ice in a thin damp cloth, and apply to the area being treated for 10–15 minutes. This can be applied every 2 hours if necessary for severe injuries, but for most postoperative indications every 3–4 hours is appropriate. Superficial tissues show the most rapid cooling and rewarming effects, but deeper tissues such as muscular layers respond more slowly and may take as long as 60 minutes to return to baseline temperature after a 10-minute application of ice, and 145 minutes after a 30-minute application.
- Commercial cold packs may contain various substances to retain the cold. Sometimes a gel is used that may be toxic. When using these packs the patient must be observed to ensure it does not bite the pack. Packs at temperatures lower than –20°C should not be used.
- Towels soaked in ice-water slush can be used but need to be changed regularly as they warm up quickly.
- Cold compression units have been used in human medicine for many years and have proven to be very effective. A sleeve is wrapped around the affected part and ice water is fed into the sleeve by gravity from a special container (Figure 4.11). The container

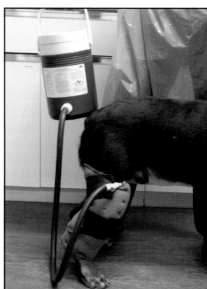

4.11

Cold therapy using a cold compression unit. Once disconnected from the water container and tubing the animal is able to exercise with the sleeve in place.

connection is removed and the animal can walk around or even exercise with the sleeve in place.

- Ice massage is appropriate for treating small areas. An ice cube may be used or water can be frozen in paper cups using a tongue depressor as a handle. The frozen water can be removed from the cup just before use and the ice is rubbed over the area for 5–10 minutes (parallel to the muscle fibres), thus providing a massage whilst cooling occurs. This technique stimulates the local mechanoreceptors, so can be useful for stimulating flaccid muscles.

Effects of cold

- Reduces pain.
- Vasoconstriction reduces blood flow and haemorrhage.
- Reduces inflammation and oedema formation.
- Reduces muscle tone (spasticity).
- Reduces metabolism and histamine release.
- Reduces nerve conduction velocity.
- Increases connective tissue stiffness.
- Increases muscle viscosity temporarily, giving reduced ability to perform rapid movements.

Contraindications to cold therapy

- Advanced systemic cardiovascular disease.
- Local areas of impaired peripheral circulation.
- Areas of ischaemia; generalized or localized vascular compromise.
- Acute febrile illness.
- History of frostbite in the area or impaired thermoregulation.
- Individuals who are cold-sensitive or have cold-urticaria (wheals and swelling occurring as a response to cold, due to histamine release).
- Radiotherapy or other ionizing radiation in the previous 6 months in the region being treated.
- Open or infected wounds (or use appropriate precautions).
- Some acute skin conditions, e.g. eczema, dermatitis.
- Malignant tissue.
- Extensive scar tissue; poor blood supply may lead to ice burns.

Precautions for cold therapy

- **Never apply ice directly to skin (ice massage is an exception); always cover ice packs with a damp towel.**
- **Take care with treatment of areas close to superficial nerves (may cause cold-induced nerve palsy).**
- **Areas of poor sensation.**

Figure 4.12 shows how to use hot and cold therapies effectively.

Cold	Hot
Use in the acute stages of inflammation	*Never* use in the first few days after injury
First 2–3 days after injury (longer if necessary)	Useful once oedema has stopped forming (usually 3–5 days after injury)

4.12 Guidelines for the effective use of hot and cold therapy following surgery or injury.

Therapeutic exercise

Therapeutic exercise is the systematic performance or execution of planned physical movements, postures or activities intended to enable the patient to:

- Prevent long-term physical impairment
- Enhance function
- Reduce risk of injury during free exercise
- Optimize overall health
- Enhance fitness and well being.

Exercise is perhaps the best known modality used in physiotherapy and represents the final element in the process of helping an animal achieve optimum function following injury, surgery or disease. In small animal practice, patients are typically discharged soon after surgery and there is often little opportunity for veterinary nurses to carry out exercise therapy. However, all animals should be given the opportunity to achieve maximum function and, if necessary, referral should be made to a veterinary physiotherapist or rehabilitation practitioner for further advice. Some animals will remain in the care of the practice for longer periods, and appropriate rehabilitation may make the difference between an animal simply coping with its disabilities and functioning normally. This section covers some of the basics of exercise therapy.

Designing an effective rehabilitation programme requires assessment of which components of a movement are not working adequately, whether normal actions can be achieved and how best to achieve them (Figure 4.13).

1. Assessment of the animal and identification of its problems:
   a) Affected structures and functional limitations
   b) Stage of recovery
   c) Desired outcome for the owners.
2. Development of a treatment plan, with realistic outcome goals.
3. Design of an exercise programme that will achieve those goals.
4. Continued evaluation of progress:
   a) Adjustment of goals
   b) Progression/alteration of exercises.

4.13 Stages in the design of an effective rehabilitation programme.

Aims and types of exercise

The aims of therapeutic exercise can be divided into four main areas:

- Strengthening
- Endurance (stamina)
- Flexibility (suppleness)
- Balance and proprioception.

Strengthening

Strength is the ability of a muscle or muscle group to produce tension and a resultant force. Exercises to improve strength create an increase in the myofibril content of the muscle and as a result increase the cross-sectional area of the muscle. Strengthening exercises include such activities as trotting, galloping, hill work (uphill and downhill), pulling weights, dancing, wheelbarrowing and swimming (see Technique 4.3).

Endurance

This is important for dogs that have to perform prolonged activities, such as long distance running (e.g. sled dogs, trailhounds, foxhounds), herding and swimming (rescue). Exercises to improve aerobic endurance usually target muscle groups for periods longer than 15 minutes and are repeated several times each week. Long-term changes occur in the muscle, including increased vascularization (which increases the amount of oxygen taken to the muscle) together with decreased resting heart rate and increased stroke volume (which allows greater time for ventricular filling), decreased resting blood pressure and increased respiratory enzymes (for generating energy more rapidly). Endurance exercises include trotting, swimming, treadmill activity and sled pulling for periods in excess of 15 minutes and progressively longer.

Flexibility

This is the ability of muscles, tendons and ligaments to stretch, allowing the joints to have a larger ROM and the animal to be able to manoeuvre through awkward spaces. Flexibility helps to protect against injury and is particularly important in cats and sporting and working dogs, although all animals require good flexibility. Flexibility exercises include any activities that make the animal reach or stretch for something, or flex the vertebral column in different directions. These include crawling under or stepping over obstacles, stair climbing, baiting and weaving.

Balance and proprioception

Balance is the ability to adjust equilibrium when standing (static balance) or during locomotion (dynamic balance), and to take account of changes in direction or ground surfaces. Proprioception is the unconscious perception of movement and spatial orientation originating from body position. Proprioception decreases with age and can also be affected by injury or surgery. It is especially affected by neurological diseases. All animals need satisfactory balance and proprioception to function normally, but many sporting and working dogs need heightened levels to cope with the demands of their work.

Balance exercises include activities requiring rapid responses to changes of the supporting surface, e.g. wobble boards, balance pads, trampolines, changes of direction when running, ball-playing, dancing and standing on the gym ball (small dogs and cats). Proprioception exercises include walking in circles or weaving, walking over obstacles or on different types of surface, and weight shifting (see Technique 4.4).

Exercise progression

Therapeutic exercise can take several forms, including:

- Assisted exercise
- Active–assisted exercise
- Free active exercise
- Resisted exercise.

Assisted exercise

When muscle strength or coordination is inadequate to perform any movement at all, an external force is applied to compensate for the deficiency. Passively moving an animal's limb through a normal walking pattern is an example of assisted exercise.

Active–assisted exercise

When muscle strength or coordination is inadequate to perform a full movement, an external force is applied to compensate for the deficiency. As the animal recovers, limb use returns to some extent but still requires some assistance from a therapist.

Free active exercise

This is used when muscle strength and coordination are adequate to perform a movement but only against the forces of gravity and bodyweight, e.g. sitting to standing.

Resisted exercise

This is used when muscle strength and coordination are adequate to perform a movement against gravity, bodyweight and additional resistance, e.g. using weights.

Rehabilitation programme

Animals commencing a rehabilitation programme will be at different points on the exercise scale, depending on current ability, but will then progress through the other stages as strength and coordination improve:

Assisted > Active–assisted > Free active > Resisted

Hydrotherapy

Hydrotherapy can be useful for fitness and fun, but in particular is one of the most useful forms of rehabilitation therapy for dogs, and has become a very popular modality used in the recovery from musculoskeletal and neurological conditions (Figure 4.14). There are several forms of hydrotherapy, including pools, underwater treadmills (UWTMs), hot tubs/spas and whirlpools.

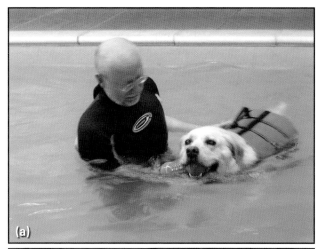

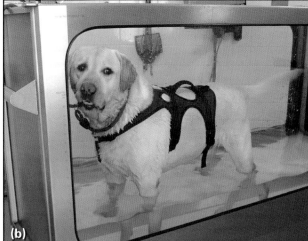

4.14 (a) In the UK hydrotherapy is most commonly carried out in a pool. Using toys can increase motivation and enjoyment of the experience for the dog. (b) Hydrotherapy can also take place on an underwater treadmill.

Other methods that can be used are bathtubs, sinks (for small dogs), plastic garden pools and ponds/lakes but for safety reasons, and to achieve better effects, a hydrotherapy facility (with trained personnel) is preferred to non-professional alternatives. When referring patients to hydrotherapy establishments, knowledge of the facility and the skill, experience and qualifications of the personnel are necessary. In the absence of personal experience of the local facilities, referral to members of an established trade organization (such as the Canine Hydrotherapy Association) should be considered.

The benefits of exercising in water include:

- Improvement in strength, endurance and stamina
- Improvement in balance and stability
- Improvement in joint ROM
- Improvement in psychological well being
- Reduction in pain
- Reduction in the weight bearing stresses on painful joints (useful for chronic conditions and obese patients)
- Gait and posture re-education
- Reduction in tissue oedema
- Improved respiratory function and strength.

Principles of hydrotherapy

It is the properties of water that provide the therapeutic value. These are:

- Buoyancy
- Hydrostatic pressure
- Viscosity
- Resistance
- Surface tension.

Buoyancy

The upward thrust of the water provides buoyancy, which means an animal in water is effectively less heavy than on land. Patients that are weak, unstable or have joint pain will be able to move more freely in the water with considerably less pain. The effects of buoyancy vary depending on the depth of water used (Levine *et al.*, 2002) (Figure 4.15).

Hydrostatic pressure

As an object is immersed deeper in water, the pressure that the water exerts on it is increased. This can be useful in helping to reduce swelling and oedema, especially in the limbs (Figure 4.16). However, this pressure will be exerted on the whole body and can make breathing difficult for patients with existing respiratory problems.

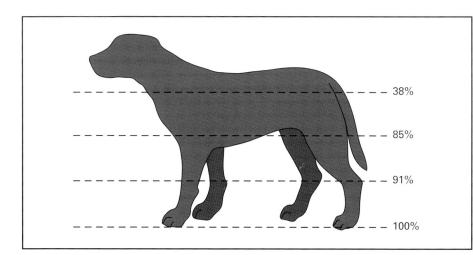

4.15 Effect of water depth on effective bodyweight. Dogs standing on dry land have an effective bodyweight of 100%. As water level rises, the effective bodyweight drops. With water at the level of the hock, the limbs are bearing 91% of the bodyweight; at the level of the stifle, the limbs are bearing 85% of the bodyweight; at the level of the hip, the effective bodyweight is reduced to 38% (Levine *et al.*, 2002). Underwater treadmills can use this principle to good effect.

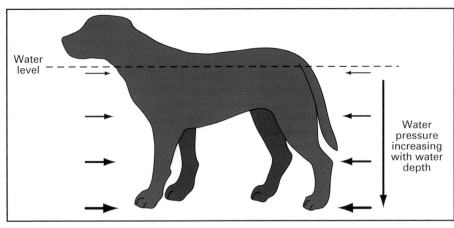

4.16 Effect of water pressure. Dogs standing or swimming in water will experience increased pressure on those parts of the body that are deeper in the water. This effectively provides an effleurage effect by pushing swellings proximally and can be a useful method of controlling oedema.

Viscosity, resistance and surface tension

The viscosity of water is much greater than that of air, so water provides resistance to an object as it moves through it. This resistance can be further increased by using jets, and working against this resistance builds muscle strength and bulk. Resistance to movement is also slightly greater on the surface of the water because of the effect of surface tension, which is the tendency of the water molecules to stick to each other, forming a 'skin' on the water surface.

The effects of buoyancy and viscosity also help to support the weak dog, as balance is easier to maintain in water than on land. Larger dogs can be encouraged into a standing position more easily and being in a normal upright position may also give the patient greater confidence. This can be done on the ramp of a hydrotherapy pool or in an UWTM.

Other effects of hydrotherapy

The water in a hydrotherapy pool should be at a temperature of between 26°C and 30°C. When warmth is applied to muscle tissue it causes an increase in elasticity of the cells, increased metabolism, increased blood flow, relaxation and pain relief. This all contributes to an overall increase in function or performance, allowing more effective and comfortable exercise. However, care should always be taken when swimming an animal that is stressed or working hard, as hyperthermia is a risk. This can be a problem especially after a hot car journey or a stressful stay in hospital.

All forms of hydrotherapy allow higher levels of exercise to be performed than on land with reduced risk of damage to joints and healing tissues. Despite their popularity, there is currently no research providing evidence that UWTMs are more beneficial than pools (Figure 4.17).

Conditions benefiting from hydrotherapy

Many conditions will benefit from the addition of hydrotherapy to a rehabilitation programme, including:

- Postoperative orthopaedic and neurological conditions
- Degenerative conditions
- Musculoskeletal conditions such as tendonitis
- Any condition where there is a lack of strength, ROM, weight bearing status or proprioceptive ability
- Obesity.

Pool	Underwater treadmill
The use of toys can improve motivation	Sensory input is provided through paw contact with the moving treadmill
The presence of the therapist in the water with the dog can improve confidence and motivation, and encourage stimulation of appropriate muscle groups	Alteration of water depth allows graduated progression of weight bearing and body support
Standing exercises are possible but only if ramps or ledges are available	Allows standing, walking and swimming to be performed (Bockstahler *et al.*, 2004)
Graduated progression of exercise levels is easy to monitor	Particularly useful in the immediate postoperative period after joint surgery

4.17 The benefits of hydrotherapy in a pool and using an underwater treadmill (UWTM). The general benefits of hydrotherapy apply to both pools and UWTMs but there are some additional benefits of each that may influence the choice of method for each patient.

Hydrotherapy can generally be started once a wound is healed, although in most postoperative cases it is started at 2 weeks. Following joint surgery, however, full swimming is generally not advisable for 4–6 weeks, because of the greater stresses placed on the joint (Millis *et al.*, 2004).

Contraindications and precautions in the use of hydrotherapy

- Fear of water.
- Open wounds.
- Faecal incontinence.
- Clinically significant cardiovascular problems.
- Infections and skin diseases.

Electrotherapy modalities

Other modalities that are available for the treatment of small animals include electrotherapy modalities. The use of all electrotherapy modalities requires specialist training, and they should only be used by trained operators who have gained a thorough understanding of the indications, contraindications, physiological effects and practical use of the modality.

Nevertheless, it is valuable for the veterinary nurse in general practice to have some knowledge of the types of electrotherapy that are commonly used within a physiotherapy treatment programme, and the effects they can have, so that referral can be made to trained operators as appropriate or training undertaken.

Laser therapy

The term LASER is an acronym for light amplification by stimulated emission of radiation. In simple terms, the laser can be considered a form of light amplifier, providing enhancement of particular properties of light energy. Many different types of laser are available but for therapeutic purposes Class 3A or 3B lasers are used. The term low-level laser therapy (LLLT) is also commonly used. Most lasers generate light in the visible red and infrared bands of the electromagnetic spectrum, with typical wavelengths of 600–1000 nm. The treatment device may be a single emitter (or probe) or a group of several emitters (cluster probe) containing a combination of lasers and light-emitting diodes (LEDs) (Figure 4.18).

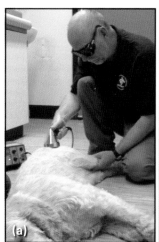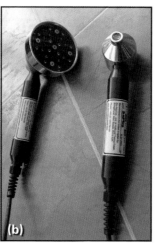

4.18 Laser therapy. **(a)** A dog receiving laser therapy, via a cluster probe, to its gluteal muscles. Note the operator's is wearing protective glasses. **(b)** A variety of single (right) and cluster (left) probes are available for most machines.

Although much of the applied laser light is absorbed in the superficial tissues, deeper effects can be achieved. Laser is generally considered to be a non-thermal energy application, although it should be appreciated that delivery and absorption of any energy to the body will result in some development of heat. The cell membrane appears to be the primary absorber of energy, which then generates intracellular effects. Laser light irradiation of tissues therefore acts as a trigger for alteration of cell metabolic processes.

Clinical applications of laser therapy

Research into the clinical effects of laser therapy has concentrated on a few key areas, including the effects on wound healing, inflammatory arthropathies, soft tissue injury and the relief of pain. There is supportive evidence for the clinical use of lasers in humans, but, as with many treatment modalities, evidence of their value in animal care remains limited at the present time.

Therapeutic ultrasound

Ultrasound waves consist of mechanical vibrations, formed by the same physical process as sound waves but at higher frequencies. These vibrations are beyond the range of human hearing, which is normally from 16 Hz to something approaching 20,000 Hz. Most of the frequencies used in speech and music are between 30 Hz and 4000 Hz. The frequencies used in ultrasound therapy are typically between 1.0 MHz and 3.0 MHz (1 MHz = 1 million cycles per second).

As the energy within the sound wave is passed to body tissue, it causes oscillations of the molecules, resulting in heat generation. Ultrasound waves can be used to produce thermal as well as non-thermal effects in the tissues to depths of 4 cm or more. As ultrasound waves pass through the body tissues, energy is absorbed. The best absorbing tissues are those with a high collagen content: ligament, tendon, fascia, joint capsule and scar tissue (ter Haar, 1999; Watson, 2000). More energy is absorbed by the superficial tissues than by the deep tissues.

Application of ultrasound therapy

Ultrasound therapy requires the use of a coupling agent between the ultrasound machine's head and the animal's skin. This can be a water-soluble gel applied to the skin, a coupling cushion (water-filled balloon) or direct transmission through water. The ultrasound machine's head must be moved continuously during treatment to ensure uniform distribution of energy to the tissues. Treatment time depends upon the size of the ultrasound machine's head and the size of the area being treated. However, treating animals with ultrasound waves presents a problem not found in humans: because of the high protein content of the hair coat, much of the energy is absorbed before reaching the underlying tissues. Even a thick layer of gel does not improve the situation and clipping is always recommended.

Therapeutic effects

The application of ultrasound waves during the inflammatory, proliferative and repair phases of tissue healing is of value because it stimulates or enhances the normal sequence of events and thus increases the efficiency of the repair process (ter Haar, 1999). It can influence the remodelling of scar tissue by enhancing the appropriate orientation of the newly formed collagen fibres and influencing the collagen profile, thus increasing tensile strength and enhancing scar mobility (Nussbaum, 1998). Recent research has also identified the benefits of using low-intensity pulsed ultrasound waves for normally healing (fresh) fractures, delayed or non-union fractures, and stress fractures (Warden *et al.*, 1999).

Electrical nerve stimulation

Electrical nerve stimulation is widely used in veterinary physiotherapy for muscle stimulation (neuromuscular electrical nerve stimulation; NMES), and also for pain relief (transcutaneous electrical nerve stimulation; TENS). Stimulators that incorporate both functions are available but in practice different models are generally used to achieve these different functions. The stimulators utilize a small control unit connected via leads to electrodes that are applied to the patient's skin. With animals, the use of an electrode gel is recommended to achieve optimal contact, and contact is further improved by clipping the hair over the area to be treated.

Neuromuscular electrical nerve stimulation

Motor nerve stimulation (Figure 4.19) can be achieved with a wide range of frequencies. Stimulation at low frequencies (e.g. 1 Hz) results in a series of twitches, whilst stimulation at 50 Hz results in tetanic contraction. Evidence exists for the 'strengthening' effect of NMES (Snyder-Macker *et al.*, 1991), which is particularly useful for animals who cannot generate useful voluntary contraction on demand and for those who find active exercise difficult, such as patients with neurological disease. There is no evidence that NMES has any significant benefit over active exercise and the use of such treatment is generally ceased once the animal is able to exercise actively.

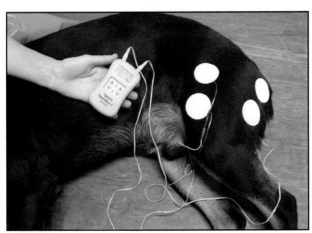

4.19 Application of neuromuscular electrical nerve stimulation to quadriceps and hamstrings, with the aim of achieving co-contraction of the two muscle groups.

Caution should be exercised when using NMES as it is possible to stimulate the muscle beyond its point of fatigue because the contractions are forced via the motor nerve. Short stimulation periods with adequate rest are preferable.

Effects of NMES

- Muscle strengthening and prevention of disuse muscle atrophy.
- Muscle re-education and facilitation of muscle control.
- Improved sensory awareness.
- Decreased spasticity and muscle spasm.
- Blood flow changes.
- Reduction of oedema.

Transcutaneous electrical nerve stimulation

This is a method of electrical stimulation that primarily aims to provide symptomatic pain relief by specifically exciting sensory nerves and thereby stimulating either the 'pain gate' mechanism and/or the endogenous opioid system. Pain relief by means of the pain gate mechanism involves activation (excitation) of the Aβ sensory fibres and reduces the transmission of noxious stimuli via the C pain fibres. The Aβ fibres respond most effectively at a relatively high rate of stimulation (90–130 Hz). There does not seem to be a single frequency that works best for every patient, but this range appears to cover the majority of individuals.

An alternative approach is to stimulate the Aδ fibres, which respond preferentially to a much lower rate of stimulation (2–5 Hz). This provides pain relief by stimulating the release of an endogenous opiate (encephalin) in the spinal cord, which in turn reduces the activation of the pain pathways.

Application of TENS

Positioning of the electrodes is not an exact science and there are many alternatives that have been found to be effective:

- Either side of the lesion or painful area
- At the appropriate nerve root(s) level
- Along the peripheral nerve
- Over the motor point
- Over trigger point(s) or acupuncture point(s)
- Over the appropriate dermatome, myotome or sclerotome.

Contraindications to electrical nerve stimulation

- Implanted pacemakers.
- Allergic responses to the electrode, tape or gel.
- Skin disease, e.g. eczema, dermatitis.
- Current or recent bleeding.
- Stimulation over infected areas or neoplasms.
- Open wounds.
- Compromised circulation, e.g. ischaemic tissue, thrombosis and associated conditions.
- Application over:
  - The ventral aspect of the neck or carotid sinus
  - The heart
  - The lower trunk, abdomen or pelvis during pregnancy
  - The eyes
  - Areas lacking sensation.

Precautions for electrical nerve stimulation

- **If skin sensation is not normal, or the skin surface is broken, it is preferable to position the electrodes at an alternative site.**
- **Avoid active epiphyseal regions in growing animals.**
- **Select stimulation parameters appropriate to the effect desired. Inappropriate stimulation parameters may cause muscle damage, reduction in blood flow through the muscle and low frequency muscle fatigue.**
- **Appropriate care should be taken to ensure that the level of muscle contraction initiated does not compromise the muscle or the joint(s) over which it acts.**
- **Patients with a history of epilepsy should be treated at the discretion of the physiotherapist in consultation with the veterinary surgeon.**

Physiotherapy in specific situations

Preoperative physiotherapy

Preoperative physiotherapy is an often neglected process that, if utilized, can be a major benefit to the eventual outcome of the surgery performed. While it is not always possible, especially when emergency surgery is required, elective surgery patients may benefit from a period of preoperative physiotherapy and rehabilitation.

Preoperative physiotherapy:

- Prepares the animal physically for the forthcoming surgery by improving muscle strength and joint stability, ROM, balance and proprioception
- Familiarizes the animal with the type of exercises required following surgery, for example, hydrotherapy. Animals familiarized with the hydrotherapy pool and surroundings, procedures and staff are less likely to react negatively when reintroduced to the pool following surgery. There is less likely to be damage to the surgical site than if the animal is unfamiliar with its surroundings
- Provides owners with a sense of involvement
- In some cases, the animal may improve to such a degree that surgery is no longer required.

Postoperative physiotherapy

Postoperative patients probably represent the major recipients of physiotherapeutic care from the veterinary nurse, and it is likely that most will have had orthopaedic or neurological surgery. Adequate and appropriate physiotherapy carried out during the first few postoperative days can have major benefits for the eventual outcome.

There are physiotherapy protocols available in a number of texts (Bockstahler *et al.*, 2004; Millis *et al.*, 2004) that provide useful guidance on the appropriate physiotherapy for most types of orthopaedic and neurological surgery. However, in practice all patients are different and will arrive with different pre-existing conditions, fitness levels and postoperative recoveries. This section does not revisit these protocols but offers the veterinary nurse a selection of therapeutic options for the majority of problems likely to be encountered in the postoperative patient. It is incumbent on the veterinary nurse, in consultation with the veterinary surgeon and/or physiotherapist, to fully assess the patient's needs (see Figure 4.13) and select the most appropriate therapeutic modalities for each patient (Figure 4.20).

Neurological disease

The veterinary nurse caring for the patient with neurological disease faces specific problems. Physiotherapeutic interventions for human patients with neurological conditions have developed greatly over recent years, with improved outcomes, and many of these can be adapted to the small animal patient. Figure 4.21 gives suggestions for a physiotherapy nursing plan for orthopaedic patients in the postoperative period, and Figure 4.22 highlights many of the problems of the neurological patient with suggestions for therapeutic interventions.

Findings on patient assessment	Aims of treatment	Therapeutic interventions
Inflammation and oedema	Control inflammatory process Reduce oedema formation	Cryotherapy; compression; elevation; effleurage; gentle active exercise; laser therapy/therapeutic ultrasound
Pain	Pain management[a]	Cryotherapy; thermotherapy; transcutaneous electrical nerve stimulation (TENS); laser therapy/therapeutic ultrasound; massage
Reduced range-of-motion (ROM)	Prevent development of contractures Restore normal ROM	Passive movements and stretches to maintain ROM
Weak muscles	Strengthen muscles	Assisted, active–assisted, active exercise as appropriate; neuromuscular electrical nerve stimulation (NMES) to appropriate muscles; hydrotherapy

4.20 Physiotherapy nursing plan for the immediate postoperative period. The options for therapeutic intervention must be selected based on the specific requirements of the individual patient. [a] Drug therapy (analgesia) is usually indicated concurrently.

Findings on patient assessment	Aims of treatment	Therapeutic interventions
Inflammation and oedema	Control inflammatory process Reduce oedema formation	Cryotherapy; compression; elevation; effleurage; gentle exercise; laser therapy/therapeutic ultrasound
Pain	Pain management[a]	Cryotherapy; thermotherapy; transcutaneous electrical nerve stimulation (TENS); massage; laser therapy/therapeutic ultrasound

4.21 Physiotherapy nursing plan for postoperative orthopaedic patients. The options for therapeutic intervention must be selected based on the specific requirements of the individual patient. [a] Analgesic medication is often indicated concurrently. (continues) ▶

Findings on patient assessment	Aims of treatment	Therapeutic interventions
Reduced range-of-motion (ROM)	Prevent development of contractures Restore normal ROM	Passive movements and stretches to maintain ROM
Weak muscles	Strengthen muscles	Assisted, active–assisted, active exercise as appropriate; neuromuscular electrical nerve stimulation (NMES) to appropriate muscles; hydrotherapy
Reduced weight bearing through operated limb	Stimulate weight bearing	Weight bearing (standing) exercises; weight shifting exercises; simulated walking (movements of limbs in normal walking patterns); NMES to appropriate muscle groups; hydrotherapy
Poor balance and proprioceptive awareness	Stimulate proprioception receptors Improve balance reactions	Sensory stimulation: sight, sound, touch; massage, passive movements and stretches; balance and proprioceptive exercises

4.21 (continued) Physiotherapy nursing plan for postoperative orthopaedic patients. The options for therapeutic intervention must be selected based on the specific requirements of the individual patient. [a] Analgesic medication is often indicated concurrently.

Findings on patient assessment	Aims of treatment	Therapeutic interventions
Hypertonicity (spasticity – upper motor neuron (UMN) lesion)	Facilitate tone normalization	Positioning of limb joints to prevent dominant pattern becoming established (e.g. if limb has dominance of extensor tone, keep one or more joints in flexed position). In recumbent patients use pillows or towels between the hindlimbs to prevent excessive adduction; moving limb through normal patterns of movement (very slowly to prevent uninhibited reflex activity); weight bearing (standing) exercises; regular passive movements and stretches to prevent contracture; massage to maintain pliability of muscle tissue and stroking massage to relax hypertonic muscles; use of warmth to help relax hypertonic muscles
Hypotonicity (flaccidity – lower motor neuron (LMN) lesion)	Facilitate tone normalization	Stimulation of joint, muscle and skin receptors: vigorous massage techniques (including ice massage), passive movements, tapping of muscles; weight bearing exercises (including assisted standing and sitting); neuromuscular electrical nerve stimulation (NMES) to stimulate neuromuscular activity (especially of extensor groups); hydrotherapy
Pain	Pain management [a]	Cryotherapy; thermotherapy; transcutaneous electrical nerve stimulation (TENS); laser therapy/therapeutic ultrasound; massage
Weak muscles	Strengthen muscles	Assisted, active–assisted, active exercise as appropriate; NMES to appropriate muscles; hydrotherapy
Reduced range-of-movement (ROM)	Prevent development of contractures Restore normal ROM	Passive movements and stretches to maintain ROM
Poor balance and proprioceptive awareness	Stimulate proprioceptive receptors Improve balance reactions	Sensory stimulation: sight, sound, touch; massage, passive movements and stretches; boots to protect feet when walking; balance and proprioception exercises
Inability to walk	Stimulate standing and walking	Weight bearing (standing) exercises; weight shifting exercises; simulated walking (movements of limbs in normal walking patterns); NMES to all muscle groups (extensor groups to assist standing and weight bearing, flexor groups to assist release, both groups to assist co-contraction); hydrotherapy; cart for patients with long-term disablement
Poor function	Stimulate transfers and functional activities	Active–assisted exercise: sit to stands, lying to sit, walking
Disorientation/depression/reduced motivation	Improve motivation	Encourage family involvement in care; regular walks outside; social contact with other dogs if appropriate

4.22 Physiotherapy nursing plan for patients with neurological conditions. The options for therapeutic intervention must be selected based on the specific requirements of the individual patient. [a] Analgesic medication is often indicated concurrently.

Senior patients

The consequences of ageing provide the small animal practice with many challenges. It is the debilitating effects of osteoarthritis, obesity and cardiovascular disease that demand most attention for physiotherapy and rehabilitation, and the veterinary nurse has an important role in the management of the senior patient (Figure 4.23).

Physiotherapy in the critical care unit

Physiotherapy for patients admitted to the critical care unit is primarily required to offset the effects of immobility, in addition to dealing with the primary reason for admission. The enforced reduction in physical activity results in significant changes in the musculoskeletal and cardiovascular systems, and with humans bed rest for even a week can lead to marked muscle atrophy, loss of ROM, exercise intolerance, increased risk of pressure sores, pulmonary complications and deep vein thrombosis (Dunning *et al.*, 2005). As soon as the animal is stable, rehabilitation procedures should be initiated to prevent the onset of these changes. A proactive approach to rehabilitation is preferable to a reactive approach to a worsening situation, and even simple physiotherapy techniques such as cryotherapy, massage, passive movements and stretching can make a huge improvement to the eventual functional outcome of the patient (Figure 4.24).

Findings on patient assessment	Aims of treatment	Therapeutic interventions
Inflammation and oedema	Control inflammatory process Reduce oedema formation	Cryotherapy; compression; elevation of the limb; effleurage; gentle exercise; laser therapy/therapeutic ultrasound
Pain	Pain management [a]	Cryotherapy; thermotherapy; transcutaneous electrical nerve stimulation (TENS); massage; pacing activities: short, frequent walks; laser therapy/therapeutic ultrasound
Reduced range-of-motion (ROM)	Prevent development of contractures Restore normal ROM	Passive movements and stretches to maintain ROM
Weak muscles	Strengthen muscles	Assisted, active–assisted, active exercise as appropriate; neuromuscular electrical nerve stimulation (NMES) to appropriate muscles; hydrotherapy
Poor balance and proprioceptive awareness	Stimulate proprioception receptors Improve balance reactions	Sensory stimulation: sight, sound, touch; massage, passive movements and stretches; boots to protect feet when walking; balance and proprioceptive exercises
Increasing weight	Weight control	Dietary advice; low impact exercise; hydrotherapy
Reduced exercise tolerance	Improve endurance	Progressive low impact exercise; hydrotherapy
Difficulty coping at home	Environmental modifications	Advice regarding suitable home environment: safe flooring, soft bedding, ramps

4.23 Physiotherapy nursing plan for senior (arthritic) patients. The options for therapeutic intervention must be selected based on the specific requirements of each individual patient. [a] Analgesic medication is often indicated concurrently.

Findings on patient assessment	Aims of treatment	Therapeutic interventions
Pressure sores	Prevent development of sores	Regular repositioning; mobilize if able
Retention of pulmonary secretions	Loosening of secretions Stimulate coughing Improve oxygenation	Postural drainage; nebulization (if appropriate); percussion massage; shaking and vibration massage; positioning; active exercise (non-recumbent patients) if able
Atelectasis	Re-expand collapsed lung segments	Postural drainage; percussion massage; shaking and vibration massage; positioning; active exercise (non-recumbent patients) if able
Reduced range-of-motion (ROM)	Prevent development of contractures Restore normal ROM	Passive movements and stretches to maintain ROM; elevation of limb to prevent oedema forming as a result of reduced muscle activity
Weak muscles	Strengthen muscles	Assisted, active–assisted, active exercise as appropriate; neuromuscular electrical nerve stimulation (NMES) to appropriate muscles

4.24 Physiotherapy nursing plan for patients in the critical care unit. The options for therapeutic intervention must be selected based on the specific requirements of each individual patient. (continues)

▶

Findings on patient assessment	Aims of treatment	Therapeutic interventions
Pain	Prevent pain and stiffness Assist in pain control	Repositioning; passive movements and stretches; stroking, effleurage, kneading massage; transcutaneous electrical nerve stimulation (TENS)
Swelling	Prevent development of oedema Reduce swelling	Use of cryotherapy (active swelling) or thermotherapy (to remove swelling); effleurage massage; elevation of swollen limb
Inability to walk	Stimulate standing and walking	Weight bearing (standing) exercises; weight shifting exercises; simulated walking (movements of limbs in normal walking patterns); NMES to all muscle groups (extensor groups to assist standing and weight bearing, flexor groups to assist release, both groups to assist co-contractions)
Disorientation/depression/reduced motivation	Improve motivation	Encourage family involvement in care; regular walks outside; social contact with other dogs if appropriate
Anxiety	Promote calmness and confidence	Calm, peaceful environment; gentle approach to treatment; stroking massage

4.24 (continued) Physiotherapy nursing plan for patients in the critical care unit. The options for therapeutic intervention must be selected based on the specific requirements of each individual patient.

The main physiotherapeutic approaches to patients in the critical care unit fall into the following categories:

- Positioning
- Chest care, including postural drainage and massage techniques
- ROM maintenance
- Control of swelling
- Pain relief
- Progressive exercise.

Positioning

Correct positioning of animals in the critical care unit is important to improve respiratory function, reduce dependent limb oedema, prevent pressure sores and prevent the development of spasticity in the hypertonic animal. The most common positioning of recumbent animals is movement between right, left and sternal recumbency every 2–4 hours using the support of pillows and foam wedges as required. This helps to prevent pressure sores and in animals with chest complications, positioning the affected side up or down allows appropriate changes in the ventilation/perfusion relationship in the lungs. In the control of limb oedema, the affected limb should be elevated above heart level using pillows or foam wedges to allow the effect of gravity to help drain the oedematous limb. Hypertonia occurs in animals with UMN lesions and the resulting spasticity causes all the muscles of the extensor or flexor groups to contract synchronously. Such patterns will be exacerbated by effort, stress and poor positioning. Treating the animal in a calm manner, moving the spastic limbs slowly and carefully, and positioning the animal in neutral positions will prevent hypertonicity from worsening and muscle stiffness/joint contracture from becoming established (Spector et al., 1982). It will also prevent the pain of permanent muscle contraction.

Chest care

Physiotherapy is particularly important to maintain bronchial hygiene, eliminate secretions from the airways, re-expand atelectatic lung segments, improve oxygenation and reduce the incidence of pneumonia. These effects can be achieved through the use of techniques such as postural drainage, massage (percussion, shaking, vibrations), positioning and exercise. Postural drainage involves positioning the body in specific ways to allow gravity to help drain secretions from specific lung segments into the larger airways, from where they can be coughed up. The animal needs to remain in the drainage position for 10–20 minutes; the use of percussion, shaking and vibration in conjunction with postural drainage can increase the effect. Animals requiring postural drainage can benefit from treatment sessions 3–4 times daily. Manning et al. (1997) have identified seven positions for postural drainage in the canine patient (Figure 4.25), but active exercise is generally more effective in mobilizing secretions than chest physiotherapy and is the treatment of choice whenever possible.

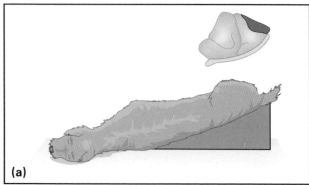

(a)

4.25 Postural drainage positions for the canine patient (area of the lung to be cleared: position to be adopted). **(a)** Lateral segment of the left caudal lung lobe: left lateral recumbency. Hind end elevated 40 degrees. (continues) ▶

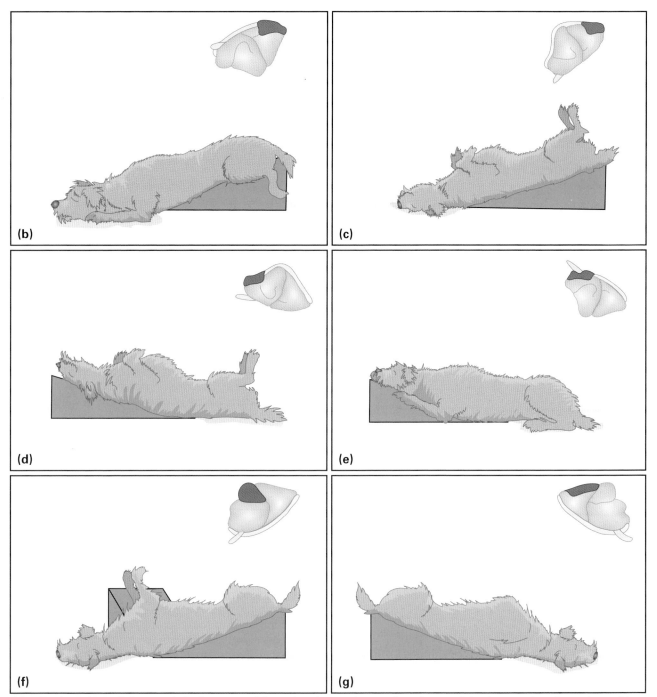

4.25 (continued) Postural drainage positions for the canine patient (area of the lung to be cleared: position to be adopted). **(b)** Left and right caudodorsal lung fields: sternal recumbency. Hind end elevated 40 degrees. **(c)** Left and right caudoventral lung fields: dorsal recumbency. Hind end elevated 40 degrees. **(d)** Left and right cranioventral lung fields: dorsal recumbency. Front end elevated 40 degrees. **(e)** Left and right craniodorsal lung fields: sternal recumbency. Front end elevated 40 degrees. **(f)** Right middle lung lobe: dorsal recumbency. A pillow under the right thorax raises the right side higher than the left. Hind end elevated 40 degrees and front end rotated one quarter turn to the left. **(g)** Lateral segment of the right caudal lung lobe: right lateral recumbency. Hind end elevated 40 degrees.

The techniques of percussion (clapping), shaking and vibration are all commonly used in respiratory physiotherapy to assist in loosening secretions by mechanical means. They are more effectively carried out in conjunction with postural drainage, but can be performed independently if necessary. It is important that the techniques (see above) are performed correctly to achieve optimum results. When percussion techniques are carried out for respiratory purposes, the hands should strike the chest wall alternately and in a regular rhythm during inspiration and expiration. The hands should not remain in the same place throughout the entire treatment, but should move around, and the treatment is continued for 30 seconds to 1 minute. Shaking and vibration also form an important element of respiratory physiotherapy. With the hands over the affected area, the chest wall is shaken or vibrated. The technique should only be performed during the expiration phase and is continued for four to six breathing cycles.

Chest care protocol

To achieve optimal results from these techniques, the patient should be placed in the appropriate postural drainage position and remain there for 10–20 minutes. During this time, percussion should be performed (30 seconds to 1 minute), followed by shaking or vibrations (four to six expirations) and a rest for 1 minute. This cycle of treatment should be repeated two to three times.

Contraindications to chest physiotherapy

■ Rib fractures or flail chest.
■ Pneumothorax or haemopneumothorax.
■ Pain.
■ Unstable cardiovascular condition.
■ Thrombocytopenia (<30,000 platelets/µl).
■ Open wounds.
■ Thoracic tumours.
■ Traumatic myocarditis.

Range-of-motion maintenance

One of the major consequences of enforced immobility such as that experienced by critical care unit patients is the development of stiffness and loss of joint and muscle ROM. This can affect all joints, especially if the stay in the critical care unit is prolonged. The use of passive movements and massage to maintain joint range and muscle pliability should form an integral part of every animal's stay in the critical care unit. Recumbent and non-ambulatory patients should receive a routine of 10 to 15 passive movements to all limb joints, moving through the full range of flexion and extension. Any joints developing contracture should receive more frequent treatment, and no animal should leave the critical care unit having lost ROM. Passive movements will have no effect on muscle strength, so it is always advisable to begin active or active–assisted exercise as soon as practical.

Control of swelling

Control of swelling is predominantly achieved through the combined use of cryotherapy, effleurage and elevation of the affected body part.

Pain relief

The primary form of pain relief in the critical care unit is likely to be prescribed medication, but physiotherapy can be effective as an adjunct. In addition to effective positioning to prevent soreness developing, the use of gentle passive movements and massage techniques will help to prevent joint stiffness, muscle tightness and the development of oedema, all of which can be a source of pain. The increase in circulation resulting from these techniques will also promote a 'feel good' factor in patients as well as helping to reduce the anxiety and stress many patients experience in the critical care unit environment.

It has been suggested recently that the use of TENS in the acute situation can generally be more effective in pain relief than when used for chronic conditions. TENS may therefore be an effective form of pain relief used either as an adjunct to, or an alternative to, other forms of pain relief.

Progressive exercise

Exercise helps to prevent many of the effects of immobilization on the musculoskeletal system. In addition to limiting loss of strength, range, balance and function, exercise can also be valuable in mobilizing chest secretions, preventing atelectasis, stimulating deep breathing and promoting coughing. Recumbent patients need to rely on the passive techniques already described, but non-recumbent patients should be helped to move every 4–6 hours. Animals that are ambulatory can be stood up and walked for 5–10 minutes and non-ambulatory animals can be assisted to stand for a few minutes. Attaining this normal upright posture can provide confidence, comfort and motivation to the animal, as well as being of benefit to other body systems. Active exercise can stimulate circulation, reduce pain and swelling, and improve strength, ROM and balance.

Physiotherapy for cats

The principles and techniques of physiotherapy described in this chapter are applicable to all species, although techniques may require modification to achieve a successful outcome in different species. Dogs represent the major patient group in small animal practice, but physiotherapy for cats is a rapidly growing area of veterinary care, and one of which the veterinary nurse should be aware.

In general terms, cats are more protective of injuries than dogs, and their lighter bulk conveys less weight bearing stress through injured limbs than with most dogs. However, the feline patient is generally less tolerant of the regular handling involved in physiotherapeutic care than most canine patients, and has reduced acceptance of new activities. To achieve satisfactory results, treatment sessions with cats should be kept short, exercises introduced more gradually, and items familiar to the cat, such as toys, used more frequently.

Massage, passive movements (Figure 4.26a), stretches, hot and cold therapy and electrotherapy can all be utilized successfully in feline rehabilitation. Many of the therapeutic exercises described in this chapter, such as dancing, wheelbarrowing and baiting (Figure 4.26bc), can be readily adapted for feline patients. In addition, cats will follow, chase and 'pat' objects such as toys dragged along the floor or waved in the air and this helps to improve strength, ROM and balance. Beams of light from torches can be moved along the floor and across walls to gain the cat's interest and encourage movement.

Leash walking and hydrotherapy can also be used to good effect with some individuals, but in most cases cats are less willing to accept these forms of physiotherapy. Because many cats are fearful of water, someone experienced in hydrotherapy should undertake the introduction of any cat into water. In some cases, cats may accept water if it is introduced in the home environment and the use of the bath may prove successful. This is especially true if the cat is already familiar with the bath and a gradual change from being washed to being rehabilitated may be achievable. However, the safety of cat and therapist is of the utmost importance and owners

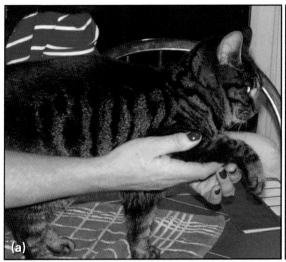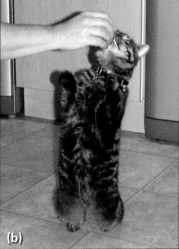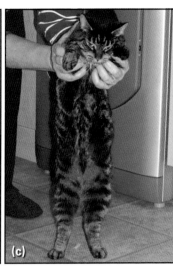

4.26 Physiotherapy for cats. **(a)** Cats can benefit from physiotherapy treatments such as passive movements and massage. **(b)** Cats are generally less tolerant of restrictive handling, but cooperation can be encouraged using toys and treats. **(c)** Exercises such as dancing can help with hindlimb strengthening.

who are inexperienced in performing hydrotherapy, and do not have appropriate harnesses or lifejackets, should always seek advice and help from a veterinary physiotherapist who can assess the risks and benefits of this form of rehabilitation.

Assistance devices

Carts

Carts (or canine wheelchairs) are available to provide support to the dog that has poor or no use of its fore- and/or hindlimbs. Carts can provide support while allowing the dog to remain active and independent. The support provided by carts varies from total support for dogs that have no use of the fore- or hindlimbs to partial support for dogs that have some use of the limbs; these carts allow varying degrees of weight bearing (Figure 4.27).

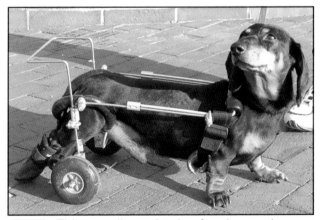

4.27 This cart allows the dog freedom and independence whilst providing support for weakened hindlimbs. (Reproduced from the *BSAVA Manual of Canine and Feline Neurology, 3rd edition*)

Carts can be particularly beneficial for dogs that are slow to recover from neurological conditions. Those that allow normal movement patterns of the limbs are especially valuable, and adjustment can be made to allow increased weight bearing as the dog regains strength. This can form an important element in the rehabilitation process. In contrast, dogs that have progressive wasting conditions such as degenerative myelopathy can also benefit from carts, as they allow the dog to function as normally and independently as possible for as long as possible, and have the facility to support the dog increasingly as further weakness and immobility occurs.

In all conditions, it is important that the animal continues to have appropriate rehabilitation in addition to the use of the cart. While it may be wonderful for an owner to see their dog moving around the park again, they must not allow the animal or themselves to become too dependent on the cart, especially if further progress is possible. If used inappropriately, carts have the potential to increase muscle wasting and weakness, stiffness and loss of range. Owners should also be made aware that not all dogs will accept carts and consideration must be given to the practicalities of being able to lift the dog into and out of the cart. Dogs using carts should be supervised at all times and should be allowed frequent rest periods out of the cart. Skin damage can easily occur and the condition of the skin should be monitored regularly.

Harnesses and slings

There is a huge variety of slings (Figure 4.28) available to help support animals and allow active–assisted exercise and walking. Slings are available that support the forelimbs, hindlimbs or whole body, and vary from simple sheepskin-lined straps to sophisticated suede or rubber harnesses with cut-outs for toileting. Using the correct size is important so that breathing, toileting and limb movement are not hampered, and there should be a soft lining to protect the skin from irritation.

Harnesses and slings can be very useful in the early stages of a rehabilitation programme, with the handler allowing increasing amounts of weight bearing as the animal's condition improves. Animals recovering from surgery and those in a critical care unit can be stood up using these devices to begin the rehabilitation process and to help with the early resumption of strength and balance.

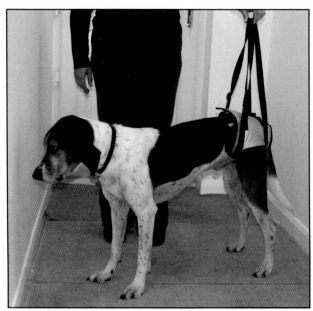

4.28 A towel or a specially designed harness can provide effective support to the weak animal.

Conclusion

The role of physiotherapy and rehabilitation in small animal care has grown rapidly in recent years. Owner expectations, the emergence of specialist physiotherapy practitioners, and recognition of the benefits that these therapies can provide has created a demand within veterinary practice that cannot be ignored. The role of the veterinary nurse in this regard is an important one, and many veterinary nurses are embracing this opportunity to extend their traditional role. Although the practice of physiotherapy encompasses many elements, the basic techniques can be integrated easily into daily nursing and can provide major benefits for the animals in veterinary care. Physiotherapy and rehabilitation should no longer be regarded as a luxury only offered by a few specialist practices, they should be regarded as valuable aspects of every veterinary nurse's role.

References and further reading

Bockstahler B, Levine D and Millis DL (2004) *Essential Facts of Physiotherapy*. BE VetVerlag, Babenhausen

Dunning D, Haling KB and Ehrhart N (2005) Rehabilitation of medical and acute care patients. *Veterinary Clinics of North America: Small Animal Practice* **35**, 1411–1426

Levine D, Millis DL, Marcellin-Little DJ and Taylor RA (2005) Rehabilitation and physical therapy. *Veterinary Clinics of North America: Small Animal Practice* **35**, 1247–1254

Levine D, Tragauer V and Millis DL (2002) Percentage of normal weight bearing during partial immersion at various depths in dogs. *Proceedings of the Second International Symposium on Rehabilitation and Physical Therapy in Veterinary Medicine*. Knoxville, Tennessee

Manning A, Ellis D and Rush J (1997) Physical therapy for critically ill veterinary patients. 1. Chest physical therapy. *Compendium on Continuing Education for the Practicing Veterinarian* **19**, 675–685

Manning AM (2004) Physical rehabilitation for the critically injured veterinary patient. In: *Canine Rehabilitation and Physical Therapy*, ed. Millis DA *et al.*, pp 404–410. Saunders, Philadelphia

Marsolais GS, Dvorak G and Conzemius MG (2002) Effects of postoperative rehabilitation on limb function after cranial cruciate ligament repair in dogs. *Journal of the American Veterinary Medical Association* **220**, 1325–1330

Millis DL, Millis DL, Levine D, Brumlow M and Weigel JP (1997) A preliminary study of early physical therapy following surgery for cranial cruciate ligament rupture in dogs. *Veterinary Surgery* **26**, 434

Millis DL, Levine D and Taylor RA (2004) *Canine Rehabilitation and Physical Therapy*. Saunders, St Louis

Monk ML, Preston CA and McGowan CM (2006) Effects of early intensive postoperative physiotherapy on limb function after tibial plateau levelling osteotomy in dogs with deficiency of the cranial cruciate ligament. *American Journal of Veterinary Research* **67**, 529–536

Nussbaum E (1998) The influence of ultrasound on healing tissues. *Journal of Hand Therapy* **11**, 140–147

Owen MR (2006) Rehabilitation therapies for musculoskeletal and spinal disease in small animal practice. *European Journal of Companion Animal Practice* **16**, 137–148

Sharp B (2008) Physiotherapy in small animal practice. *In Practice* **30**, 190–199

Snyder-Mackler L, Laden Z, Schepsis AA and Young JC (1991) Electrical stimulation of the thigh muscles after reconstruction of the anterior cruciate ligament. *The Journal of Bone and Joint Surgery* **73-A**, 1025–1036

Spector SA, Simard CP, Fournier M *et al.* (1982) Architectural alterations of rat hind limb skeletal muscle immobilized at different lengths. *Experimental Neurology* **76**, 94–110

ter Haar G (1999) Therapeutic ultrasound. *European Journal of Ultrasound* **9**, 3–9

Warden S, Bennell K, McMeeken JM and Ward JD (1999) Can conventional therapeutic ultrasound units be used to accelerate fracture repair? *Physical Therapy Review* **4**, 117–126

Watson T (2000) Masterclass. The role of electrotherapy in contemporary physiotherapy practice. *Manual Therapy* **5**, 132–141

Technique 4.1
Passive movements

Technique

The movement of a joint in a rhythmical manner through the full pain-free range.

Preparation

- The procedure is best carried out in a quiet, calm environment, so the animal is fully relaxed. A muzzle may be required for some animals, especially if they are in pain.
- Gentle massage (stroking, effleurage, kneading) should be carried out on the muscles around the area for 2–3 minutes to help the patient relax. Heat may also be used to relax muscles and other soft tissues, but should *not* be used during the first 2–3 days after surgery or when there is acute swelling or inflammation present.
- The patient should be in a comfortable position (normally in lateral recumbency) with the limbs fully supported.
- The other joints of the limb should be left in a neutral position (as if the animal were standing) and their movement minimized during the procedure. It may be necessary to position other joints to allow full ROM of the affected joint, e.g. full hock flexion also requires the stifle to be flexed.

Application

- Position yourself comfortably.
- Grasp the limb and hold the bones above and below the joint to be moved.
- Take the joint slowly into full flexion until initial resistance is felt, or until the animal shows signs of discomfort.
- Maintaining the hand holds, move the joint slowly into full extension until resistance or discomfort is felt.
- Repeat in a rhythmical manner 15 to 20 times. This should be carried out three to four times daily, or more frequently if joints have already lost range.

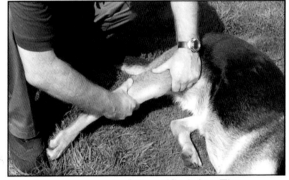

Passive movement of the stifle joint. The therapist takes the joint into full extension.

- Repeat the process on the other joints of the limb, especially if the animal is immobile and unable to actively move the limb. When treating the small joints of the digits, it is possible to move each joint individually or all the digits simultaneously.

Technique modifications

- In cases where there has been neurological damage or enforced immobility, it is also beneficial to carry out passive movements in functional patterns. This involves moving all the joints of a limb simultaneously, thereby simulating a normal gait pattern.
- When carrying out passive movements to the joints with long levers, such as the hip and shoulder joints, it can be difficult to maintain the hand hold through the full movement. In these cases it is beneficial to divide the full range into two halves (e.g. flexion half and extension half) and treat each half as if it is one passive movement.
- In cases where there is hypertonicity present, it is important that all passive movements are performed very slowly so as not to stimulate reflex muscle activity.

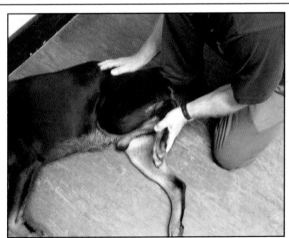

Passive movements in functional patterns. The limb is moved around in a bicycling fashion, simulating the normal gait pattern.

Technique 4.2
Stretching

Technique

The joint(s) to be stretched is placed in a position in which the muscles and other soft tissues are at their greatest length. A low-intensity stretch is then applied.

Preparation

For information on preparation see Technique 4.1.

Application

- Position yourself comfortably.
- Grasp the limb and hold the bones above and below the joint to be moved.
- Take the joint through the full pain-free range until resistance to motion is felt (generally the distal bone is moved relative to the proximal bone).
- Hold the stretch for 30 seconds and if possible try to increase the range gently during the stretch, especially if the resistance eases. Take care not to increase discomfort. *Do not* 'bounce' at the end of the range.
- Release the pressure gently and repeat several times (two to three repetitions is recommended).
- Generally, three to four sessions of stretching should be performed each day, and it may take several weeks to see any marked improvement.
- If muscles that cross two joints have become restricted, it is advisable initially to stretch each joint separately until flexibility improves. Then stretch both joints together to increase the functional range of the muscle.

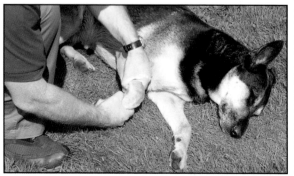

Stretch being carried out to the carpal extensor muscles.

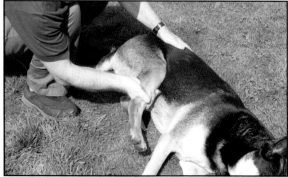

Two-joint muscle stretching. Combined stretch into hip flexion and stifle extension being carried out to the hamstrings.

Technique 4.3

Strengthening exercises

Overview

These exercises will increase the animal's muscular strength for standing, walking and playing. The assisted exercises will be of benefit to animals that are unable to stand and walk independently, and the active exercises are designed for animals that are more able.

Assisted exercises

Gym balls and physiotherapy rolls

These can be very effective in helping disabled animals assume a normal standing posture. By positioning the animal over the ball or roll, it will be able to bear some weight through its limbs.

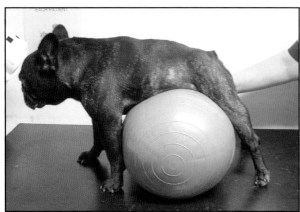

Gym balls and physiotherapy rolls can help an animal achieve functional postures and movements, such as standing.

Several additional exercises can also be carried out:

- After rolling the animal down into a sitting position, it can be encouraged and assisted to stand
- Rocking the ball forwards and backwards, or side-to-side, and alternating the weight bearing through the limbs can enhance balance and weight shifting
- Bouncing the ball provides dynamic weight bearing through the limbs.

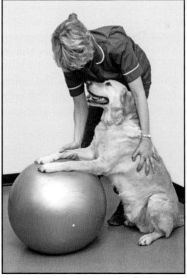

Sit to stand for a large dog.

➡

Technique 4.3 *continued*
Strengthening exercises

Active exercises

Leash walking

Slow leash walks form the basis of most rehabilitation programmes. They provide the owner with suitable control over the activity of the animal.

■ In the early stages of rehabilitation, all walks should be performed *slowly* to encourage the animal to bear weight on all limbs.
■ The owner can praise the animal when it bears weight on the affected limb.
■ It is easy to monitor and increase walks in a graduated manner, starting with two to three walks each day of 5 minutes' duration and increasing on a weekly basis by 5 minutes each walk.
■ Additional exercises can be incorporated into the daily walks as the animal's condition improves:
  – Slopes and stairs
  – Stepping over and around obstacles
  – Changes of direction
  – Walking over different surfaces: pavement, grass, gravel
  – Transitions: slow/fast/slow, walk/stop/walk, walk/sit/walk.

Sit to stand

A functional exercise that also helps to strengthen the hip and stifle extensor muscles that are vital for standing. The therapist should ensure that the sit is done correctly and the limbs are folded symmetrically underneath. Assistance may be required to position the limbs correctly and ensure that the push off is also performed symmetrically. It may be helpful to sit the animal in a corner or with its affected limb against a wall if it persistently sits with the limb out to the side.

Start with 6 to 10 repetitions twice daily and progress by increasing repetitions or adding small weights to the animal's hindquarters.

Slopes and stairs

These can be very helpful as they help to strengthen the hindlimb muscles. It is important to encourage *slow* and *controlled* ascent and descent, to ensure that the animal is using all limbs independently.

■ To strengthen hindlimb muscles, walk the animal straight up and zigzag down.
■ To strengthen forelimb muscles, zigzag the animal up and walk straight down.
■ Start with small gentle slopes (or a few steps) and progress to steeper, longer inclines (several flights of stairs).

Wheelbarrowing

A good exercise to strengthen the forelimbs. The hindlimbs are lifted from the ground and the animal encouraged to walk forward.

As the animal's strength improves it can be walked:

■ Up and down inclines
■ Over low obstacles
■ In different directions and around obstacles.

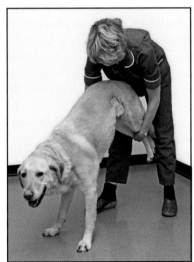

Wheelbarrowing: a good exercise for forelimb strengthening.

Technique 4.3 *continued*
Strengthening exercises

Dancing

A good exercise to strengthen the hindlimbs. The forelimbs are lifted from the ground and the animal encouraged to step around.

As the animal's strength improves it can be walked:

- Up and down inclines
- Over low obstacles
- In different directions and around obstacles.

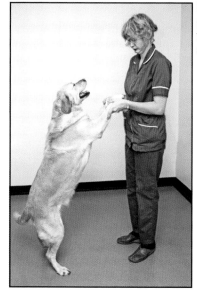

Dancing: a good exercise for hindlimb strengthening.

Weights

The use of weights to provide increased resistance can be very beneficial for the animal that requires higher levels of muscular strength. Weights can be applied in a variety of ways:

- Leg weights
- Backpacks with added weights
- Sleds or carts attached to harnesses. These must be pulled by the animal.

Technique 4.4
Balance and proprioception exercises

Overview

These exercises will improve the animal's ability to maintain good standing and walking balance. They will help the animal cope with the various changes of body position required during normal activity. The assisted exercises will be of benefit for animals that are unable to stand and walk independently, and the active exercises are designed for more able animals.

Assisted exercises
Standing

- With the animal standing four-square, and supported by a towel or harness, it is encouraged to stand and bear weight as much as able. The therapist can assist by providing the minimum support required. Initially, the animal may only be able to stand for 1–2 minutes, but this should be increased as necessary, and support gradually reduced.
- Whilst in the standing position, the therapist can slowly rock the towel from side to side to simulate the alternate weight bearing performed during gait and stimulate balance mechanisms.

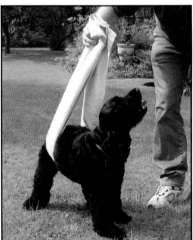

Assisted standing. A towel or harness can provide a weak animal with the opportunity to mobilize. Assisted standing and walking can help with motivation in addition to strengthening limb muscles and improving balance.

Walking

- With towel or harness support as necessary, the animal is encouraged to walk short distances. Support is gradually removed as the animal becomes able to walk without support.

Active exercises
Weight shifting

Exercise 1:
- With the animal standing four-square, gently push at hips or shoulders to encourage it to maintain balance. Push to sides/forward/back. After applying the push, quickly release pressure so the animal sways back to the starting position. Initially only use enough force so that the animal can correct its balance without having to take a side step. As the animal gets stronger and more able, slightly stronger pushes can be applied so it has to step to maintain its balance.
- Initially start by standing the animal on the floor.
- Progress to standing on a balance pad/wobble cushion/pillow.
- When the animal is able to walk, these pushes can be applied during movement.

Exercise 2:
- With the animal standing four-square, gently lift one leg off the ground so more weight is borne on the supporting legs. Hold for a count of 5 seconds. Lift a different leg each time the exercise is performed, so the animal's balance mechanisms are fully tested.
- Gently push in different directions, as in the previous exercise.
- Progress from standing on the floor to standing on a balance pad/wobble cushion/pillow.
- Progressively increase hold time and repetitions.

Technique 4.4 *continued*

Balance and proprioception exercises

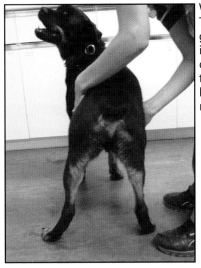

Weight shifting. The dog is gently pushed in different directions to stimulate balance reactions.

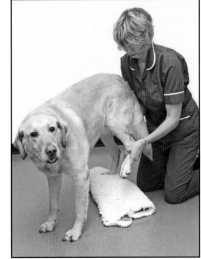

Three-leg standing. Raising one limb forces the dog to adjust its weight bearing through the remaining limbs, and helps with strength, balance and proprioception.

Treating/baiting

- With the animal standing four-square, treats are given in different positions to encourage weight bearing on all limbs. This will also encourage spinal mobility and help to improve balance.

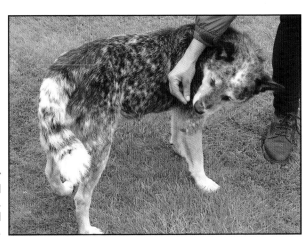

Treating/baiting. Treats can be used effectively to improve spinal mobility, balance and weight bearing. With the treat held to the side, the spine laterally flexes and weight is shifted to the contralateral limbs.

Balance pads and wobble cushions

- Balance exercises can be carried out whilst the animal is stood on an unsteady surface such as a balance pad, wobble cushion or trampet. Just one limb may be positioned on the pad, or both fore- or hindlimbs, or even all four limbs to create unsteadiness throughout the whole body (small dogs and cats may be stood on top of a gym ball but take care to prevent falling).

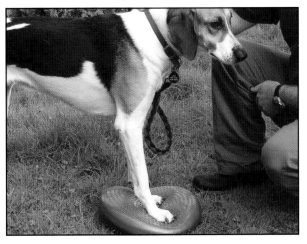

Balance pads/wobble cushions. Very useful equipment for the re-education of balance and proprioception.

Technique 4.4 *continued*

Balance and proprioception exercises

- Gently push the animal in different directions in a random manner.
- Lift one limb and allow the animal to regain its balance, and then push gently in different directions.
- Set up several foam pads, wobble cushions or pillows in a line at least 3 feet long. Walk the animal over them slowly.
- Progressively increase repetitions and depth of the foam/pillow surface.

Weaving

- Place several cones in a random fashion. The animal should be walked *slowly* around the cones in various directions.
- Progressively increase repetitions and the numbers/nearness of the cones.

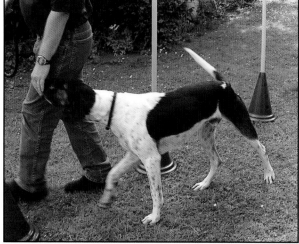

Weaving around obstacles helps improve balance, weight shifting and spinal lateral flexion. Increasing the difficulty of the course improves the animal's ability to cope.

Step overs

- Place three poles in a line, approximately 0.5–1.0 m apart. The animal should be walked *slowly* down the line of obstacles, and encouraged to step carefully over each one. Once the last obstacle has been cleared, make a circle, and come back in the opposite direction.
- If poles are difficult, use any type of low obstacle that can quite easily be stepped over.
- The distance between poles and the starting height will be dependent on the size of the animal.
- Progressively increase the number and height of poles/obstacles, but make sure the animal is still able to *step* over them and does not have to jump.
- Using two poles close together will encourage the animal to increase its stride length.

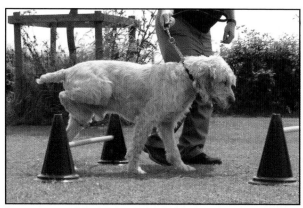

Step overs. Stepping over obstacles is a useful exercise to improve stride length, balance and joint ROM. The height and width of the obstacles can be increased to encourage greater joint flexion and extension, but take care not to raise them too high or the animal may simply jump over them.

5

Management of the critical care unit

Belinda Andrews-Jones and Amanda Boag

This chapter is designed to give information on:

- The definition and philosophy of a critical care unit
- Identification of patients requiring critical care
- Organization of a critical care unit, including necessary equipment and staffing
- Monitoring of patients within a critical care unit
- Infection control within a critical care unit

Introduction

This chapter provides information for qualified veterinary nurses on how to establish and run a critical care unit or area within a practice. Committed and diligent nursing plays an essential part in the successful treatment of critically ill patients. This can best be provided in an area dedicated for the higher level of care required for the critically ill.

The philosophy of the critical care unit and management

Critical care is a unique specialty that involves treatment of patients with both medical and surgical diseases. A factor common to all critical patients is the potential to develop problems that can be rapidly life-threatening. The aim of a critical care unit is to facilitate early recognition of these problems. Action can then be taken to prevent problems progressing to the point where the animal's life is at risk. In critical care, the body systems focused on most closely are the cardiovascular, respiratory and neurological systems (sometimes called the major body systems), because problems in these systems are most likely to result in death. Other body systems, especially the renal system, do however need to be considered, along with general nursing care. Critically ill patients may also be on multiple drugs, some of which can themselves lead to side-effects. The critical care veterinary nurse needs to have a thorough and well rounded knowledge and understanding of both medical and surgical disease processes, as well as a good knowledge of possible complications and treatments.

What is a critical care unit?

A critical care unit or intensive care unit is an area of a veterinary practice or hospital where patients with life-threatening conditions or the potential to develop them can be hospitalized. This area should be designed to allow the close monitoring required by the critically ill. Equipment and drugs to support normal function of the major body systems should be available. By their nature, critical care units require a greater level of nursing care and staffing than general wards. In some larger hospitals it is possible to have a specific room dedicated for this purpose; however, in smaller practices a critical care area can still be designated within the main kennel area.

Identification of patients requiring critical care

There are many reasons why a patient may need critical care. These include diseases and conditions affecting the major body systems (e.g. heart failure, pneumonia, seizures) but also severe diseases affecting other organs (e.g. pancreas, liver, kidneys) with secondary effects on the major body systems. Some patients may be admitted directly to the critical care unit following trauma or another acute incident (e.g. toxicity). Others may be admitted following deterioration of a pre-existing medical condition and yet others may be admitted for postoperative monitoring following major surgery. The list of potential patients is endless and the critical care veterinary nurse needs to be familiar with the pathophysiology of many illnesses as well as a wide range of diagnostic and therapeutic procedures. When admitting a patient to a critical care unit the veterinary nurse should always obtain the following information:

- Patient signalment (age, breed, sex, neuter status)
- Diagnosis
- Severity of illness
- Coexisting disease
- Prognosis
- Treatment plan and response to treatment up to this time
- Risk of cardiopulmonary arrest and owner's wishes regarding resuscitation should this occur.

The veterinary surgeon in charge of the case will also need to discuss with the owner the anticipated future quality of life of the pet if it survives the hospitalization period, the availability of the necessary equipment, drugs and staff to provide the level of support the patient needs, and the owner's ability (both financial and emotional) to support their pet through a period of critical illness with an uncertain outcome.

Some patients may only require critical care support for a short period of time, whereas others may need prolonged care. The amount of time a patient spends in a critical care unit is dependent on the extent of its illness or injury. As the patient's condition improves, it will require less intensive care, and when the standard of care is able to be met in a general ward, the patient can be discharged from the critical care unit. The requirement for a patient to remain within the critical care unit should be reviewed on a daily basis by the veterinary surgeons and veterinary nurses caring for the pet.

Challenges and rewards of critical care

Providing nursing care for the critically ill patient can be challenging, not only from the veterinary medical perspective but also emotionally. Each case is different; even patients with similar illnesses will have subtle differences from each other. As the ability to treat these critically ill patients grows, the critical care veterinary nurse must keep abreast of developments in treatment options; the learning process is never complete.

Due to the severity of the illness (Figure 5.1), critical care patients have a high mortality rate. Critical care veterinary nurses work closely with these patients and the owners, and can develop strong bonds. It can be very emotionally demanding and upsetting to see a patient deteriorate or die that the team have spent a large amount of time nursing.

Issues surrounding euthanasia of the critically ill patient can also be challenging. Sometimes owners may want to prolong their pet's life, whereas the veterinary staff may feel this is not in the pet's best interests. Conversely, owners may request euthanasia when the veterinary team feel that there is a realistic

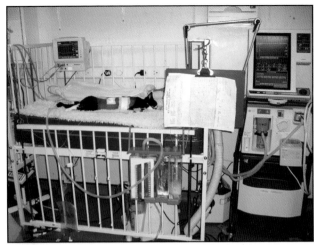

5.1 A critically ill cat in the critical care unit on mechanical ventilation with continuous suction thoracic drainage.

chance of a successful recovery. Ultimately the decision as to whether to euthanize is the owner's. It is the critical care team's job to guide the owner at this difficult time and support them and their pet, whether or not the team agree with their decision. Critical care veterinary nurses need to be optimistic and positive about the chosen treatment plan. As complications of treatment are not uncommon in the critical care unit, the critical care veterinary nurse must also learn not to become despondent at setbacks. These emotional challenges are helped by being part of a strong veterinary team, with open communication between all members of staff and owners encouraged and supported.

Organization of the critical care unit

The site of the critical care unit within the practice should be carefully considered. Ideally it should be in a central position with easy access to imaging areas and operating theatres. However, it should be possible to limit access to essential staff only; therefore, it cannot be part of a major thoroughfare. The area should be well lit, well ventilated, spacious and tidy. Items and equipment should be organized in an orderly and methodical fashion. There should be a mobile crash box or trolley (see Figure 5.5) that is well stocked and ready for use at all times. It should be the responsibility of one person in the practice (commonly a veterinary nurse) to ensure that the crash box is checked at least once weekly, as well as after every use. It is useful to have a chart of emergency drug doses for different weights of patients (see *BSAVA Manual of Practical Veterinary Nursing*) displayed in the designated emergency area or in the crash box/trolley itself. During a cardiopulmonary arrest, it is essential that the correct drug dosages can be drawn up and administered rapidly without the need for prolonged or complex calculations. Check lists for suggested equipment for a critical care unit, a resuscitation box/trolley and for drugs can be found in Figures 5.2, 5.3 and 5.4.

Equipment	Essential	Desirable
Crash cart/box (Figure 5.5)	✓	
Electrical defibrillation		✓
Oxygen source with various delivery attachments	✓	
Crash alarm (not necessarily commercial)	✓	
Humidified oxygen	✓ (if oxygen to be used for more than a few hours)	
Commercial oxygen cage		✓
Intensive care ventilator		✓
Patient incubator		✓
Human paediatric cot		✓
Clippers	✓	
Contact telephone numbers	✓	
Multiple electrical sources	✓	
Electrocardiographic monitor	✓	
Blood pressure measuring device:		
■ Doppler	✓	
■ Oscillometric		✓
■ Direct		✓
Multiparameter monitor		✓
Selection of intravenous catheters, including central lines	✓	
Selection of fluid therapy bags	✓	
Rapid infuser	✓	
Intravenous fluid pumps	✓	
Syringe drivers		✓
Access to blood products		✓
Access to blood gas machine		✓
Access to electrolyte analysis	✓	
Access to biochemistry analysis		✓
Access to microscope	✓	
Centrifuge and refractometer	✓	
Access to haemoglobin analysis	✓ (if using oxyglobin)	✓
Pulse oximeter	✓	
Capnography		✓
Patient weighing scales	✓	
Examination table/trolley	✓	
Kennels and bedding	✓	
Covered mattresses	✓	
Sink for hand washing	✓	
Storage for equipment and consumables		✓
Adequate clean facilities	✓	

5.2 Suggested equipment for a critical care unit.

Oxygen supply (piped or cylinder)	Anaesthetic machine or oxygen supply Anaesthetic circuits, ideally: modified T-piece for patients <10 kg; Bain for patients >10 kg 'Ambu' bag
Airway	Cuffed endotracheal tubes of varying sizes (all cuffs checked regularly) Stylet to facilitate intubation (e.g. proprietary stylet, rigid plastic male urinary catheter) Syringe for inflation of endotracheal tube cuff White open-weave tape for securing (tying-in) of the tube Laryngoscope with blades of varying size Large-bore over-the-needle catheter for tracheal oxygen delivery Tracheostomy kit with tubes of varying size Artery forceps Suction equipment: syringe with urinary catheter attached; handheld suction; suction pump
Drugs	Adrenaline (epinephrine)[a] Atropine[a] Lidocaine[a] Calcium gluconate (10%) Dextrose (glucose) (50%) Dobutamine Dexamethasone Doxopram Diazepam Furosemide Glyceryl trinitrate (2%) paste Sodium bicarbonate Mannitol Multiple syringes of heparinized saline should be available Emergency drug dosages chart should be readily available
Catheters	Over-the-needle catheters of varying sizes for intravenous access Intraosseous needles Tape to secure catheters Butterfly catheters for thoracocentesis Equipment for placement of intravenous catheters (see Chapter 6)
Fluid therapy	Isotonic replacement crystalloid (e.g. Hartmann's solution, 0.9% saline) Colloid
Equipment	Scalpel blades Syringes (multiple sizes) Electrocardiograph Electrode gel Defibrillator with external and internal paddles Defibrillator dosage chart Stopwatch/clock Pen and paper for recording information
Asepsis	Surgical scrub and surgical spirit Sterile surgical gloves of appropriate sizes

5.3 Suggested equipment for a crash box or trolley. [a] Syringes can be preloaded and clearly labelled with strength and date.

Cardiorespiratory	Adrenaline (epinephrine) Atropine Digoxin Diltiazem Dobutamine Dopamine Furosemide Glyceryl trinitrate Lidocaine Procainamide Propranolol Sotalol
Gastrointestinal	Maropitant Metoclopramide Omeprazole Ondansetron
Antimicrobial	Range to allow broad-spectrum coverage: Amikacin Amoxicillin/Clavulanate Ampicillin Cefuroxime Metronidazole Sulfadoxine/trimethoprim
Antiseizure	Diazepam Phenobarbital
Analgesia	Buprenorphine Carprofen Fentanyl Meloxicam Methadone Morphine Ropivacaine Medetomidine
Reversal agents/ antidotes	Acetylcysteine Chlorphenamine Naloxone Neostigmine
Anaesthesia/ sedation	Acepromazine Butorphanol Ketamine Midazolam Propofol
Steroids	Dexamethasone Hydrocortisone
Electrolytes and hormones	Glucose (50%) Calcium gluconate (10%) Soluble/neutral insulin Potassium chloride Sodium bicarbonate
Other	Mannitol Phytomenadione/Vitamin K1
Fluid therapy	Selection of crystalloids and colloids including: Isotonic replacement crystalloid (e.g. Lactated Ringer's, 0.9% sodium chloride) Hypertonic saline Colloid (e.g. pentastarch, tetrastarch)

5.4   Suggested list of drugs that should be stored in the critical care unit.

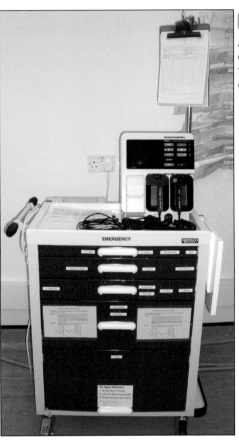

5.5   A crash cart/trolley for a critical care unit.

Stock level and control

All stock levels should be checked frequently. The amount of stock should be regularly adjusted to take into account the needs of the patients in the unit. A basic level should be maintained, but further amounts should be able to be obtained promptly when required.

Staffing

The single most important criterion for a critical care unit is the availability of sufficient adequately trained staff. The unpredictable condition of the critically ill patient means that a critical care unit cannot only run during normal working hours but must be suitably staffed 24 hours a day, 365 days a year, or whenever a patient is hospitalized in it. Staff are a much more important resource than any equipment. A veterinary surgeon should be available at all times, although they may not necessarily be in the unit continuously. Contact details for all veterinary surgeons with patients in the unit must be readily available. It is ideal that there are two suitably qualified veterinary nurses in the unit at all times as some tasks require two people for completion; however, one qualified veterinary nurse and another member of staff working under their direction may be sufficient.

Due to the necessity for continuous staffing, critical care departments require a team approach. All members of staff must be valued for their role. Each member of staff should be supported and should develop the capability to handle stress well and flourish under pressure. All veterinary nurses may need to make responsible decisions quickly and act on them promptly, and training must be given such that they develop the confidence to do this. It is also essential that all members of staff communicate well, both with other staff and with clients. The critical care veterinary nurse needs to remain calm and controlled at all times and be enthusiastic and motivated despite the demands of the role.

Admission of a new patient

Whenever a new patient is admitted to the critical care unit, the veterinary nurse responsible for the patient should familiarize themselves fully with the case. The familiarization should include a review of the patient's history and pertinent problems as well as a basic physical examination. Although a physical examination will have been performed already by the clinician, it is vital that the individual veterinary nurse involved with the case is also aware of the patient's physical status. It is impossible to monitor changes in patients accurately if the initial parameters are not known. A minimum evaluation of mentation, pulse rate and quality, mucous membrane colour and capillary refill time, respiration rate and effort and rectal temperature should be performed and recorded on admission.

Following a physical assessment, the veterinary nurse should review the clinician's orders and formulate a nursing care plan. A good critical care veterinary nurse will think ahead and anticipate problems and complications before they arise. It is important that any instructions on the patient's orders are clarified, and the veterinary nurse should feel confident to ask the clinician questions to ensure the best nursing care. The following factors may need to be clarified:

- What is the patient's resuscitation status?
- When were any catheters (intravenous or urinary) placed and last checked? Are there any concerns with the catheters, e.g. sterility during placement?
- When did the patient last urinate and defecate?
- When did the patient last eat and drink?
- Is the patient to be offered food and water at this time? If they can be offered food, are there any special dietary requirements? If the patient is allowed to eat normally, what kind of food does it usually eat at home?
- Are there any special nursing requirements such as padded bedding, physiotherapy or barrier nursing?

The patient's specific problems should also be reviewed. Potential problems and complications should be considered and the clinician asked for instructions on what to do in certain scenarios. For example, if a patient has a thoracostomy tube, would the clinician like the tube to be drained automatically if the patient is becoming more dyspnoeic or would they like to be contacted prior to this? Consideration should also be given to the parameters that the clinician has requested are monitored and how they should be interpreted. Specific 'Notify if...' criteria should be defined for each patient and agreed to by the veterinary surgeon and nursing staff.

> ## Procedures on admission of a patient to the critical care unit
>
> - **Familiarize yourself with the patient and previously collected information.**
> - **Assess the patient: previous history and physical examination.**
> - **Review the clinician's orders.**
> - **Think ahead: anticipate problems and complications.**
> - **Formulate a nursing care plan.**

Owners' visits and communication

When a patient is hospitalized in a critical care unit, this can be a stressful and worrying time for the owners. A policy on owner visits should be created for each unit. Generally visits should be encouraged, to build a positive working relationship between staff and owners. Visits are often of great benefit to the patient, although on rare occasions they may be to the patient's detriment (e.g. a patient who becomes very distressed when the owner leaves, or a patient with respiratory distress that gets worse when it sees the owner and becomes excited). In these rare cases, future visits should be gently discouraged after explaining to the owners why this is the case.

It is necessary to establish boundaries so that owner visits do not interfere with the care of either the individual patient or others hospitalized in the unit. It can be difficult to predict a good time for an owner to visit their pet in advance, and owners should be made aware that they may need to wait or to curtail the visit abruptly. It should also be remembered that it can be very distressing for an owner the first time they see the patient. Critically ill patients often have a number of different catheters and tubes attached to them that an owner may not understand. It is important to have an honest discussion with the owner and to explain to them what to expect when they see their pet.

In order for the client to make rational decisions regarding their pet's care, it is important that they trust the veterinary team and that time is spent explaining the nature of the animal's problems, possible treatment options, complications and prognosis. The owner should be made to feel at ease and to have confidence that their pet is in good hands and will be well cared for in a pleasant environment. The veterinary nurse can be a vital part of that communication and can give the owners a valuable link to their pet's progress during a difficult time. It is essential that the veterinary nurse and veterinary surgeon in charge of the case communicate well so that the owners receive the same information from all members of the veterinary team. Should the patient undergo any deterioration, it is important that the situation is communicated honestly and as soon as possible to the owner. Although this is usually the responsibility of the veterinary surgeon, they may delegate that role to the veterinary nurse, especially if the veterinary surgeon is involved with necessary treatment measures for the patient at the time.

Cost of treatment

Critical care can be very costly, not just because of the use of expensive drugs and equipment, but because these patients are very demanding of both veterinary nurses' and veterinary surgeons' time. Bill updates should be prepared regularly and communicated to the clinician for ongoing discussion with the owner. Cost does sometimes become an issue in patient management and this must be recognized and respected.

Protocols

Performance of regular tasks can be improved by the development of protocols. This can help with staff training as well as representing current best practice. Each critical care unit should have a set of protocols for frequently performed patient tasks. This ensures that all staff are working to the same guidelines and standards. It is suggested that protocols are developed for:

- Intravenous catheter (peripheral and central) care
- Recumbent patient care
- Urinary catheter care
- Thoracostomy tube (chest drain) care
- Tracheostomy tube care
- Feeding tube care
- Parenteral nutritional care
- Transfusion administration
- Ventilation patient care.

The protocols should represent current best practice, as appropriate to the local environment, and should be reviewed regularly.

Rounds and shift handovers

As discussed above, critical care is a task that continues for 24 hours a day, 7 days a week, therefore, it cannot be performed by one person. Continuity of care is also vitally important, and detailed case handover rounds are therefore an important part of the work of a critical care unit. Rounds should be performed every time there is a change of nursing shift cover and should ideally involve both veterinary surgeons and veterinary nurses at least once daily. Rounds are most valuable when there is open communication and questioning is welcome (Figure 5.6). Team work is the key element.

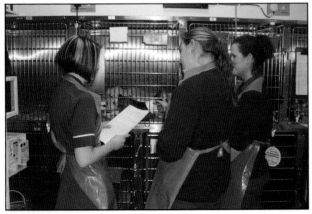

5.6 Critical care unit veterinary nurses discussing patient care during rounds at shift change.

During rounds much of the same information should be covered as when the patient is admitted. This should include:

- Signalment of the patient (name, breed, age, sex, neuter status)
- Patient's major problems
- Reason for admission
- Brief review of medical history
- Review of physical examination and parameters that are being monitored, especially highlighting any parameters that have changed during the previous shift
- Review of patient's status with regard to food and water intake, and defecation and urination
- Update on any new diagnostic results
- Update on prognosis and current concerns
- Events or interventions during the previous shift
- Suggestions or special advice for the new shift.

Other factors that should be considered at the time of shift changeovers include the checking and signing of dangerous drug logs, the need to restock any drugs or equipment (especially those required for cardiopulmonary–cerebral resuscitation) and any expected owner visits.

Once the previous shift have left, the critical care veterinary nurse should briefly review all the patients' charts and note any further information, including the intensity of treatments and any procedures which need to be performed during the shift that will take a long time. This will allow the veterinary nurse to plan the time they are on shift effectively and to achieve all the requested tasks.

Recumbent patients deserve special consideration. Generally recumbent patients require turning every four hours and, especially with larger patients, this can best be achieved when additional help is available. Shift changeover can be a good time to do these tasks as there will be more people present.

Clinical notes

Clinical notes are a vital part of patient care and it is a legal requirement to keep accurate records. The notes give a written review of how the case was managed, including the rationale for treatment decisions. It is vital, especially with critical care cases, that as much information as possible is noted, so that every shift can review earlier notes fully.

Every time the patient is handled, even for a minor procedure, a note should be made on the hospitalization sheet. Every entry on the notes should be initialled to allow the member of staff making the note to be identified and so that further information can be obtained if required. Administration of medications should also be recorded and initialled, as should any changes to the hospitalization sheet. The clinician in charge of the patient should be responsible for writing the patient's orders daily and signing them once written.

Nursing care plans

Critical care veterinary nurses are encouraged to develop written nursing care plans for their patients, taking into account the unique requirements of that patient and considering its physical, physiological and psychological well being. Care plans are an essential part of nursing and if done well help to ensure that important issues in the patient's medical treatment orders are not overlooked.

Nursing care plans need not take a long time to create and most veterinary nurses will already be considering all the issues, if in a less systematic way. When creating a nursing plan for a critically ill patient the following should be considered:

- What are the daily nursing goals for each patient?
- Is the patient clean, dry and comfortable?
- Is the patient's pain relief adequate?
- When did the patient last defecate/urinate?
- Is the patient consuming/receiving adequate water and nutrition?
- Is the patient's mental status being stimulated; for example, fresh air, walks outside, owner visits, grooming and affection?
- How are nosocomial infections being prevented?

Seemingly small details of care may lead to a huge improvement in the patient's well being. For instance, spending time encouraging an inappetent animal to eat, and succeeding, may prevent the necessity of placing an invasive feeding tube.

Patient care

It is essential that critical care veterinary nurses, and the unit itself, are organized at all times. In a busy critical care unit, tasks will need to be prioritized so that all patients are treated appropriately. Generally, treatments for and monitoring of the most severely ill or most unstable patients should be performed first, followed by analgesia for all other patients that require it. The prioritization process is performed best by veterinary nurses who are familiar with the patients and the treatments, including how long various procedures will take and whether help from other staff members is required. Good time management is an essential skill for a critical care veterinary nurse to develop.

The status of critically ill patients may change rapidly either in response to therapy or to the underlying disease. The critical care veterinary nurse must be flexible and be prepared to change their plan and priorities on an ongoing basis. Monitoring of patients is one of the major roles of a critical care unit. Changes in patients should be recorded and acted on rapidly. Early detection of deterioration or complications gives the best chance of successful intervention to address the problem. For example, if a patient is losing blood postoperatively, it is much better that this is recognized when the patient is showing signs of only mild hypovolaemia rather than when the patient is showing signs of severe hypovolaemic shock. The early stages of shock may be quite subtle and consist of just a mild increase in heart rate and an alteration in pulse quality.

Monitoring will need to be tailored to the individual patient; however, there are certain parameters (Figure 5.7) that should be recorded regularly regardless of the patient's disease, including:

- Perfusion parameters:
  - Heart rate
  - Pulse quality
  - Mucous membrane colour
  - Capillary refill time.
- Respiratory rate and effort
- Thoracic auscultation
- Demeanour
- Rectal temperature
- Bodyweight (every 12 hours).

Body system/assessment	Parameter	Intervals
Cardiovascular	Pulse rate and quality Mucous membranes Capillary refill time Arterial blood pressure Central venous pressure (if central catheter present)	Every 1–6 h
Respiratory	Respiratory rate and effort Oxygen saturation (pulse oximeter)	Every 1–6 h
Demeanour	Patient appearance and behaviour	Every 2–6 h
Temperature		Every 2–12 h
Urination assessment	Walk, check tray, check bladder and drain urinary collection bag Calculate ml/kg/h and specific gravity when obtainable	Every 2–4 h
Wounds/dressings/intravenous catheters	Tension, swelling and discharge	Every 4–12 h
Intravenous catheters	Flush	Every 4 h
Arterial catheters	Flush	Every 1 h
Recumbent patients	Ensure patient is turned	At least every 4 h

5.7 Routine patient parameter assessments in the critical care unit.

The frequency of assessment of the various parameters will vary between patients and should be reviewed on a daily basis. In very unstable patients these parameters may need to be monitored up to every 30 minutes, reducing to every 2–4 hours as the patient becomes more stable, and to every 8–12 hours just prior to discharge from the critical care unit.

Other physical examination findings that should be noted include details of the status of any wounds or bandages. For recumbent patients, there should be regular checks for any signs of decubitus ulcers or urine or faecal scald, with action taken if necessary. The patient's mental well being should also not be overlooked.

Other monitoring techniques

Repeated physical examination is the most important monitoring tool and does not require expensive equipment. However, the physical examination can be supplemented by a number of further monitoring tools. The use of modern technology to aid patient monitoring should never replace the physical examination, and values generated by machines should always be interpreted carefully, especially if they do not agree with the physical assessment. In most circumstances, the monitoring of trends provides much more useful information than measurement at a single time point. Prompt action should be taken in response to any unexpected findings; there is no point in performing monitoring if the findings are not going to be acted upon.

Further monitoring tools include:

- *Continuous electrocardiography:* this is useful for patients with dysrhythmias or those with rapidly changing heart rates. It may also be useful for monitoring patients with intracranial disease or certain electrolyte abnormalities such as hyperkalaemia
- *Arterial blood pressure:* this can be measured by either indirect (Doppler or oscillometric) or direct (arterial catheter) methods. The information provided is dependent on the method used and whether a systolic, diastolic or mean pressure is obtained. Arterial blood pressure represents the driving force for tissue perfusion. Prolonged hypo- or hypertension should be avoided
- *Central venous pressure:* this is a measure of the blood pressure in the central venous compartment and is usually obtained via a catheter in the jugular vein. It provides the best indication of vascular filling and is especially useful in patients at risk of volume overload, such as those with heart failure or renal failure that also require fluid therapy
- *Pulse oximetry:* this provides a measure of haemoglobin saturation. It is easy to perform although it can be unreliable, especially in conscious patients. It is not sensitive to early hypoxia, but identification of subtle trends can be an important clue that the patient's oxygen status is altering and should prompt a more accurate assessment, such as arterial blood gas analysis
- *End-tidal carbon dioxide:* this provides a measure of the amount of carbon dioxide present in exhaled air and is closely related to the patient's arterial carbon dioxide and ventilation status

- *Blood tests:* the ability to perform regular in-house monitoring tests of certain parameters is important. Which parameters are monitored will depend on the nature of the patient's disease and the facilities available. Consideration should be given to regular monitoring of packed cell volume (PCV)/refractometric total solids (TS), blood glucose, electrolytes, venous and arterial blood gases, clotting parameters and blood smear examination.

Accurate and diligent monitoring is arguably the most important aspect of critical care nursing. The critical care veterinary nurse should be continually reassessing the patient's status, response to treatment and the need for any alterations to the patient's management plan.

Psychological requirements

Amongst all the medical care a critically ill patient needs, it can be easy to overlook the patient's psychological needs, although it is essential that these are considered. Time should be spent talking to and grooming the patients. The alternative is that the patient will learn that the only attention it receives is when a relatively unpleasant task, such as blood sampling, is performed. This can be distressing to the patient and make the animal harder to handle and nurse in the long term.

Where possible, it can be encouraging for dogs to experience fresh air, so regular visits outside are important once the patient is able to tolerate this. Cats should be given the opportunity to exercise if possible. Toys can be given to stimulate the pet, and an owner's familiar possession can bring consolation.

Allowing patients to rest is another important consideration. As a critical care unit must run 24 hours a day, lights can be on and the environment may be noisy throughout this time. Where possible (and taking into account the needs of all the patients) the lights may be turned down during quiet periods overnight to allow the patients to rest. Grouping treatments together is also a useful technique to prevent sleep interruption.

Analgesia

The critical care veterinary nurse is the person who normally spends the most time with the patient, and is often in an ideal position to comment on the patient's analgesic requirements and response to therapy. The critical care veterinary nurse should be encouraged to be proactive in informing the veterinary surgeon if they believe the patient's analgesic regime is not sufficient. Pre-emptive analgesia is generally considered desirable to avoid the 'wind-up' phenomenon seen with pain. Pain assessment scores can be used to allow a more objective assessment of the patient, especially between different shifts and veterinary nurses. As some critically ill patients will have undergone surgery, it is vital that adequate analgesic drugs are provided, and this should be considered when the critical care unit is being set up. A range of pure and partial opioid agonist, non-steroidal anti-inflammatory and local anaesthetic drugs should be available for use and it is recommended that a multimodal approach to analgesia be adopted.

Although the legislation associated with the provision of pure opioid drugs, such as morphine or methadone, may reduce the willingness of some practices to stock them, in patients with severe pain (e.g. after trauma) these drugs are the only ones that will have sufficient effect and it is strongly recommended that all critical care units have access to these drugs.

Progress and assessments

Assessment sheets are an ideal way to formalize a patient care plan. Subjective, objective, assessment and plan (SOAP) (Figure 5.8) schemes are a well used medical and veterinary form of assessment.

Infection control

Infection control is very important throughout the whole practice but nowhere more so than in a critical care unit. Critically ill patients are particularly susceptible to hospital-acquired infections (HAIs). Factors predisposing to HAIs include:

- Age (paediatric and geriatric)
- Immunosupresion from drug therapy or disease processes
- Antimicrobial therapy
- Invasive equipment such as intravenous catheters, urinary catheters and thoracostomy tubes
- Open wounds
- Long-term hospitalization.

HAIs (previously known as nosocomial infections) are infections that the patient acquires once hospitalized that it did not have prior to admission. HAIs may be endogenous or exogenous. Endogenous infections are infections acquired from the patient's own normal flora. Exogenous infections are mainly acquired from infected patients or healthy carriers and transmitted to the patient via medical equipment (fomites) or personnel. The goal should be to reduce the incidence of HAIs to zero and, although this goal may be unobtainable, protocols should be in place to get as close to it as possible. Areas for consideration when designing protocols to reduce HAIs include environmental factors, staff factors and patient factors.

Subjective	Opinion of how the patient seems, rather than objective facts	Seems depressed today, but bright outside when walked Pain assessment: seems fully controlled with methadone q4h and carprofen
Objective	Physical examination findings that can be measured	TPR: WNL Cardiovascular: WNL Respiratory: thoracic drain removed yesterday, auscultation chest seems clear, veterinary surgeon agreed Neurological: WNL Gastrointestinal: eating and drinking only very small amounts, some diarrhoea today Cutaneous: faecal staining on fur adjacent to anus Urogenital: has not urinated for 12 hours, medium bladder size Musculoskeletal: WNL Temperature: WNL
Assessment	Personal evaluation of the patient based on the subjective and objective findings	Doing quite well but: - Not eating adequately - Urine output reduced? - Cutaneous faecal scalding needs to be prevented
Plan	What are your intentions for the patient?	Respiration: continue to monitor respiratory rate and effort, and auscultate Depression: continue with regular visits outside for fresh air. Maybe owners could visit today? Groom at least once today Diet: Calculate calorific requirements, water requirements and the amount the patient is taking; if the amount is deficient talk to clinician regarding nutritional support Offer more palatable foods, but keep bland due to diarrhoea, hand tempt Cutaneous: wash, dry, clip fur around anus and apply barrier cream. Cover tail with dressing to keep clean. Check cleanliness q3h Continue to monitor urine output: take outside regularly. If not improved shortly, talk to clinician regarding placement of indwelling urinary catheter, and collection system, and monitoring output and specific gravity Analgesia: continue to provide thick soft bedding and prescribed analgesia

5.8 Care plan for a terrier, 2 days following a thoracotomy. TPR = Temperature, pulse and respiration; WNL = Within normal limits.

Environmental factors

All practices should have a strict cleaning protocol that is reliably enforced and regularly reviewed. Consideration should be given to environmental monitoring for bacterial load as well as gross contamination. All equipment should be cleaned and wiped with disinfectant after each use, including equipment leads, pulse oximeters, clipper blades and breathing circuits. All staff should be aware of the risk of transmission of microorganisms between patients on fomites. Fomites include any inanimate objects, such as leads and muzzles, which may be used with multiple patients. 'Hand touch' sites (i.e. sites that are touched regularly) should be wiped with disinfectant at least twice a day. These sites may vary between critical care units but might include the phone, computer, door handle and pens. Patient accommodation should be disinfected regularly and thoroughly, especially after a patient is discharged, and bedding should be changed regularly. There should be a protocol to ensure all work surfaces and floors are cleaned and disinfected frequently. Sticky mats at the entry and exit points of the critical care unit may help to reduce the transmission of dirt and microorganisms. Alternatively, shoe covers or designated footwear can be used.

Staff factors

Good hand hygiene is one of the most important aspects of controlling HAIs. The objective of hand washing is to remove both dirt and microorganisms. The hands of personnel represent the major route of transmission of exogenous infections. Proper use of an antiseptic hand wash, such as chlorhexidine, will kill transient skin flora and reduce the multiplication of resident flora. All staff must be trained in the importance of diligent hand hygiene, which should be performed before and after every patient interaction. Hand washing should be encouraged by the presence of easily accessible hand washing facilities, including sinks with mixer taps. Hand drying should be performed using disposable towels, and a pedal-operated bin should be available. To ensure adequate hand washing, rings (other than a plain wedding band) should not be worn in the critical care unit and short-sleeved clothes should be worn. Nails should be kept short and clean. Regular hand washing with an antiseptic solution can irritate and dry out sensitive skin; provision of a pump dispenser for skin moisturizer close to the sink can reduce this problem. Signs should be placed around the clinic to remind people of the importance of hand washing and all visitors should be expected to comply with the hand washing policy. A 'critical culture' should be encouraged in which all staff members feel able to remind each other of the importance of this simple measure.

In a busy environment such as a critical care unit, where it may be difficult to perform a thorough hand wash between all patient interactions, alternative methods of hand hygiene, such as alcohol hand rubs, may be used in some circumstances. The use of alcohol hand rubs can improve compliance with hand hygiene and reduce the amount of time spent washing hands. They can be less irritating to the skin than frequent washing with antiseptic scrubs and they dry quickly without the need for paper towels. Staff should be encouraged to carry alcohol hand rubs attached to their protective clothing. They can also be attached to each kennel door to act as a reminder that hands should be cleaned prior to touching the patient. Alcohol hand rubs are very effective as long as there is no gross contamination of the hands with biological material. In this situation, a thorough hand wash should be performed.

Gloves may be worn for patient interactions such as handling open wounds or tubes that enter body cavities. However, glove use does not substitute for hand washing. When non-sterile gloves from box packaging are used, the hands should be washed (or sprayed with an alcohol rub) before and after putting the gloves on as a precaution in case the outside of the gloves has been contaminated.

Patient factors

Patients with multiple catheters (intravenous and other) are at particular risk for infection, and great care and attention must be paid whenever catheters entering a vessel or body cavity are handled. Intravenous catheters should be disconnected from fluid lines as infrequently as possible and injection ports should be swabbed with alcohol prior to administration of any intravenous medication. Hands should be thoroughly washed and gloves worn whenever urinary catheters or thoracostomy tubes are handled. Similarly, scrupulous hand hygiene should be observed and gloves worn whenever an open wound is examined. If the patient has an open wound when admitted to the critical care unit, it is recommended that a microbiological swab is taken and submitted at the time of admission. Open wounds should be covered at all times. Equipment should be carefully cleaned before use on a new patient, and disposable equipment (e.g. thermometer sheaths) should be used where possible to limit the risk of patient cross-contamination. Overuse of antibiotics is associated with an increase in multidrug-resistant infections, so the need for antibiotic therapy should be carefully considered for each patient.

Hand hygiene

Hand hygiene should be carried out:

- **Before and after examining a patient**
- **Before and after touching catheters, drains and wounds**
- **After removing gloves**
- **When the hands are visibly soiled**
- **On arrival at and before leaving work**
- **Before and after eating or smoking**
- **Before and after visiting the toilet.**

Antibiotic-resistant bacteria

Any bacteria can cause a HAI, including those sensitive to all antimicrobials. Unfortunately, however, many HAIs are caused by bacteria that have developed resistance to many of the commonly used antimicrobial drugs. This includes methicillin-resistant *Staphylococcus aureus* (MRSA) and extended spectrum beta-lactamase producing *Escherichia coli*. Some animals and humans are colonized with these bacteria, and although they are not a risk to a healthy individual they can become a risk if that individual becomes ill. Alternatively, healthy colonized animals or humans can act as a source of infection for critically ill patients. It is not practical to screen and decolonize all staff and patients for these bacteria and so it is likely they will continue to be introduced to critical care units. This emphasizes the importance of diligent hygiene measures, especially hand hygiene, to reduce the transmission of these organisms from healthy individuals to critically ill patients. Inappropriate use of antimicrobials is a factor in the development of antimicrobial resistance and can promote colonization by these bacteria. Indiscriminate use of antimicrobials should therefore be avoided, especially with those antimicrobials, such as enrofloxacin, which have been particularly associated with the development of resistance.

Barrier nursing

Barrier nursing is a technique that should be used with some patients in critical care units. A patient may need to be barrier nursed if it is particularly susceptible to HAIs, in an effort to further reduce the risk of becoming infected. This category may include patients with profound immunosuppression (either from drug therapy or disease), patients with open wounds and unvaccinated patients. Other patients may be known or suspected to be suffering from a contagious, transmissible or zoonotic disease. In such cases, barrier nursing is required for the safety of other patients and staff. Although full isolation in a separate room would be ideal for these patients, on occasion the severity of the condition requires that they are nursed in an environment set up for critical care. When this is necessary, the infected patient should be placed as far from other patients as possible, and strict precautions should be used to prevent cross-contamination.

Barrier nursing involves the wearing of a plastic gown or apron, shoe covers, gloves, mask and sometimes goggles whenever the patient is handled (Figure 5.9). Equipment that could act as a fomite should be kept for the sole use of this patient. Such items include thermometers, pens and stethoscopes. A note should be clearly placed on the patient's kennel and clinical record stating that the patient must be barrier nursed and giving the reason why. If the animal needs to be moved to another area of the hospital (such as for imaging procedures or to go outside to urinate), the veterinary nurse and clinician should liaise and discuss what precautions should be taken at this time. Barrier nursing can be very demanding

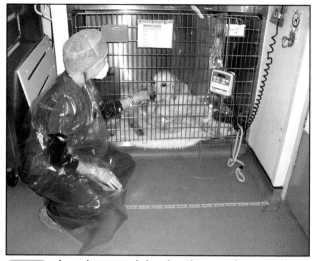

5.9   A patient receiving barrier nursing care in the critical care unit.

of staff time but if performed diligently can result in a better outcome both for that patient and for all other patients in the critical care unit.

Conclusion

Critical care nursing can be both physically and psychologically demanding, but the personal rewards can be vast. The critical care veterinary nurse works to a very high standard as part of a close-knit team alongside the veterinary surgeon and owners, as well as other veterinary nurses. Knowledge and skills are constantly challenged and developed, and the work is never monotonous. Ultimately, helping to save the lives of the most severely ill patients is the best reward of all.

References and further reading

Andrews-Jones B and Boag A (2007) Triage and emergency nursing. In: *BSAVA Manual of Practical Veterinary Nursing*, ed. E Mullineaux and M Jones, pp. 105–126. BSAVA Publications, Gloucester

Battaglia A (2000) *Small Animal Emergency and Critical Care: A Manual for the Veterinary Technician*. WB Saunders, Philadelphia

King L and Boag A (2007) *BSAVA Manual of Canine and Feline Emergency and Critical Care, 2nd edition*. BSAVA Publications, Gloucester

6

Advanced fluid therapy

Paula Hotston Moore and Jo Murrell

This chapter is designed to give information on:

- Advanced fluid therapy
- The properties of different crystalloid solutions and the factors influencing selection of the appropriate crystalloid solution for the individual patient
- The pharmacokinetics of colloid solutions and the characteristics of the different colloid solutions that are commercially available
- Collection of blood from donors, blood typing and administration of blood to recipients, including the use of the blood substitutes
- The technique to measure central venous pressure as a guide to fluid therapy
- Potassium homeostasis and management of hyper- and hypokalaemia
- Acid–base homeostasis and common acid–base disorders

Introduction

Provision of fluid therapy is a common task for veterinary nurses. The area is covered in all standard texts for veterinary nurses and technicians but often the background information provided uses simple models of understanding that may be inadequate for experienced veterinary nurses or those seeking a deeper understanding of the subject. This chapter provides greater detail in many areas that will meet this need and allow veterinary nurses managing fluid therapy to care for these patients with a greater insight into the underlying physiological abnormalities.

Crystalloid-based fluid therapy

Crystalloids are solutions containing electrolyte and non-electrolyte solutes that are capable of entering all body fluid compartments. They are as effective as colloids in expanding the plasma compartment (blood volume), but a much greater volume of crystalloid fluid is required to produce equivalent plasma expansion because the crystalloid is also distributed to other sites (e.g. interstitial and intracellular compartments).

Crystalloid solutions can be classified as either balanced or unbalanced, and as either maintenance or replacement solutions.

Choice of crystalloid solution

The choice of fluid to administer is dependent on the nature of the disease process and the composition of the fluid lost. However, in most circumstances it is important to remember that severe deficits in circulating blood are life-threatening and intravenous administration of any fluid type is better than none. Lactated Ringer's (or Hartmann's) solution is a good first choice while waiting for laboratory results to confirm abnormalities in electrolyte concentration.

- Losses should be replaced with a fluid that is similar in volume and electrolyte composition to that which has been lost from the body.
- If clinical assessment of hydration status indicates hypovolaemia, a replacement solution should be administered rapidly (administration of a colloid solution should be considered).
- Once fluid and electrolyte deficits have been replaced and ongoing losses stabilized, a maintenance solution can be given.

Types of crystalloid solution

- *Balanced solutions*: the composition of the fluid resembles that of extracellular fluid (e.g. lactated Ringer's solution).
- *Unbalanced solutions*: the composition does not resemble that of extracellular fluid (e.g. normal saline solution).
- *Replacement solutions*: the composition of replacement solutions resembles that of extracellular fluid (i.e. balanced crystalloid solutions are also replacement solutions). They are used to replace fluid deficits due to excessive fluid loss caused by conditions such as diarrhoea, vomiting or severe haemorrhage.
- *Maintenance solutions*: these solutions contain more potassium and less sodium than replacement fluids and are used for ongoing fluid therapy in animals that are unable to meet their daily fluid and electrolyte requirements through drinking. The sodium and potassium concentrations in maintenance fluids reflect the relative losses of these electrolytes in normal animals that require ongoing fluid therapy because they are unable to drink. Maintenance solutions can be purchased commercially or can be made by mixing together replacement solutions and adding potassium.

Characteristics of common crystalloid solutions

Lactated Ringer's solution

Lactated Ringer's (or Hartmann's) solution is a balanced electrolyte solution that contains lactate. The lactate is metabolized in the liver by gluconeogenesis or oxidation, and both of these processes consume hydrogen ions. Therefore, administration of lactate-containing solutions has an alkalinizing effect. This prevents the dilutional acidosis that can otherwise occur due to dilution of plasma bicarbonate by exogenously administered fluids that do not contain lactate. The solution is suitable for routine fluid therapy in anaesthetized patients. The solution contains calcium and cannot be given through the same intravenous line as blood products because of the risk of clot formation. In patients with severe liver disease or hyperlactataemia, there is potential for lactate accumulation and an increase in blood lactate concentration following administration of lactated crystalloid solutions, which is due to the inability of the liver to metabolize lactate. Acetated polyionic solutions may be more suitable than lactated crystalloid solutions for this patient group, but these are not widely used in the UK.

Normal saline

Normal saline (0.9% NaCl) solution contains higher amounts of chloride than does plasma. It will dilute plasma bicarbonate and provides chloride for reabsorption from the glomerular filtrate, leading to hyperchloraemic acidosis. The degree of acidosis is unlikely to be a problem in healthy patients; therefore, normal saline is used for routine fluid therapy during anaesthesia. The solution is ideal for patients with a hypochloraemic metabolic alkalosis due to vomiting of stomach contents.

Dextrose

Dextrose (5%) solution contains no electrolytes so when it is metabolized only water remains. The amount of dextrose is inadequate to meet calorific requirements because the volume of fluid required to provide sufficient calories would far exceed maintenance fluid requirements. The solution is suitable for patients that have suffered from pure water loss (e.g. they have been denied access to water). It is not suitable for routine administration during anaesthesia and surgery.

Dextrose saline

Dextrose saline (2.5% dextrose and 0.18% NaCl) solution is designed to increase the free water content of the body and may be of use in the management of patients with hypernatraemia. Serum electrolyte concentrations should be monitored carefully to ensure that excessive dilution does not occur.

Acetated polyionic solutions

Acetated polyionic solutions (e.g. acetated Ringer's solution) use acetate as an alkalinizing agent in place of lactate. Acetate is metabolized rapidly throughout the body, so the alkalinizing effect of this solution is more readily available and does not rely on adequate liver function. Acetate can cause vasodilation when given rapidly, which may be detrimental to unstable and hypotensive patients. Acetate-containing solutions are also contraindicated in patients with diabetic ketoacidosis because they may theoretically result in increased ketone body production. Some commercial solutions do not contain calcium and can be administered through the same intravenous line as blood products.

Hypertonic saline

Solutions of hypertonic saline (7.2% NaCl) are used to provide rapid resuscitation and plasma volume expansion in animals with hypovolaemic shock. They are useful in large-breed dogs where the infusion of large volumes of colloids or replacement crystalloid solutions would otherwise be required. Hypertonic saline must be followed by the administration of isotonic fluids for several hours to ensure stable plasma volume expansion and to prevent hypernatraemia. The rate of administration of hypertonic saline solution must be carefully monitored; rapid administration can result in hypotension, bradycardia and bronchoconstriction. The dose administered should not exceed 4 ml/kg.

Colloid-based fluid therapy

Plasma colloid osmotic pressure

The strict definition of a colloid is a solution containing atoms or molecules that resist sedimentation, diffusion or filtration. By contrast crystalloid solutions are freely diffusible. Oncotic pressure is the osmotic pressure exerted by colloids in solution, although the osmotic pressure of colloids in plasma is greater than that calculated for an ideal solution. This discrepancy occurs because negatively charged proteins (such as albumin) retain cations in the intravascular space by electrostatic attraction. These cations also contribute to the osmotic pressure because osmotic pressure is proportional to the number of molecules present rather than their size. Albumin accounts for about 60–70% of plasma colloid osmotic pressure, with globulins making up the remainder.

Pharmacokinetics and pharmacodynamics

The principle of using colloids for fluid therapy relies on the fact that, in the absence of increased microvascular permeability, the increased molecular size of colloids means that colloids are retained within the vasculature to a greater extent than crystalloids. Therefore, smaller volumes of colloid will result in greater plasma volume expansion compared with crystalloids, allowing a more rapid effect to be achieved.

In contrast with natural colloid solutions such as albumin, in which all molecules are the same size, artificial colloid solutions contain molecules that vary in molecular weight, leading to complex pharmacokinetics after administration.

- The smaller molecules pass rapidly into the urine or interstitium and are rapidly eliminated from the circulation.
- Larger molecules remain in the circulation and are gradually eliminated by hydrolysis or removed by phagocytosis.
- This pattern of molecule removal from the circulation (initial rapid loss of molecules followed by a slower decline) results in an exponential decline in intravascular volume expansion.
- Manufacturers' data sheets describing the duration of volume expansion from an artificial colloid solution can be misleading because they imply that the major proportion of the plasma volume expansion lasts for 24–36 hours, when in reality it is much shorter (6–12 hours, depending on the solution).

Adverse effects

Volume overload

As colloid solutions are retained in the intravascular space for longer than crystalloids, the risk of volume overload following injudicious administration of colloids is greater than with crystalloids.

Abnormalities in coagulation

All artificial colloid solutions can have an effect on coagulation. The effects on coagulation appear to be directly related to the intravascular concentration of artificial colloid. Higher plasma concentrations of colloid, resulting from administration of larger or repeated doses or reduced intravascular degradation, have the greatest effect. The exact mechanism of the effect on coagulation is unknown, although a reduction in the concentration of factor VIII and von Willebrand factor (vWF) has been recognized following administration of artificial colloid solutions. There appears to be significant individual variation in the clinical relevance of changes in coagulation status, but in some animals administration of artificial colloids can lead to potentially life-threatening bleeding.

Acute renal failure

Colloids should be used with caution in patients with oliguric or anuric renal failure because the kidneys are the major route of excretion of all artificial colloids.

Anaphylactic reactions

Anaphylactic reactions have been reported following administration of most types of artificial colloid, but the incidence of serious complications is extremely low. Anaphylaxis may manifest as urticaria, pruritus, vomiting, diarrhoea, acute circulatory collapse or seizures. Administration of the colloid solution should be stopped immediately and supportive treatment instigated.

Characteristics of different colloid solutions

Colloid solutions are now described in terms of the *number molecular weight* (M_n), which is the total molecular weight of all molecules divided by the number of molecules. Use of M_n allows recognition of the smaller molecular weight particles in the solution. The oncotic pressure exerted by the solution depends on the total number of molecules, whereas the duration of effect is determined by the size of the particles.

Hetastarch

Hetastarch (hydroxyethyl starch, HES) is a synthetic polymer of glucose with an M_n of 69,000. It contains larger particles than any other artificial colloid solution currently available. Hetastarch can increase plasma volume by 71–172% of the administered volume, and generally increases plasma volume by at least the volume given. The duration of effect is relatively long, with an effect on plasma volume expansion generally persisting 24 hours after administration.

Pentastarch

Pentastarch is a synthetic polymer of glucose with a lower molecular weight than hetastarch and an M_n of 63,000. This colloid is more rapidly metabolized than hetastarch and has a shorter half-life (2.5 hours). Approximately 70% of pentastarch is excreted after 24 hours, compared with 38% of a hetastarch solution. Pentastarch is considered to have limited effects on coagulation.

Gelatin solutions

These solutions are prepared by degradation of bovine collagen. The two solutions currently used in the UK are succinylated gelatin (Gelofusine) and urea-linked gelatin (Haemaccel). These solutions have lower molecular weights than the other artificial colloid solutions and have a relatively short duration of effect. The average M_n of gelatin solutions is 24,500. The magnitude of plasma expansion is unlikely to be greater than the infused volume, so the risk of volume overload is low compared with other artificial colloid solutions. Although some effects on coagulation have been reported, serious adverse effects on coagulation are rare.

Dextrans

The dextran molecule is a linear polysaccharide that is produced by bacteria growing on a sucrose-containing medium. Dextrans are available in high molecular weight (Dextran 70) and low molecular weight (Dextran 40) forms (the M_n values are 41,000 and 26,000, respectively). Dextrans are not commonly used in the UK because of concerns about clinically significant effects on coagulation and the risk of anaphylactic reactions.

Dosage

It is recommended that the dosage of artificial colloid solutions should not exceed 20 ml/kg/day. Recommendations for the volume to be administered as a single bolus for blood pressure support during anaesthesia vary depending on the status of the patient and the cause of hypotension. Administration of a 5 ml/kg bolus followed by re-evaluation of the patient is a good starting point for a resuscitation protocol involving a colloid solution. This dose can be repeated if necessary.

Blood therapy

The aim of fluid therapy is both to replace losses and to maintain the fluid and electrolyte balance of the body. Fluid is generally replaced on a 'like for like' basis: whichever type of fluid is lost from the body is replaced with fluid of the same sort. If water and electrolytes are lost, then they should be replaced with water and electrolytes. If blood is lost, then the patient should ideally receive blood to replenish that loss.

During blood loss, the blood circulating volume, oxygen-carrying capacity and perfusion are decreased. In an ideal situation, blood is given to the animal to replace these losses. In order for this to be possible, blood has to be taken from a donor animal.

Blood donors

There are numerous clinical situations in general veterinary practice when administration of blood is necessary. According to RCVS guidelines (January 2008), taking blood from a donor, with the owner's permission, with the intention of administering it to a recipient is an acceptable and recognized procedure. This should be carried out within a veterinary establishment or between local practices. If this is done on a larger commercial scale for the purpose of storage, then a licence is required under the Animals (Scientific Procedures) Act 1986.

Veterinary practice staff commonly identify potential donor animals in order to keep a practice register of available donor candidates. This also means that the practicalities can be discussed with the owners in advance. A record of the donors is kept in the practice in order to enable a donor to be contacted speedily when necessary. Some veterinary practices offer a goodwill arrangement in that the donor receives annual vaccinations at cost price in recognition of being on the donor register.

Blood donors

Animals that are blood donors should:

- **Be in good general health**
- **Be of a reliably good temperament and feel at ease in the veterinary environment**
- **Be free from infectious disease**
- **Be blood typed (particularly cats)**
- **Be regularly tested for feline infectious anaemia (FIA) and feline immunodeficiency virus (FIV) (cats)**
- **Be vaccinated against common infectious diseases (and cats should have been tested for feline leukaemia virus (FeLV) infection before primary vaccination)**
- **Have a minimum weight of 25 kg (dogs) or 4.5 kg (cats)**
- **Be between 1 and 8 years of age**
- **Not have received a blood transfusion previously**
- **Not currently be receiving any medication**
- **Have tested negative for blood-borne diseases found abroad or have not travelled outside the UK.**

Owners of blood donors need to:

- **Be available within a 10–15-minute drive from the practice to allow for speedy donation of blood in emergency situations**
- **Agree to try to bring their animal to the practice at short notice whenever possible**
- **Notify the practice if they are on holiday**
- **Contact the practice should their animal become unwell or be receiving medication so that it can be temporarily removed from the register**
- **Continue with regular vaccination of their animal.**

It is advisable to perform a routine haematology and biochemistry blood analysis on all potential donors prior to being admitted on to the practice donor register, and then repeat this annually. In addition, donor animals must be blood typed and this information kept on record for future donations. Thirteen blood groups have been described in the dog; these comprise the dog erythrocyte antigen (DEA) system. A reaction in the recipient to any type of donor blood is possible; however, the severity is increased with donors who are DEA1.1 and DEA1.2. Ideally all donors should be DEA 1.1 and DEA 1.2 negative.

Three blood groups are classified in cats: A, B and AB. It is reported that a recipient of blood type B that receives type A blood is likely to suffer a severe reaction. It is essential that cats receive donor blood of the same type as their own. All cats should have a blood type test carried out before donating blood. Commercially available test kits can be used for in-house blood typing of all donors. In addition to blood typing, a cross-match test can be performed. This determines the compatibility of the donor's and the recipient's blood. The test measures agglutination: no clotting occurs if the blood is a true match. Cross-matching is undertaken if:

- The recipient has received another recent transfusion (within the last 72 hours)
- A transfusion reaction has occurred previously
- It is not known whether the recipient has received a prior blood transfusion and therefore any associated problems are unknown.

Blood collection

Dogs

The donor must undergo a full clinical examination to ensure excellent physical health immediately prior to giving blood. The blood can be collected into a human blood collection set via the jugular vein. The set consists of a blood collection bag containing an anticoagulant, citrate phosphate dextrose (CPD). Leading from the collection bag is a length of tubing with a 14-gauge needle attached to the end. The donor is restrained either in lateral recumbency, in a sitting position or in sternal recumbency. It is important that the donor adopts a comfortable position because it will need to remain fairly still for a short while to allow blood collection.

The venepuncture site (jugular vein) is clipped and prepared aseptically and sterile gloves are worn. A local anaesthetic gel can also be applied; sufficient time should be allowed for this to take effect before venepuncture. The sterile needle is introduced into the jugular vein and blood flows from the needle, into the tubing and directly into the blood collection bag. The collection bag is gently inverted to mix the anticoagulant with the blood. The maximum amount of blood to be taken from a dog is 16–18 ml/kg. The human blood collection bag holds 430–520 g of blood.

Once the required amount of blood has been collected, the tubing is clamped and the needle removed from the jugular vein. Direct digital pressure must be applied to the venepuncture site for several minutes to prevent bleeding and formation of a haematoma. The donor is then given a small meal and hard exercise is withheld for 24 hours after donation. Because donors must be of a good temperament and feel at ease in the veterinary environment it is not usual practice to sedate dogs for donation of blood. The owners must check the venepuncture site for haematomas or excessive bruising during the 48 hours after donation; any concerns should be brought to the attention of the veterinary surgeon.

Cats

As a much smaller amount of blood is collected from a cat, and the large gauge attached needle in a human collection set is unsuitable, a different collection method is used for feline donors. Only 11–13 ml/kg of blood is taken from a cat at one time.

Blood is collected from the jugular vein using a standard sterile 21-gauge needle or butterfly needle with a short extension set and a 10 ml syringe. One millilitre of anticoagulant (CPD can be withdrawn from a human blood collection set) is added to the syringe for every 9 ml of blood to be collected. Small blood collection bags that contain no anticoagulant are commercially available. A three-way tap should be placed between the extension set or butterfly needle and the syringe to minimize the number of times the jugular vein is punctured and for the blood to be collected in a sterile manner. The disadvantage of this collection technique is that it is not a completely closed system and the risk of contamination is greater.

The cat is restrained either sitting, in lateral recumbency or upside down in the handler's lap. A strict aseptic technique is employed for venepuncture. The collection syringe is gently rotated in order to mix the blood and anticoagulant together. Sedation is sometimes used for feline donors to minimize stress levels. Some veterinary surgeons avoid the use of sedatives in non-essential cases while others use a combination of ketamine and midazolam, which has a minimal effect on the animal's cardiovascular and respiratory systems.

Direct digital pressure is applied to the venepuncture site immediately after blood collection and the cat is fed a small meal afterwards. Intravenous crystalloid fluids are often given to the donor after donation to replace the lost volume of blood. It is recommended that cats be kept indoors for 24 hours after blood donation; this allows the owner to maintain close observation. The owners must check the venepuncture site for haematomas or excessive bruising during the 48 hours after donation; any concerns should be brought to the attention of the veterinary surgeon.

Administration of collected blood

If blood has been collected into a blood collection bag it can be administered to the recipient through a blood giving set; this has a filter in place to remove any blood clots prior to administration to the recipient. Blood that has been collected into a syringe can be transferred into a low volume collection bag (without anticoagulant) and administered in the same way. Alternatively, a new needle is used to administer blood to the recipient.

The jugular or cephalic vein of the recipient is used; the area is clipped and prepared aseptically. Blood is warmed to 37°C prior to administration. Warming can be carried out by placing the collected blood in a heated jacket or in warmed water. Overheating of the blood results in agglutination and protein breakdown. Blood is administered at an initial rate of 0.25 ml/kg/h for the first 15 minutes. The patient is monitored closely during this time for any possible transfusion reactions. If no problems occur the transfusion rate is then increased to 20 ml/kg/h. The total volume of blood required is administered over 2–4 hours.

Monitoring the patient during blood transfusion

Incompatibility reactions are most likely to occur in the first hour following transfusion and the patient must be monitored closely. There are numerous signs that indicate a transfusion reaction, which vary from very mild to a serious life-threatening situation. If the patient is showing any abnormal clinical signs the veterinary surgeon should be informed immediately and the transfusion stopped. The usual treatment for a blood transfusion reaction is administration of crystalloid fluids, antihistamines, antibiotics and corticosteroids. Some transfusion reactions do not occur immediately; they can manifest themselves at any time up to 2 weeks after the transfusion.

Blood transfusion reactions

Immediate clinical signs associated with blood transfusion reactions include:

- Urticaria
- Hypersalivation
- Muscle tremors
- Tachycardia
- Vomiting/nausea
- Restlessness
- Jaundice
- Dyspnoea
- Haemoglobinuria
- Pyrexia
- Facial oedema
- Tachypnoea
- Convulsions.

Delayed clinical signs associated with blood transfusion reactions include:

- Jaundice
- Haemoglobinuria
- Any immune response.

Use of whole blood and blood products

At the time of writing (March 2008) there is one commercial 'blood bank' in the UK, selling both canine blood and blood products. This organization has a licence to take and store blood and circulate it on a commercial basis. Its aim is to extend this service to include feline blood in the future.

Whole blood

Blood is taken from the donor and administered to the recipient (see above). Whole blood is used in cases of acute haemorrhage and in bleeding and clotting disorders. Whole blood contains cells, clotting factors and platelets. Whole blood has a relatively short shelf-life (20–25 days) and the quality of the blood decreases over this time period as cells become damaged and clotting factors are inactivated. In particular, clotting factors and platelets become inactive within hours to a few days, and therefore whole blood cannot be considered a suitable source of these unless administered within the first few hours following collection.

Fresh frozen plasma

Plasma is useful in cases of severe burns or severe hypoproteinaemia (e.g. protein-losing enteropathy or nephropathy). Whole blood is centrifuged to separate the plasma, which is then frozen at –30°C. The freezing process preserves the clotting factors in plasma. This process is usually done commercially and the plasma is purchased from a commercial organization. The plasma arrives at the veterinary practice frozen and is defrosted immediately prior to use. Plasma is administered directly through a blood giving set. Cryosupernatant has similar characteristics to fresh frozen plasma but does not contain clotting factors.

Isolated clotting factors

These are rarely used because they are very expensive. Artificially produced clotting factors can be used as an alternative and are available commercially. Cryoprecipitate contains a range of clotting factors (rather than individual clotting agents) and can be used to manage patients with inherited disorders of clotting or bleeding (e.g. von Willebrand's disease and haemophilia A).

Packed red blood cells

These are used in cases of severe anaemia and acute haemorrhage. The packed red blood cells are separated from whole blood by centrifugation; this is done commercially. Packed red blood cells need to be stored at between 1°C and 6°C. When packed red blood cells are given to the patient, normal saline is often also administered intravenously by 'piggy backing' the saline into the giving set used to administer the red blood cells. The purpose of this is to reduce the viscosity of the red blood cells and also to ensure that all the red blood cells are administered and none remain in the giving set.

Alternatives to blood

A synthetic alternative to blood is a product called Oxyglobin™. This is a plasma volume expander that contains cross-linked bovine haemoglobin and circulates freely in the plasma. It improves oxygen delivery by increasing the oxygen content of the blood and expanding intravascular volume. It is only authorized for use in dogs and for the management of severe anaemia.

The main advantages in using Oxyglobin™ rather than whole blood are that:

- No blood typing or cross-matching is necessary because a transfusion reaction is unlikely
- The product is known to be free from infectious diseases
- There is no need for a donor animal to be used, thus saving time
- Oxyglobin™ has a long shelf-life, allowing it to be constantly available.

The cost of Oxyglobin™, together with the recent introduction of a canine blood bank in the UK, currently discourages regular use of the product as the purchase of blood products is generally preferred. The use of Oxyglobin™ also has a number of side-effects:

■ Administration can interfere with biochemical blood and urine tests that rely on colorimetry because of discoloration of the patient's urine and plasma. There is a transient red–brown discoloration of the patient's urine, a yellow–red discoloration of the skin, mucous membranes and sclera, and yellow/orange/red spots on the skin. These side-effects usually last for 3–5 days

■ Oxyglobin™ has a higher viscosity and colloid osmotic pressure than blood; therefore, volume overload can occur when a large volume is administered rapidly or when the product is administered in conjunction with other crystalloid or colloid fluids. It must also be used cautiously in patients that are prone to circulatory overload (e.g. dogs with congestive heart failure).

Oxyglobin™ is warmed to 37°C prior to use and is administered via a standard giving set and intravenous catheter. Oxyglobin™ must not be administered in conjunction with any other fluids. The recommended dose of Oxyglobin™ is 30 ml/kg i.v. at a rate of up to 10 ml/kg/h.

Central venous catheters

Central venous catheters are routinely placed into the jugular or saphenous veins and end in the cranial or caudal vena cava. As an alternative, the medial saphenous or femoral veins can be catheterized.

Central venous catheters

Central venous catheters are used for:

■ **Administration of large volumes of fluids**
■ **Administration of large volumes of drugs**
■ **Administration of chemotherapy and other irritant drugs**
■ **Repeated collection of blood samples**
■ **Continuous administration of drugs**
■ **Measurement of central venous pressure**
■ **Administration of parenteral nutrition**
■ **Administration of drugs during cardiac arrest**
■ **Intravenous access when a peripheral vein is not accessible.**

Central catheters have a larger lumen than those used in peripheral veins; this allows a large volume of fluid to be administered over a shorter period of time. Multi-lumen central catheters allow administration of drugs with simultaneous measurement of central venous pressure, or administration of different drugs through separate lumens. However, it has been reported that multi-lumen catheters are associated with a higher incidence of infection because of increased opportunities for bacteria to enter the catheter.

Central catheters should not be placed in patients with coagulation problems because it is difficult to apply sufficient pressure to the site of insertion should bleeding occur, which may lead to a jugular haematoma. Patients with suspected raised intracranial pressure are not ideal candidates for central catheters because the catheter can obstruct drainage from the head region and lead to a further increase in intracranial pressure.

There is a variety of techniques for placing central venous catheters. The most common is the Seldinger technique, which uses an over-the-guidewire catheter (Figure 6.1). An introducer needle is introduced into the vein, a soft-tipped guidewire is passed through the needle and the needle is then removed. A dilator is passed over the guidewire, the dilator is removed, the catheter is passed over the wire and the wire is then removed, leaving the catheter in place. The advantage of this particular method is that a soft, long and very flexible catheter can be used.

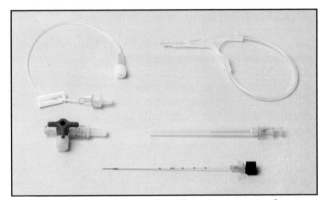

6.1 Equipment required for placement of a jugular catheter using the Seldinger technique. The kit comprises a needle through which the guidewire is introduced, a dilator and the catheter. A three-way tap and extension set to attach to the catheter hub are also shown.

The 'Peel Away' catheter is an alternative method of central catheter placement that is simpler than the Seldinger technique. At present it is only suitable for medium- to large-sized dogs, owing to the range of catheter sizes available (Figure 6.2).

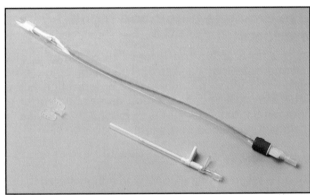

6.2 'Peel Away' catheter suitable for placement in the jugular vein of medium- to large-sized dogs (bodyweight >15 kg).

Central venous catheters are typically made from polyvinylchloride (PVC) or Teflon™ material. The soft material causes less tissue response and reduces trauma during catheter placement. The smooth exterior is less likely to allow accumulation of bacteria and therefore infection. Figure 6.3 shows a central

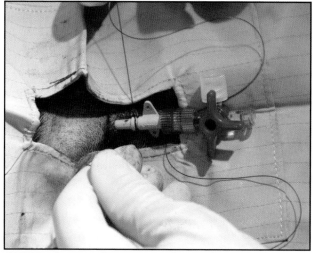

6.3 A central venous catheter placed in the jugular vein of a dog is secured to the skin using a suture. Note that the area has been covered with a sterile drape to maintain asepsis during catheter placement and that the person placing the catheter is wearing sterile gloves. A three-way tap has been attached to the end of the catheter to control fluid administration through the catheter and prevent air embolism.

venous catheter in position. A central catheter can be left in place for 7 days; removing the catheter before this time period is not associated with a lower incidence of infection.

Problems associated with central venous catheter placement include:

- Excessive bleeding from the catheter insertion site
- Infection at the catheter site
- Leakage of fluids or drugs from around the catheter or the catheter hub
- Septic thrombophlebitis
- Pneumothorax
- Air embolism if the catheter is not capped while in the vein due to air being sucked into the vascular system through the open-ended catheter.

The catheter can become infected in several ways:

- At the time of insertion from bacteria on the patient's skin
- Contaminated drugs or fluids entering the catheter
- Contamination of the catheter port.

If a catheter is removed because obvious infection is present, a bacterial swab taken from around the catheter insertion site should be sent for culture to determine the appropriate antibiotic regime for the patient. In addition, the tip of the catheter should be collected aseptically and submitted for bacteriological culture.

The following can be employed to minimize the likelihood of catheter contamination:

- Aseptic preparation of site and patient (sterile gloves, drape patient)
- Skin preparation with chlorhexidine scrub

- Dressing of the catheter once in place. A standard bandage may be preferable to an occlusive dressing to prevent bacterial accumulation and 'trapping' of bacteria and fluid under the adhesive dressing
- Preventing patient interference; this prevents bacteria entering the catheter and prevents the catheter moving in the vein, which may lead to thrombus formation
- Wearing gloves when administering drugs and fluids via the catheter
- Securing the catheter in place by using zinc oxide tape and a light dressing.

Nursing considerations

- **Check the catheter frequently (at least three times daily) for signs of infection, perivascular administration of fluid, leakage of fluid from the catheter and giving set junction or 'blowing' of the vein.**
- **Flush twice daily with sterile heparinized saline. Use an extension set to minimize handling of the catheter connection.**
- **Change dressing daily.**
- **Ensure aseptic handling of catheter at all times.**

Measurement of central venous pressure

The measurement of central venous pressure (CVP) can be used to estimate and monitor circulatory volume. CVP is the pressure in the right atrium of the heart, therefore its measurement requires placement of a catheter in the jugular vein. Placement of jugular catheters is a technique that many veterinary surgeons are unfamiliar with and consequently CVP is not often measured in general veterinary practice. However, once mastered, measurement of CVP is relatively straightforward and it can provide useful information to assist in the management of fluid therapy, particularly in critically ill patients.

The equipment required to monitor central venous pressure is:

- A jugular catheter
- Crystalloid fluids
- A standard fluid giving set
- A three-way tap
- An extension set
- A manometer (usually consists of a ruler with a length of extension tubing attached to it along a centimetre scale).

The animal is placed in lateral recumbency to expose the jugular vein. It can be useful to place a small sandbag under the neck to facilitate exposure of the jugular vein and catheter placement. Either a long over-the-needle intravenous catheter or a through-the-needle catheter (for example, one that requires the Seldinger technique) is placed in the jugular vein in order to measure CVP.

The catheter must be placed using strict aseptic technique in order to avoid contamination and infection. The skin of the animal is prepared as if for aseptic surgery: the hair is clipped using a size 40 blade and the skin is cleaned with diluted surgical scrub. The veterinary surgeon scrubs up and wears sterile gloves for placement of the catheter. The long catheter is advanced into the right jugular vein, ideally until the tip of the catheter lies in the vena cava within the thoracic cavity. The length of catheter that needs to be inserted should be measured before the start of placement. If the catheter is too long and the tip lies in one of the chambers of the heart it may cause cardiac complications such as arrhythmias. The catheter should then be carefully secured in place and connected to the CVP monitoring system.

- The giving set is attached to the bag of crystalloid fluid and a three-way tap is attached to the Luer end of the giving set.
- The extension set and the manometer are also connected to the three-way tap.
- Fluid from the bag of crystalloid fluid is run through the giving set and the extension set to ensure that no air is in the tubing. Any air will result in an air embolism if the system is connected to the animal.
- Fluid is then run through the manometer tubing until the fluid level is above 14–15 cmH$_2$O on the centimetre scale.
- The equipment is now ready to be connected to the catheter and the extension set is connected to the jugular catheter in the usual way.
- To measure CVP the three-way tap is turned off towards the crystalloid fluids. The catheter is then in direct communication with the fluid column in the manometer. The level of fluid in the column will slowly fall until the pressure in the fluid column (in cmH$_2$O) is the same as the CVP. The height of the fluid column can be measured against the centimetre scale on the manometer. By convention CVP should be measured with the zero of the manometer scale level with the base of the heart. Once settled there will be small oscillations in the fluid column as CVP changes slightly during inspiration and expiration. CVP is measured and recorded on the patient's records (Figures 6.4 and 6.5).
- Between CVP measurements the jugular catheter can be used to administer fluids. The crystalloid fluids in the CVP arrangement can easily be administered to the animal by altering the flow of fluid via the three-way tap. To administer fluid to the animal the three-way tap is turned off towards the manometer.
- The normal range of CVP is 3–7 cmH$_2$O. Repeated measurements of CVP can give an accurate picture of the circulatory volume status of the animal. A high CVP can indicate over-administration of fluid, occlusion of the catheter or right ventricular heart failure. A low CVP may indicate reduced blood volume. Changes in CVP are more important than absolute values; these changes give an indication of the status of the animal.

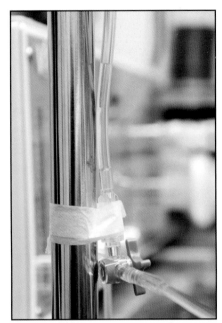

6.4 To measure central venous pressure (CVP) using the manometer technique a three-way tap is attached to the jugular catheter. One connection port on the three-way tap is attached to an open-ended fluid-filled length of drip tubing held vertically. The other connection port is attached to a bag of crystalloid fluid. The height of the column of fluid supported in the open-ended tubing is equivalent to the CVP of the patient.

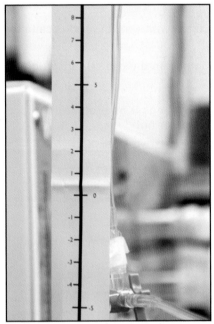

6.5 A centimetre ruler scale can be attached to the open-ended drip tubing to facilitate measurement of central venous pressure (CVP). The three-way tap should be at the level of the patient's heart. The CVP in this patient is 8.5 cmH$_2$O (measured above the three-way tap, which has been placed at the height of the heart base).

Jugular catheters must be carefully monitored and checked daily for signs of infection, swelling or pain around the site of catheter insertion. There is potential for life-threatening haemorrhage or air embolism if the system should become disconnected.

Potassium-related disorders

Potassium is the major intracellular cation. Maintenance of normal intracellular and extracellular concentrations of potassium is essential for:

- Maintenance of a normal resting cell membrane potential
- Generation of action potentials and maintenance of electrical activity of the heart
- Maintenance of normal cell volume
- Normal cell growth.

Normal potassium concentrations are tightly regulated by ensuring that potassium loss (mainly in the urine) is matched to potassium gain (absorption from the diet in the gastrointestinal tract).

Hypokalaemia

Figure 6.6 details the primary causes of hypokalaemia and gives examples of conditions that can result in hypokalaemia by the different mechanisms.

Mechanism 1:
decreased intake of potassium

Administration of potassium-free fluids or fluids such as lactated Ringer's solution during fluid therapy
Decreased intake through aberrant diet (unlikely)

Mechanism 2:
translocation of potassium from the extracellular fluid to the intracellular fluid

Administration of insulin and glucose-containing fluids, promoting uptake of potassium by cells
Alkalaemia

Mechanism 3:
increased loss of potassium

Urinary loss:
- Chronic renal failure (cats)
- Chronic administration of loop and thiazide diuretics
- Cushing's disease
Gastrointestinal loss:
- Vomiting of stomach contents
- Diarrhoea

6.6 Primary causes of hypokalaemia.

Clinical signs of hypokalaemia

- Muscular weakness.
- In cats, weakness of the neck muscles and ventroflexion of the head are commonly seen.
- Polyuria and polydipsia.
- Anorexia.
- Impaired urinary concentrating ability.
- Electrocardiographic changes and cardiac arrhythmias may develop due to delayed ventricular repolarization.
- Many animals will show no overt clinical signs of hypokalaemia.

Management of hypokalaemia

Hypokalaemia is managed by potassium supplementation. Potassium chloride (KCl) is the additive of choice for parenteral administration. The calculated dose of KCl can be added to a bag of the fluid being administered to the patient. It can be difficult to estimate the dose of potassium required to correct hypokalaemia from the serum potassium concentration because potassium is primarily an intracellular cation. Regular monitoring of serum potassium concentration is essential.

- Potassium should not be administered intravenously at rates >0.5 mmol K^+/kg/h to avoid potential adverse cardiac effects. Use of infusion pumps or syringe drivers will improve the accuracy of the rate of fluid administration and reduce the risk of overdose.
- The solution should be mixed carefully when KCl has been added to a fluid bag to prevent inadvertent overdose.
- It should be ensured that the concentration of potassium in the solution for infusion does not exceed 60 mmol/l. High concentrations of potassium may cause pain during infusion through peripheral veins.
- Careful potassium supplementation is essential when using insulin to treat diabetic ketoacidosis because of the effect of insulin on the uptake of glucose and potassium by cells.

The guidelines indicated in Figure 6.7 can be used to calculate the amount of potassium that should be added to 0.9% NaCl for intravenous fluid therapy to correct hypokalaemia. The stock KCl solution (typically 15% KCl solution) must be diluted with at least 25 times its own volume before intravenous administration, therefore concentrated solutions must be diluted prior to use. Intravenous doses must be titrated for each patient and the rate of infusion must not exceed 0.5 mmol K^+/kg/h.

Serum potassium concentration	Amount of K^+ to add to 250 ml 0.9% NaCl
<2 mmol/l	20 mmol
2.0–2.5 mmol/l	15 mmol
2.5–3.0 mmol/l	10 mmol
3.0–3.5 mmol/l	7 mmol

6.7 Guidelines for potassium supplementation.

Potassium gluconate (e.g. Tumil-K) is recommended for oral supplementation in patients who require chronic potassium supplementation (e.g. cats with chronic renal failure) and is safer than intravenous administration owing to the lower risk of overdose.

Dosage guidelines for oral potassium supplementation

- Cats: 2–6 mmol/cat/day orally.
- Dogs: 0.2–0.5 mmol/kg orally q8h.

Hyperkalaemia

Hyperkalaemia is life-threatening and must be managed appropriately and quickly. It is uncommon in animals with normal renal function because excess potassium is excreted through the kidneys. The most common causes of hyperkalaemia in cats and dogs are:

- Decreased urinary excretion due to urethral obstruction, ruptured bladder or oliguric renal failure
- Addison's disease (hypoadrenocorticism)
- Massive tissue breakdown
- Diabetic ketoacidotic crisis (hypokalaemia may alternatively be seen in this condition)
- Translocation of potassium from the intracellular fluid to the extracellular fluid caused by mineral acids such as ammonium chloride (NH_4Cl) or hydrochloric acid (HCl).

Clinical signs of hyperkalaemia

Clinical signs associated with hyperkalaemia arise because of changes in cell membrane excitability. Changes in the electrocardiogram are characteristic and can be used to confirm hyperkalaemia if laboratory testing of the serum potassium concentration is not immediately available. Muscle weakness can also occur when potassium concentrations are >8 mmol/l.

Electrocardiographic changes (Figure 6.8) include:

- Impaired conduction through the atria, leading to a decrease in the amplitude and widening of the P wave
- Narrowing and tenting of the T waves, reflecting abnormal repolarization
- Widening of the QRS complex because of slowing of conduction through the atrioventricular system.

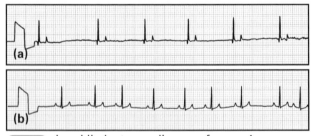

6.8 Lead II electrocardiogram from a 4-year-old Bearded Collie with hyperkalaemia associated with Addison's disease taken **(a)** before and **(b)** after treatment (1 mV/cm and 25 mm/sec). In (a) the P waves are absent, the T waves are peaked and there is profound bradycardia. (Reproduced from the *BSAVA Manual of Small Animal Endocrinology, 2nd edition*)

In severe hyperkalaemia:

- Atrial conduction ceases and the P wave disappears
- Pronounced bradycardia develops
- The QRS complex may merge with the T wave
- Ventricular fibrillation may develop because of slow intraventricular conduction and decreased duration of the refractory period.

Treatment of hyperkalaemia

- Management of the underlying cause.
- Encouragement of renal excretion of potassium. Fluid therapy with lactated Ringer's solution improves renal perfusion and can increase renal excretion of potassium. This assumes that urine can be excreted normally or with assistance, e.g. by cystocentesis or by peritoneal drainage in the case of a ruptured bladder.
- Encouragement of movement of potassium from the extracellular fluid to the intracellular fluid:
  - Administration of glucose increases endogenous insulin secretion and causes movement of potassium into cells. The combination of glucose with insulin may result in a greater reduction in serum potassium concentration
  - Administration of sodium bicarbonate also encourages potassium to move into cells, as hydrogen ions leave the cells to titrate the administered bicarbonate in the extracellular fluid.

Adjunctive therapy

Calcium gluconate can be administered to antagonize the effects of hyperkalaemia on cell membranes. Hyperkalaemia decreases the resting membrane potential of cells. Administration of calcium gluconate increases the extracellular fluid calcium concentration and reduces the threshold resting membrane potential of cells. This normalizes the difference between the resting and the threshold cell membrane potential that is otherwise increased by hyperkalaemia, and reduces the likelihood of hyperkalaemia resulting in serious cardiac arrhythmias. This is only used in life-threatening situations.

Acid–base disorders

A basic understanding of the physiological processes involved in maintenance of acid–base balance and normal body pH is required in order to interpret and manage acid–base disorders in clinical patients. The Henderson–Hasselbalch equation describes the relationship between the pH of the extracellular fluid and the components of the bicarbonate buffer system, which is the largest buffer system in the extracellular fluid.

Henderson–Hasselbalch equation

$$pH = pK + \log \frac{HCO_3^-}{0.03(P_aCO_2)}$$

where:

pH = the negative logarithm of the hydrogen ion (H^+) concentration

pK = 6.1, the negative logarithm of the dissociation constant for carbonic acid (H_2CO_3)

HCO_3^- = the concentration of bicarbonate (mmol/l)

P_aCO_2 = the partial pressure of carbon dioxide (CO_2) in arterial blood (mmHg)

0.03 = the solubility coefficient for PCO_2 in plasma (mmol/l/mmHg)

From this equation it is evident that any change in the ratio of the concentrations of HCO_3^- and P_aCO_2 will result in a change in the pH of the extracellular fluid and body tissues, resulting in an acid–base disturbance. If the change in ratio occurs because of a change in the concentration of HCO_3^-, it is termed a metabolic event. A metabolic acidosis occurs when the concentration of HCO_3^- falls relative to P_aCO_2; a metabolic alkalosis occurs when the concentration of HCO_3^- increases relative to P_aCO_2. Respiratory acidosis and alkalosis occur due to changes in P_aCO_2 relative to the concentration of HCO_3^-, because carbon dioxide tension is determined by respiratory function.

Acid–base disorders include:

- Acidaemia: present when blood pH <7.35
- Acidosis: a primary physiological process that, occurring alone, tends to cause acidaemia
- Alkalaemia: present when blood pH >7.45
- Alkalosis: a primary physiological process that, occurring alone, tends to cause alkalaemia
- Primary acid–base disorder: one of the four acid–base disturbances manifested by an initial change in either HCO_3^- or P_aCO_2
- Compensation: the body tries to compensate for any change in pH in order to maintain homeostasis. Therefore, primary changes in HCO_3^- or P_aCO_2 are accompanied by compensatory changes in the concentrations of these compounds in order to try and restore the correct concentration ratio. However, the compensation is often not sufficient to return the pH to normal values.

Common causes of acid–base disorders

Respiratory acidosis

The respiratory system is tightly regulated in order to maintain the arterial carbon dioxide tension between 35 mmHg and 45 mmHg. Respiratory system dysfunction can lead to increased carbon dioxide tension and a respiratory acidosis. Respiratory causes of acid–base imbalance occur most commonly in animals during anaesthesia:

- Central nervous system depression leads to inadequate ventilation, e.g. depression caused by anaesthetic agents
- Re-breathing during anaesthesia, e.g. caused by use of an inappropriate breathing circuit for the patient or exhausted soda lime in a re-breathing circuit
- Respiratory disease leading to inadequate ventilation, e.g. flail chest, severe pneumonia, severe pulmonary oedema.

Respiratory alkalosis

Causes of respiratory alkalosis include:

- Voluntary hyperventilation
- Hypoxaemia leading to increased ventilation due to a hypoxic drive
- Iatrogenic, due to excessive intermittent positive pressure ventilation during anaesthesia.

Metabolic acidosis

The traditional approach to acid–base imbalance divides metabolic acidosis into increased and normal anion gap types of acidosis. Increased anion gap acidosis occurs when excess acid that has an unmeasured anion is added to the blood (e.g. during ketoacidosis). Normal anion gap acidosis occurs when chloride, which is routinely measured, is added to the blood (e.g. during administration of NH_4Cl) or when there is loss of bicarbonate from the blood that is replaced by the chloride ion (e.g. during severe diarrhoea).

Increased anion gap acidosis

This can be caused by:

- Diabetic ketoacidosis
- Chronic renal failure (retention of sulphates, phosphates and organic anions)
- Lactic acidosis
- Ethylene glycol poisoning.

Normal anion gap acidosis

This can be caused by:

- Diarrhoea
- Excess NH_4Cl administration.

Metabolic alkalosis

Probably the most common cause of metabolic alkalosis seen in veterinary practice is loss of HCl from stomach acid owing to acute vomiting. Other causes are:

- Exogenous administration of HCO_3^-
- Excess renal reabsorption of HCO_3^- caused by administration of diuretics.

Clinical approach to acid–base disorders

- The existence of an acid–base disorder can be determined from analysis of an arterial blood gas sample or serum electrolyte measurements.
- The presence of an abnormal pH and/or P_aCO_2 indicates the presence of at least one primary acid–base disorder (Figure 6.9).

Acid–base disturbance	Primary event
Metabolic acidosis	$\downarrow pH = \dfrac{\downarrow HCO_3^-}{P_aCO_2}$
Metabolic alkalosis	$\uparrow pH = \dfrac{\uparrow HCO_3^-}{P_aCO_2}$
Respiratory acidosis	$\downarrow pH = \dfrac{HCO_3^-}{\uparrow P_aCO_2}$
Respiratory alkalosis	$\uparrow pH = \dfrac{HCO_3^-}{\downarrow P_aCO_2}$

6.9 Changes in bicarbonate (HCO_3^-) concentration and the partial pressure of carbon dioxide in arterial blood (P_aCO_2) leading to changes in blood pH.

- Coexisting clinical conditions resulting in more than one acid–base imbalance may lead to opposing acid disorders. This is a complex field but such conditions may result in a high pH when there is an obvious acidosis or a low pH when there is an obvious alkalosis.
- The initial approach to an acid–base disorder should be to treat the underlying clinical disorder leading to the acid–base imbalance. In many cases, treatment of the underlying condition alone is sufficient to correct the acid–base imbalance. The acidaemia or alkalaemia should only be treated to correct the abnormal pH if the abnormality in pH is very severe.

Use of serum electrolytes in the interpretation of acid–base disorders

An electrolyte abnormality is often the first sign of an acid–base disorder, therefore, it is always useful to measure the electrolytes used to calculate the anion gap in any patient with a suspected acid–base abnormality. This does not require specialist laboratory equipment and should be possible in most veterinary practices.

Anion gap measurement

The anion gap is the sum of routinely measured cations minus the routinely measured anions:

Anion gap = $(Na^+ + K^+) - (Cl^- + HCO_3^-)$

where HCO_3^- is measured as serum CO_2.

However, because the serum concentration of K^+ is a numerically small value it is usually omitted from the equation; therefore, the anion gap is usually calculated as:

**Anion gap =
$Na^+ - (Cl^- + HCO_3^-)$ or $Na^+ - (Cl^- + serum\ CO_2)$**

The normal anion gap measured using this equation is 12 ± 4 mEq/l. An anion gap always exists because there are other anions in the plasma that are not included in this equation (such as proteins and organic acids), which leads to an 'artificial' imbalance in electrochemical neutrality.

Interpretation of the anion gap

- *Normal anion gap*: there is no laboratory evidence to support an anion gap acidosis.
- *Low or negative anion gap*: this may occur due to:
  - Excess unmeasured cations
  - Reduction in unmeasured anions (e.g. hypoproteinaemia).
- *Elevated anion gap*: the patient may have an anion gap metabolic acidosis.

Treatment of metabolic acidosis by administration of sodium bicarbonate

Administration of sodium bicarbonate to correct a metabolic acidosis should be reserved for cases when blood pH is between 7.1 and 7.2. Sodium bicarbonate should only be administered in an amount sufficient to increase the pH to 7.2, in order to avoid inadvertent overdose and iatrogenic alkalaemia. Severe acidosis (pH <7.2) can result in impaired cardiac contractility, impaired pressor response to catecholamines and ventricular arrhythmias, so treatment with bicarbonate is justified. Sodium bicarbonate must be given cautiously and blood pH measured repeatedly during treatment in order to prevent overdose.

The dose of sodium bicarbonate required to treat a severe metabolic acidosis can be calculated using the following equation:

mmol HCO_3^- = volume of distribution of bicarbonate
x bodyweight x HCO_3^- deficit per litre

which can also be stated as:

mmol HCO_3^- = 0.3 x bodyweight x base excess

Half of the calculated dose should be given slowly over approximately 30 minutes and blood gas analysis should be repeated. Further doses of bicarbonate can be given slowly, titrated to effect by repeated measurement of blood pH.

Potential complications of sodium bicarbonate therapy include:

- Volume overload due to the administration of sodium ions and associated retention of water
- Paradoxical central nervous system acidosis. The bicarbonate ions react with hydrogen ions (to correct the metabolic acidosis), producing water and carbon dioxide:

$$HCO_3^- + H^+ \Leftrightarrow H_2CO_3 \Leftrightarrow H_2O + CO_2$$

  Carbon dioxide is able to diffuse rapidly across the blood–brain barrier into the cerebrospinal fluid and may cause central nervous system acidosis. This is most likely to occur if the sodium bicarbonate is given very quickly
- Hypokalaemia: as hydrogen ions are consumed by bicarbonate in the extracellular fluid they will be replaced by hydrogen ions from the intracellular fluid. Hydrogen ions are exchanged for potassium ions across the cell membrane, potentially leading to hypokalaemia.

Conclusion

Advanced fluid therapy is a complex area, requiring knowledge of the normal physiology of fluid homeostasis and a good working knowledge of the acid–base and electrolyte derangements that occur in pathological conditions. Use of blood gas analysis and anion gap measurements will allow fluid therapy to be individually tailored to meet the needs of each patient, so that a more rapid return to normal physiological status can be achieved. However, acute deficits in circulating blood volume leading to hypovolaemia (e.g. resulting from haemorrhage or sepsis) are life-threatening, and implementation of fluid replacement therapy with any type of fluid (crystalloid or colloid) is paramount. Fine tuning of the type of fluid and electrolytes required to restore homeostasis can be instigated once the acute crisis in circulating blood volume has been controlled.

References and further reading

Boag A and Hughes D (2007) Fluid Therapy. In: *BSAVA Manual of Canine and Feline Emergency and Critical Care, 2nd edn*, ed. L King and A. Boag, pp. 30–45 BSAVA Publications, Gloucester

Day M, Mackin A and Littlewood J (2000) *BSAVA Manual of Canine and Feline Haematology and Transfusion Medicine*. BSAVA Publications, Gloucester

DiBartola S (2000) *Fluid Therapy in Small Animal Practice*. WB Saunders Company, Philadelphia

Hotston Moore P (2004) *Fluid Therapy for Veterinary Nurses and Technicians*. Elsevier, Oxford

Martin L (1999) *All You Really Need to Know to Interpret Arterial Blood Gases*. Lippincott Williams and Wilkins, USA

Pet Blood Bank UK (Accessed January 2008) http://www.petbloodbankuk.org/

7

Advanced anaesthesia and analgesia

Kathy Challis and Chris Seymour

This chapter is designed to give information on:

- Establishing an anaesthetic service in veterinary practice
- The definition and application of balanced anaesthesia
- The rationale for selection of anaesthetic, sedative and analgesic agents
- The use of mechanical ventilation
- Application of aids to monitor patients during anaesthesia

Establishing an anaesthesia service in practice

If fortunate enough to be designing a practice from scratch, the first thing to consider is the layout of space to facilitate safe anaesthesia. The mortality rate in veterinary anaesthesia is much higher than in human anaesthesia (Figure 7.1) and when designing a new practice it is important to look at the reasons for this, and how this situation might be improved.

Species	Deaths per 10,000 anaesthetics (healthy patients)
Dog	5.4
Cat	11.2
Human	0.05

7.1 Anaesthetic death rates in veterinary and human patients. (Data from Arbous *et al.*, 2001; Brodbelt *et al.*, in press)

It is usually considered that the greatest risks of anaesthesia are during induction and recovery. At induction, there are two simple measures that can help to reduce anaesthesia risk. Firstly, it is vitally important that the induction area is sited in a position to minimize stress, not only to personnel but also (and especially to) the patient. Stress to the patient at

induction may result in the release of catecholamines, increasing the risk of cardiac arrhythmias and even death. Ideally, it should be possible to enclose an induction area, keeping non-essential personnel out, and keeping other animals out of sight, sound and smell of the patient (Figure 7.2). Noise also increases stress levels, so this should be kept to a minimum. Secondly, an induction area should have easy and swift access to emergency facilities (i.e. help from other personnel, emergency drugs and endotracheal

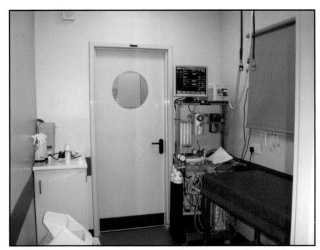

7.2 Provision of a separate enclosed area can minimize disturbance and distress during induction.

(ET) tubes). However, it is rare to be able to design a practice from scratch and thus be able to achieve an ideal design, but with imaginative use of screens, blinds and notices, much can be done to reduce noise and stress levels in an induction area.

Designing an ideal recovery area is probably more difficult as there are contradictory factors at work. For instance, the patient should be kept in a quiet and stress-free environment for its recovery, but it is even more important that a recovering patient is observed closely until it has fully recovered. At this stage it is important to consider the use of personnel in the practice. Ideally, a recovering patient should be observed constantly by a competent trained person who is not distracted by other tasks. In practice, this may not be possible and a patient is left in its cage and checked intermittently. This is one of the most dangerous situations and occasionally results in animals dying unattended in recovery. Constant observation of recovering patients can be difficult to achieve but it may be helpful if the recovery area is sited in a busy, well observed position, such as a preparation room.

Wherever the recovery area is sited, it should contain the following:

- Oxygen supply
- Suction machine
- ET tubes, needles, syringes and emergency drugs
- Electrical sockets
- Equipment for warming the patient
- Appropriate monitoring equipment, including pulse oximeter and electrocardiogram (ECG) machine.

Significant pollution of the atmosphere in recovery areas occurs from anaesthetic gases expired by recently anaesthetized patients. Good ventilation is therefore essential: extrapolating from the Department of Health guidelines, 15–20 air changes an hour are recommended.

Equipment
Gas supplies

Providing piped gases requires a greater initial capital outlay, but this is outweighed by the advantages. These include significant health and safety benefits from reducing the amount of cylinder handling and movement, improved convenience, and general patient safety in reducing the risk of operator error. When considering gas supplies, it makes sense to plan the waste gas scavenging at the same time (see below). It is also important to remember that the area will need to be thoroughly and regularly cleaned. Planning with regard to the location of drains, sloping of floors and portability of equipment is essential. Surfaces should be chosen for floors, walls and ceilings that can be washed without damage.

Anaesthetic machines

Advanced planning is also desirable when choosing anaesthetic machines. In particular, it is necessary to consider whether movable machines are needed. Wall-mounted units (Figure 7.3) are space-saving and convenient but have reduced flexibility in where they are used.

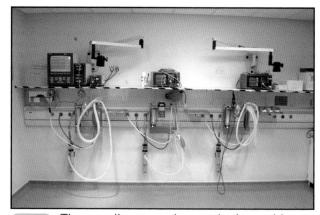

7.3 Three wall-mounted anaesthetic machines in a busy preparation room. (Reproduced from the *BSAVA Manual of Canine and Feline Anaesthesia and Analgesia, 2nd edition*)

The practice should aim to acquire machines with safety features, e.g. low oxygen warning devices (ideally including automatic cut-out of nitrous oxide in the case of a failing oxygen supply), over-pressure valve and emergency air-intake valve.

Machines can often be bought cheaply from human hospital sales and many veterinary practices make use of these successfully. However, in these cases there may be problems in procuring spare parts for repairs. One significant advantage of purchasing new, or professionally refurbished, anaesthetic machines is the availability of service contracts.

Breathing systems

For a description of individual breathing systems see the *BSAVA Manual of Practical Veterinary Nursing*. A variety of breathing systems should be available, including those suitable for controlled ventilation and for use in all sizes of animals treated by the practice. The Humphrey ADE system (Figure 7.4) fulfils almost all these criteria and is becoming increasingly popular in practice. The stock of breathing systems will need to be augmented by a variety of masks and induction chambers.

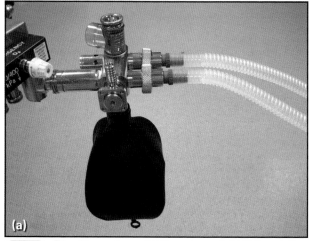

7.4 The Humphrey ADE system. **(a)** Without the canister and with parallel breathing tubing and reservoir bag. (Reproduced from the *BSAVA Manual of Canine and Feline Anaesthesia and Analgesia, 2nd edition*) (continues) ▶

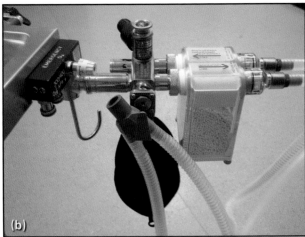

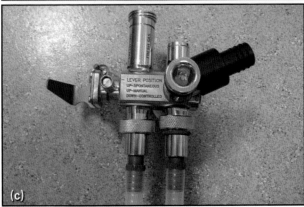

7.4 (continued) The Humphrey ADE system. **(b)** With soda lime canister attached. **(c)** Top view. (Reproduced from the *BSAVA Manual of Canine and Feline Anaesthesia and Analgesia, 2nd edition*)

Ventilators

The type of cases seen in a practice, as well as the number of staff, will determine whether it is necessary to have mechanical ventilators or not. For example, a practice that performs a significant number of thoracotomies or uses neuromuscular blocking agents (NMBAs) will benefit from owning mechanical ventilators (see below).

Monitoring equipment

Pulse oximeters and oesophageal stethoscopes for monitoring patients under anaesthesia are commonly seen in practice. Some practices have Doppler detectors for indirect arterial blood pressure measurement in the assessment of hypertension in medical cases and ECG machines may be available, but they are not necessarily used in the operating theatre. However, they are invaluable monitoring devices for general anaesthesia and Doppler detectors are relatively inexpensive. Direct blood pressure monitoring, capnography and arterial blood gas measurement are being increasingly used in practice.

Temperature monitoring should be standard for all anaesthetized patients and is not expensive or difficult to provide. Some anaesthetic monitoring units incorporate oesophageal or rectal probes for continuous temperature monitoring, but standard digital or mercury thermometers can be used for intermittent monitoring.

Other equipment
Warming equipment

These include hot air blankets (e.g. Bair Huggers®), water blankets and bubble wrap. Microwaveable heating devices (e.g. SnuggleSafe) and heat pads should be used with care as there have been reports of serious burns being inflicted by these devices. A patient loses heat especially through its extremities, so wrapping its paws and tail in bubble wrap or bandages can help to counter this. It is important to note that some drugs used for premedication may affect a patient's ability to maintain its temperature. Therefore, patient temperature and monitoring should commence at the time of premedication.

Laryngoscopes

These should be available with a full set of blades (Macintosh, Miller or Wisconsin). It is worthwhile investing in well made models where the bulb is situated in the handle and light is projected to the blade via a fibreoptic bundle. If the bulb is mounted on the blade itself, the bulb can become very hot and cause burns to the oral mucosa.

Examination lights

Good lighting should not be overlooked in the induction areas, as well as in the operating theatres.

Endotracheal tubes

Red rubber tubes are easy for intubation and relatively cheap, but are not to be recommended as they are more irritant to the patient's airway than plastic polyvinylchloride or silicone tubes. In addition, the cuff on rubber tubes is spherical in shape and creates a less effective seal than the rectangular shape of the plastic or silicone tube cuffs. These provide greater contact with the tracheal mucosa at a lower pressure and are less likely to result in tracheal damage (including tracheal rupture).

Many people prefer to use uncuffed ET tubes for cats to avoid the incidence of tissue necrosis in the trachea. However, there may be occasions where use of a cuffed tube is necessary, for instance when performing intermittent positive pressure ventilation (IPPV) or to protect the airway from fluids generated by oral surgery. If using a cuffed tube with a cat, the safest way is to inflate the cuff gently, listening for gas escaping round the tube, while an assistant gently squeezes the bag on the breathing system (with the expiratory valve closed). By only inflating until the sound of gas escaping ceases, over-inflation can be avoided.

Emergency supplies

Emergency boxes or trolleys need to be sited conveniently, their contents clearly listed (Figure 7.5) and regularly checked. Some practices choose to have some emergency drugs already drawn up to pre-calculated doses. This is a matter for personal preference, but it can be very helpful in a stressful emergency situation. Any drawn up drugs must obviously be clearly labelled with the drug, the dose and the date, and must be regularly checked and replenished.

Drugs
Adrenaline
Atropine
Glycopyrrolate
Propranolol
Lidocaine
Sodium chloride
Equipment
Needles
Syringes
Catheters
Three-way taps
Stethoscope
Tape
Optional (depending on practice layout)
Endotracheal tubes
Laryngoscope and blades
Tracheotomy kit
Resuscitation ('Ambu') bag

 Overview of the contents of an anaesthetic emergency ('crash') box.

Scavenging

Most veterinary nurses are aware of some of the adverse effects of waste anaesthetic gases on operating department personnel. These effects may include drowsiness, giddiness, problems with coordination, liver and kidney disease and, for pregnant staff, an increased rate of spontaneous abortion and birth defects. Working practices (Figure 7.6) are important to reduce pollution by waste gases, but crucial to a safe working environment is the anaesthetic gas scavenging system in all areas where inhalation anaesthesia is carried out. Broadly, these systems can be described as passive or active.

Good working practices will do much to reduce waste gas contamination:

- Turn off vaporizers when not in use
- When using masks, make sure that they are well fitting
- Inflate endotracheal tubes sufficiently
- Empty the breathing system before disconnecting the patient
- Avoid spillages of anaesthetic substances and have protocols in place if this does happen
- Check all anaesthetic equipment at the beginning of each working day, including leak testing of anaesthetic machines
- Whenever possible, fill vaporizers at the end of the day and always use the correct key filling device
- Use a rota to ensure that it is not always the same person who refills the vaporizers
- Ensure that all anaesthetic machines and the scavenging system are checked and serviced regularly

 Good working practices to minimize environmental contamination by volatile anaesthetic agents.

Passive

A passive system may consist simply of a collection system that conveys waste gases from the exhaust valve ('pop-off' or APL valve) of the breathing system (using the expiratory effort of the patient), out of the building via either a hole in the wall or an open window. This system is easy and inexpensive to set up but is not necessarily appropriate, depending on the design of the building. The wall outlet must be lower than the expiratory valve and the tubing leading to the outside of the building must not be too long or vulnerable to kinks or occlusion. If the gases are vented through an open window, windy conditions outside may affect the efficiency of the system.

A commonly used alternative form of passive scavenging involves the use of activated charcoal canisters (e.g. 'Aldasorber') (Figure 7.7). These are connected to the outlet of the breathing system or ventilator and remove halogenated anaesthetics by absorption on to the porous surface of the charcoal. The canister must be positioned below the exhaust valve. This is another easy system to use and involves minimal set up costs. However, the effectiveness declines as the charcoal becomes exhausted. The canister must be checked daily by weighing on scales accurate to 0.1 kg. The charcoal canister releases vapours when heated, so they must not be placed near a source of heat and must be disposed of appropriately, as chemical waste. A charcoal canister does not scavenge nitrous oxide and is therefore unsuitable for use with this gas.

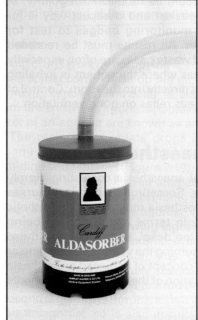

An activated charcoal anaesthetic agent scavenger cylinder ('Aldasorber') with scavenging tubing attached. (Reproduced from the *BSAVA Manual of Canine and Feline Anaesthesia and Analgesia, 2nd edition*)

Active

In active scavenging (Figure 7.8), the waste gases are scavenged from the exhaust valve by negative pressure created by an extractor fan or the hospital vacuum system. For scavenging to be effective, it must be used with correctly installed air-break receivers on the anaesthetic machines. Initial set up costs are high but active scavenging is effective for all anaesthetic gases and is easy to use.

Drug	Classification	Route of administration	Onset of action	Duration of action	Comments
Morphine	Mu agonist	Dogs: i.v., i.m., s.c. (slow i.v. only) Cats: i.m., s.c.	10–15 min	1–4 h (longer in cats)	May cause vomiting. Profound bradycardic and respiratory depressant effects from i.v. injection. If giving intravenously, administer very slowly
Methadone	Mu agonist	i.m.	20 min	4 h	Similar to morphine but less likely to cause vomiting
Pethidine	Mu agonist	i.m.	10–15 min	30–60 min	Causes increased heart rate
Fentanyl	Mu agonist	i.v.	2 min	20–30 min	Likely to cause bradycardia and respiratory depression
Alfentanil	Mu agonist	Slow i.v.	15–20 seconds	10–20 min	Likely to cause longer period of apnoea than fentanyl. Reduces dose requirements of other anaesthetic drugs by at least 50%
Buprenorphine	Partial mu agonist/ antagonist	i.v., i.m., s.c.	30–45 min	4–12 h	Fewer respiratory depressant and bradycardic effects
Butorphanol	Kappa agonist/ mu antagonist	Dogs: i.v., i.m., s.c. Cats: i.m., s.c.	15 min	2–3 h	Less potent analgesic

7.10 A comparison of commonly used opioid analgesic agents.

from a dark cage or carrier into a brightly lit induction room is likely to cause it discomfort and distress. Opioid drugs may also cause behavioural changes pre- and post-anaesthesia, including excitement, restlessness and panting (dysphoria). Monitoring the patient's temperature is always important during anaesthesia, but particularly after opioid administration in cats as the patient's ability to regulate its temperature may be adversely affected.

Non-steroidal anti-inflammatory drugs

This class of drugs has a quite different mechanism of action to the opioids and works well with them to complement their analgesic effects. NSAIDs work by inhibiting the cyclo-oxygenase (COX) enzymes that are responsible for the production of prostaglandins. Prostaglandins are involved in inflammatory pain but also have beneficial roles throughout the body, such as protective effects within the gastrointestinal system and maintaining blood flow to the kidneys. The side-effects often seen with NSAIDs are a result of inhibition of such 'beneficial' prostaglandins. Although work is continuing to produce NSAIDs that are increasingly selective in their action, at present all NSAIDs have the risk of producing undesirable effects in addition to their valuable analgesic qualities.

The prostaglandins that it is desirable to inhibit with the use of these drugs are those involved in inflammation at the site of an injury, and which increase sensitivity of pain receptors. Most of the desirable effects are mediated by the COX enzyme known as COX-1, with the generally more undesirable inflammatory and pain sensitizing effects produced by COX-2. The newer NSAIDs aim to work predominantly by inhibiting COX-2, but this has not been perfectly achieved yet, so care must be taken with the use of NSAIDs.

Selection of these drugs is the responsibility of the veterinary surgeon but an understanding of the risks is relevant to the veterinary nurse in anaesthesia. In particular, when NSAIDs are used during anaesthesia, care must be taken to maintain good blood perfusion to the kidneys. Fluid therapy should be employed and blood pressure carefully monitored. If the blood pressure is low, the first action should be, if at all possible, to reduce the delivered concentration of volatile anaesthetic on the vaporizer. Volatile anaesthetics have hypotensive effects, so a balanced anaesthetic regime, including the use of other analgesic drugs such as opioids, will enable the vaporizer setting to be kept as low as possible. If the blood pressure continues to be low, other measures may be necessary to avoid damage to the kidneys.

Other analgesics

Nitrous oxide

This gas is often used during anaesthesia for its analgesic qualities. It inhibits the N-methyl-D-aspartate (NMDA) receptors, which are involved in the hypersensitivity to pain phenomenon known as 'wind-up' or central sensitization. The analgesic qualities of nitrous oxide allow for the concentration of volatile anaesthetic delivered to be kept as low as possible, but in fact it is also a sympathetic stimulant, tending to support the cardiovascular system. Despite its useful qualities, care must be taken with its use.

Nitrous oxide must always be used with at least 33% oxygen to ensure the patient is not breathing a hypoxic gas mixture. If using a rebreathing system it is safest to use 50% oxygen, unless agent monitoring is employed. Pulse oximetry should be used in any case. Its tendency to move to gas-filled spaces is well known, so nitrous oxide should not be used in conditions where this would constitute a danger, such as gastric dilatation or pneumothorax. If using a cuffed ET tube, nitrous oxide can move into the cuff, so the inflation should be checked every 30 minutes when nitrous oxide is used. At the end of the anaesthesia nitrous oxide moves rapidly into the alveoli, diluting oxygen levels; this can cause hypoxia (diffusion hypoxia). To avoid this, 100% oxygen should be administered for 5–10 minutes after the discontinuation of nitrous oxide.

Trace levels of nitrous oxide in the environment are potentially more dangerous than those of volatile agents, especially to pregnant women, and the gas should only be used with a well functioning active scavenging system and not with activated charcoal canisters. Nitrous oxide is odourless, increasing the risk that accidental exposure will be undetected. Unfortunately, it is also a significant greenhouse gas. For these reasons, it is possible that the use of nitrous oxide may be reduced in the future. However, it remains useful for its analgesic and anaesthetic-sparing qualities.

Ketamine

This also inhibits NMDA receptors and is therefore useful in preventing central pain sensitization. Although it can be given as an anaesthetic in combination with other drugs, it is often used at sub-anaesthetic doses to provide analgesia either by bolus or by constant rate infusion (CRI). Ketamine can cause an increase in blood pressure, central eye position, cardiac arrhythmias and excitement on recovery. However, these effects are less likely to be seen at low analgesic doses. Ketamine is not suitable for use as a sole anaesthetic agent in dogs as it causes undesirable levels of excitement.

Medetomidine

This drug is often used in practice for its sedative qualities, but its analgesic effects are not always recognized. Like ketamine, it can be used successfully as an analgesic at low doses either by bolus or by CRI. Medetomidine causes vasoconstriction, which may create difficulties with monitoring, but blood pressure tends to be increased because of greater vascular resistance. As the blood pressure increases, the heart rate lowers as a reflex response. However, as with ketamine, at low analgesic doses these effects will tend to be much less noticeable. It should be noted that by using atipamezole to reverse the sedative effects of medetomidine, the analgesic effects are also reversed.

Local and regional anaesthesia

Local and regional anaesthesia for small animal surgical procedures are generally used as an adjunct to general anaesthesia, due to the difficulty of restraining these patients and the relative safety of general anaesthesia. These techniques can provide an extremely useful contribution to the analgesia component of balanced anaesthesia. An effective nerve block with local anaesthetic can provide a complete block to nociceptive responses, and so help not only by enabling the anaesthetic to be kept as light as possible, but also by avoiding the sensitization of the pain pathways and minimizing postoperative pain.

Local and regional anaesthetic techniques can be employed to good effect for a variety of different procedures, including mandibular and maxillary blocks for dental procedures (Figure 7.11), brachial plexus blocks for forelimb surgery and intercostal blocks for thoracic surgery. Local anaesthetic drugs can be used, with care, in conjunction with a tourniquet to provide intravenous regional anaesthesia. For all nerve blocks it is necessary to know the relevant anatomical landmarks and the position of nerves and blood vessels, as well as specific risks such as entering the chest cavity during a brachial plexus block. Further details can be found in the *BSAVA Manual of Canine and Feline Anaesthesia and Analgesia, 2nd edition*.

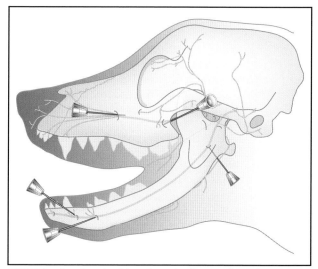

7.11 Anatomical landmarks for performing maxillary, infraorbital, inferior alveolar and mental nerve blocks in dogs. (Reproduced from the *BSAVA Manual of Canine and Feline Anaesthesia and Analgesia, 2nd edition*)

Selection and dosage of the drugs is the responsibility of the veterinary surgeon, but if the anaesthesia nurse is involved in the calculation, it should be borne in mind that the dose should be worked out according to the lean weight of the animal, not necessarily the actual weight. Toxicity can arise from using these drugs, as a result of miscalculation, by using the wrong dose for a particular route, or by accidental intravenous administration. Signs of toxicity can include ataxia, sedation and convulsions in the conscious patient, hypotension and, in extreme cases, ventricular arrhythmias. The anaesthesia nurse should know the time of onset and duration of the local anaesthetic drugs being used (Figure 7.12).

Drug	Onset of action	Duration of action
Lidocaine	5 min	1–2 h
Bupivacaine	10–20 min	4–6 h
Ropivacaine	10–20 min	3–5 h
Mepivacaine	5–15 min	1.5–2.5 h

7.12 Comparison of drugs used in local anaesthesia.

Epidural and spinal anaesthesia and analgesia

The epidural route is very effective for the administration of analgesic and anaesthetic drugs. It can be used for surgery on the hindlimbs, abdomen and perineum, potentially providing analgesia before, during and after surgery.

- Epidural anaesthesia refers to the administration of local anaesthetic drugs by the epidural route.
- Epidural analgesia refers to analgesic drugs, usually an opioid such as preservative-free morphine, given epidurally.

Very commonly, and effectively, a combination of local anaesthetic and analgesic drugs will be given. The local anaesthetic drugs may provide a partial or complete nerve block, and morphine can provide analgesia for 12–24 hours after administration.

The usual site for epidural injection is the junction between the seventh lumbar vertebra (L7) and the sacrum. The landmarks may be easier to locate if the patient is placed in sternal recumbency with the hindlegs drawn forward. Alternatively, the animal can be placed in lateral recumbency with the hindlegs drawn forward. Whichever position is used, it is important to have the legs placed symmetrically.

The injection site must be clipped (Figure 7.13) and the area checked. If any sort of skin infection or inflammation can be seen, the epidural should not be attempted. The most prominent parts of the iliac wings should be located and, by drawing an imaginary line between them, locating the midline, and then moving caudally, the depression between L7 and S1 can be felt (Figure 7.14). This is the where the epidural injection should be given and the skin should be prepared aseptically.

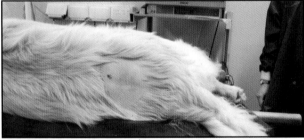

7.13 The epidural site is clipped and prepared aseptically.

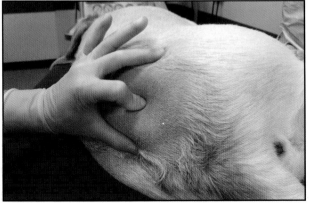

7.14 Palpating the depression between L7 and S1.

The patient must be carefully monitored during the procedure, including its arterial blood pressure. Local anaesthetics can cause vasodilation and hence a decrease in blood pressure. Epidural injection should not be attempted until the patient is properly anaesthetized and stable.

It is best to use a spinal needle or a Tuohy needle (Figure 7.15) rather than a normal hypodermic needle. Both types have a stylet, which prevents occlusion with a core of tissue as the needle is inserted. The Tuohy needle is preferred because it has a blunt bevel and a gentle curve at the tip. These features allow the needle to pass through the ligamentum flavum with much less chance of puncturing the dura mater.

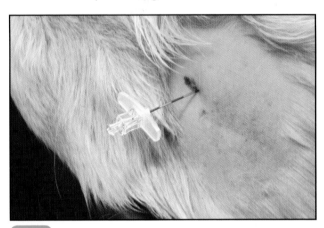

7.15 Correct placement of a Tuohy needle.

The needle should be placed perpendicular to the skin in each dimension and introduced slowly. As the needle passes through the ligamentum flavum a 'pop' may be felt, giving a helpful hint that the needle has entered the epidural space. It may be easier to feel the 'pop' when using a Tuohy needle. The stylet is removed from the spinal needle and a test injection can be made. If the needle is correctly in the epidural space, there should be no resistance to injection. By injecting sterile saline with an air bubble behind, the air can be observed for compression. If there is no compression and the saline injects easily, it is likely that the needle is placed correctly. An alternative to using the saline and air bubble injection is to inject air with a low-resistance syringe (Figure 7.16). If any resistance is felt with this technique, the needle is not placed correctly.

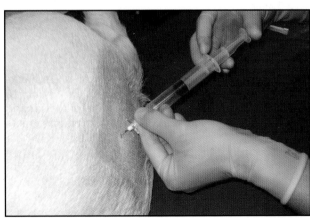

7.16 Use of a low-resistance syringe to test for correct needle placement.

Once correctly placed, the spinal needle is observed to ensure there is no evidence of blood or cerebrospinal fluid (CSF). In most dogs, the spinal cord only extends to the level of L6 so it is unlikely CSF will be seen. The spinal cord in cats extends to L7 so CSF is more likely to be seen. If blood is seen, the needle should be withdrawn and the injection attempted again with a new spinal needle. If blood continues to be seen it is best to abort the procedure. If CSF is seen, the needle can be withdrawn slightly, tested again, and closely observed for any more CSF. Alternatively, the drugs can still be injected turning it into a spinal injection. For spinal anaesthesia and/or analgesia, smaller doses and volume must be given. It is generally safe to continue the procedure, using only a quarter of the volume that had been drawn up for epidural injection.

Once the needle has been correctly placed (see Figure 7.15), the test syringe can be carefully removed and replaced with the syringe containing the drugs for injection. The injection should be administered slowly. If a successful epidural or spinal injection has been achieved, it should be possible to maintain the patient on a lower setting of the vaporizer. Depending on which local anaesthetic drugs have been used, and the length of the procedure, there may be some loss of motor function on recovery and the patient may require some sedation until this is regained.

This procedure has been considered in-depth here because it is perhaps underused in practice considering what a useful contribution to analgesia it makes, and that it can be performed without large amounts of specialized equipment.

Muscle relaxation

Muscle relaxation is the third component of balanced anaesthesia. As discussed above, some anaesthetic drugs do provide a degree of muscle relaxation, for example, the inhalation anaesthetics. However, for procedures where a greater degree of muscle relaxation is required, it would be undesirable to provide this by just turning up the vaporizer because of the depressant effects this would have on the cardiovascular and respiratory systems. Other drugs such as the benzodiazepines or local anaesthetic drugs also provide some muscle relaxation. For surgical procedures that require a great level of muscle relaxation (Figure 7.17), NMBAs should be used.

Neuromuscular blocking agents

NMBAs cause paralysis of all muscles, including those associated with breathing, so IPPV must be employed. A breathing system suitable for IPPV must be used, along with a cuffed ET tube, and there must be a mechanical ventilator suitable for the size of the patient or an appropriately skilled person dedicated to the patient's ventilation.

NMBAs do not cross the blood–brain barrier and do not produce unconsciousness; however, they produce a degree of immobility that mimics unconsciousness. This means that the patient's anaesthesia must be extremely carefully monitored to ensure that the animal is unconscious. Although NMBAs do decrease the anaesthetic requirements, care must be taken not to reduce the anaesthetic level too much. The patient must be watched constantly and vigilantly for any signs of returning consciousness. These could include some or all of the following: increased heart rate, hypertension, salivation, mydriasis and lacrimation.

The two types of NMBAs used in veterinary practice, depolarizing and non-depolarizing, both work at the neuromuscular junction to inhibit the neurotransmitter, acetylcholine (ACh). ACh enables neurons to communicate with each other, diffusing across the synaptic junction between nerve and muscle cells and binding to receptors. ACh only remains bound to the postsynaptic receptors very briefly before being broken down by the enzyme, acetylcholinesterase.

Most of the NMBAs in veterinary use are non-depolarizing (also known as competitive; see Figure 7.20). They cause muscle relaxation by competitively binding to the receptors, blocking the activity of ACh. The only depolarizing (also known as non-competitive) NMBA used clinically is suxamethonium, which causes muscle relaxation in a different way. Suxamethonium molecules occupy the ACh receptors and depolarize the plasma membrane of the skeletal muscle fibre, causing an initial muscle contraction. However, as suxamethonium is not metabolized by acetylcholinesterase, the molecules continue to occupy the receptors, blocking any further muscle contractions. After administration of suxamethonium fine muscle twitches just before paralysis may be seen. The initial muscle contraction caused by depolarizing NMBAs is associated with postoperative pain.

Procedure	Comments
Thoracotomy	Muscle relaxation may facilitate the veterinary surgeon's access, allowing for easier retraction of the chest Surgery on relaxed muscles tends to reduce postoperative pain
Abdominal surgery	Easier access for veterinary surgeon through abdominal muscles Reduction of postoperative pain
Joint reductions	May make it easier for veterinary surgeon to reduce the joint Possible reduction of postoperative pain (debatable)
Ophthalmic surgery	Central eye position caused by NMBA facilitates corneal surgery Complete immobility of patient during microsurgery
Neurosurgery	Complete immobility of patient
Intubation	Sometimes given in cats for difficult intubation
Whilst using ventilators	Enables ventilation to be controlled if the patient is 'fighting' the ventilator

7.17 Indications for the use of neuromuscular blocking agents (NMBAs).

Monitoring the neuromuscular blockade

The neuromuscular blockade must be monitored throughout:

- At the outset, to ascertain when the blockade is complete
- As the blockade wears off to decide whether further NMBAs should be given
- At the end of the procedure to ensure it is safe to wake the patient up.

Muscle paralysis does not happen at the same time throughout the body. The muscles controlling respiration are among the last to be affected, and the first to regain their function. So it is not safe to assume that because a patient is able to breathe on its own, the neuromuscular blockade has been completely reversed. The usual way of monitoring the neuromuscular blockade is with the so-called 'train-of-four'. This involves using a peripheral nerve stimulator (PNS) to send a series of four electrical pulses to electrodes attached to the skin over a peripheral nerve (Figure 7.18).

The PNS should be placed and tested before the NMBA has been administered. In the non-paralyzed patient, when the 'train-of-four' nerve stimulation is instigated, the muscle will be seen to give four equal twitches. Once the NMBA has been given, the nerve should be stimulated again and the twitches observed. As the blockade starts to become effective, the twitches will be seen to diminish in strength, until when the blockade is complete there will be no twitches at all (Figure 7.19).

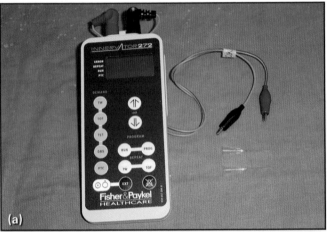
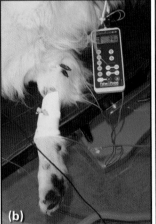
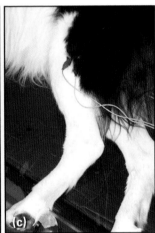
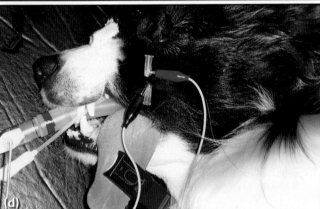

7.18 **(a)** Peripheral nerve stimulator with needle electrodes. **(b)** Placement of needle electrodes over the ulnar nerve on the medial aspect of the elbow. **(c)** Stimulation of the peroneal nerve can be achieved by electrode placement over the lateral head of the fibula. **(d)** Needle electrodes placed over the facial nerve as it exits the infraorbital foramen. (Reproduced from the *BSAVA Manual of Canine and Feline Anaesthesia and Analgesia, 2nd edition*)

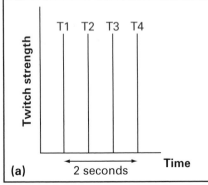
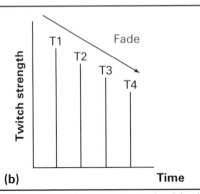
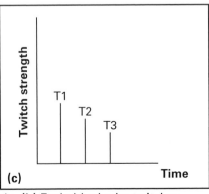

7.19 **(a)** Four equal twitches before the onset of neuromuscular blockade. **(b)** Early blockade: twitches diminishing. **(c)** More profound blockade: twitches diminished or absent. (Reproduced from the *BSAVA Manual of Canine and Feline Anaesthesia and Analgesia, 2nd edition*)

If a PNS is not available, the best way to monitor the blockade is to observe the diaphragm for twitching movements. As the respiratory muscles are more resistant to NMBAs, respiration will be one of the last functions to be lost as the blockade becomes effective, and later, some twitching of the diaphragm may be one of the first signs to herald the end of the blockade.

Reversal of neuromuscular blocking agents

The two types of NMBA are quite different in the way their action is reversed. Suxamethonium (depolarizing) only lasts about 5 minutes before it is metabolized by the body, so reversal of this drug is not required. Non-depolarizing NMBAs work by competing with ACh for occupation of the ACh receptors. Acetylcholinesterase-inhibiting (anticholinesterase) drugs can be administered to reverse these NMBAs; ACh is degraded by acetylcholinesterase, so by inhibiting acetylcholinesterase, more ACh is available to reoccupy its receptors, enabling normal muscle function to return.

It may not always be necessary to reverse the blockade, depending on the length of the procedure and duration of action of the drug. Anticholinesterase drugs may cause muscarinic side-effects such as bradycardia, excessive secretions in the airways and cardiac arrhythmias, so they are only given in combination with an antimuscarinic drug. The anticholinesterase drug must be matched with an antimuscarinic of a similar onset and duration time, so the combinations used are edrophonium with atropine, or neostigmine with glycopyrrolate (Figure 7.20).

Close observation during the recovery period is vital after the use of NMBAs. In case of a problem with an airway, the patient must be recovered in an area with quick access to ET tubes, breathing systems and a source of oxygen. If a reversal drug has been used, it is necessary to be aware of the danger of the NMBA recycling; in other words, if the NMBA used has a longer duration of action than the reversal agent, the neuromuscular blockade could recur when the reversal agent has worn off.

Ventilators

Indications for ventilation

Mechanical ventilation may be desirable for a variety of reasons:

- Hypoventilation: this may be caused by the anaesthetic drugs administered (e.g. a fentanyl or ketamine infusion) or be a result of lung disease, obesity or positioning of the animal, and is likely to cause hypercapnia
- Intrathoracic surgery
- Use of NMBAs
- If the patient's respiration is inadequate to take in enough inhalation anaesthetic to keep a steady and suitable level of anaesthesia, e.g. during panting or irregular breathing
- Raised intracranial pressure (ICP): to avoid hypercapnia, which can cause an increase in ICP. Ventilation may also be desirable in patients with a brain tumour, or suspicion of one, when raised ICP may cause the tumour to herniate.

Use of a mechanical ventilator

It is for the individual practice to decide whether the advantages outweigh the disadvantages, but ventilators are not the most expensive items of veterinary equipment and the indications for using them are quite common.

Advantages

In practices without ventilators, the above situations can be, and are, managed with hand-ventilation. However, ventilating a patient during a thoracotomy is a skilled technique and one that ties the anaesthetist effectively to one job. A mechanical ventilator frees the anaesthetist for other important tasks during a difficult anaesthetic. In addition, mechanical ventilators enable the anaesthetist to control the level of ventilation much more easily than with hand-ventilation.

Drug	Duration of action	Comments
Neuromuscular blocking agents		
Suxamethonium	5 min (cats) 15–20 min (dogs)	Not generally recommended in dogs. Use generally restricted to facilitating intubation in cats
Atracurium	30–40 min	Can cause histamine release if given rapidly
Vecuronium	20–25 min	Metabolized by the liver, so duration of action may be prolonged with liver disease
Pancuronium	45–60 min	May cause tachycardia
Rocuronium	15 min (cats) 30 min (dog)	Fast onset time
Reversal agents		
Neostigmine and glycopyrrolate	30 min	
Edrophonium and atropine	Transient	

7.20   Comparison of neuromuscular blocking agents and reversal agents.

Disadvantages

An animal breathing naturally inhales in response to negative pressure in its chest. Mechanical ventilation works by positive pressure in the chest. This positive pressure can cause a decrease in venous return through the vena cava, resulting in a drop in arterial blood pressure.

Incorrect use may cause lung damage, e.g. by the use of excessive pressures. A patient with low compliance, meaning that its lungs are rigid and difficult to ventilate, may need a much higher pressure for adequate ventilation. Whereas a young animal, with high compliance may suffer lung damage from high pressures.

Ventilation removes the means of monitoring a patient by respiratory rate. By controlling ventilation, increases or decreases in the respiratory rate cannot be seen. With conscientious monitoring of the patient this should not be a problem, but it could be argued that mechanical ventilators encourage inattentiveness. The patient's regular respiratory rate may give a misleading impression of stability. In addition, the ventilator may spread infection by harbouring respiratory pathogens. Bacterial filters (Figure 7.21) should always be used to prevent the ventilator becoming an agent for spread of infection. Another disadvantage is the initial financial outlay.

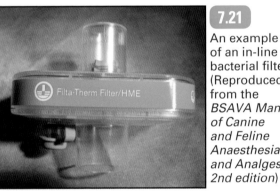

7.21
An example of an in-line bacterial filter. (Reproduced from the *BSAVA Manual of Canine and Feline Anaesthesia and Analgesia, 2nd edition*)

Types of ventilator

There are different ways of classifying ventilators but perhaps the simplest method is by the way they work. Firstly, the adjustable parameters should be considered. Generally, one or more of these parameters are unable to be adjusted, but depending on the ventilator it is possible to set:

- Tidal volume (usually calculated as 10–15 ml/kg bodyweight)
- Inspiratory time
- Expiratory time
- Inspiratory airway pressure (usually set at 10–20 cmH₂O) but this is quite variable.

Ventilators can be divided into whether they are controlled by volume or by pressure. Within these two groups, they can be subdivided into categories depending on 'cycling'. This term refers to how the ventilator is prompted to move from inspiration to expiration (i.e. by time, pressure or volume).

For example, a volume controlled ventilator with time cycling allows the operator to set the tidal volume and the inspiratory and expiratory times. The ventilator will deliver the selected volume over the selected inspiratory time and then move to its expiratory phase. In a healthy patient, if the tidal volume has been set correctly, the ventilator will probably deliver the gas at the correct pressure. However, in the case of decreased compliance, or of an incorrect tidal volume setting, it is possible to deliver an inadequate or a damagingly large tidal volume. Whichever type of ventilator is used, it is essential to watch the patient's chest excursions to ensure a suitable pressure has been selected.

For detailed descriptions of the different types of ventilator available, see the *BSAVA Manual of Canine and Feline Anaesthesia and Analgesia, 2nd edition*.

Managing a patient on a ventilator

While a patient is on a ventilator, it will sometimes be seen to 'fight' or breathe against it. Sometimes this is temporary, at the start of ventilation. It could also be an indication that the patient's level of anaesthesia has become light. However, if it persists it may be necessary to take steps to stop this happening. Sometimes simply increasing the tidal volume, the pressure or the respiratory rate may work. If not, it may be necessary to suppress the patient's ventilation by the use of drugs (NMBAs or short-acting opioids, such as fentanyl).

Anaesthetic depth

Use of a ventilator may have an effect on anaesthetic depth. The ventilator tends to increase the efficiency of delivering the inhalation agent to the patient, so if a previously hypoventilating patient is put on a mechanical ventilator, the increased rate and depth of respiration may cause the animal to become too deeply anaesthetized. Careful monitoring of arterial blood pressure (which may drop in any case due to mechanical ventilation), heart rate, eye position and jaw tone should enable the anaesthetist to prevent the patient becoming 'too deep'.

During mechanical ventilation it is particularly desirable to measure the adequacy of ventilation. This is most simply achieved using capnography and aiming to set ventilation levels that result in an end-tidal carbon dioxide level of 30–35 mmHg (4.6–6.6 kPa). Blood gas analysis, if available, is a very valuable monitoring tool.

When setting up the ventilator, parameters that are physiologically normal should be aimed for; chest excursions should look natural and a respiratory rate should be set that looks natural for an anaesthetized animal. It may in fact be desirable to set the respiratory rate slightly lower. The efficiency of the ventilator may hyperventilate slightly compared with the patient's own efforts.

Taking the patient off the ventilator is not usually a problem. If ventilation has been controlled for some time, it may take a while for the patient to start breathing on its own. The situation can generally be managed by reducing the level of ventilation (i.e. the respiratory rate or the tidal volume) or by taking the patient off the ventilator and using hand ventilation until the patient is spontaneously breathing again. Although turning down the vaporizer slightly may help the situation, it is not advisable to turn it off completely until an adequate level of spontaneous respiration has been restored.

Aids to monitoring

The anaesthetist may be distracted by the colours and numbers generated by electronic monitoring devices, and there is a danger of spending so much time looking at and fiddling with the monitoring equipment that direct monitoring of the patient may be forgotten. The veterinary nurse's senses (sight, hearing, touch and smell) are invaluable for gaining information about the patient's condition. This section looks at some of these monitoring devices and their strengths and limitations.

Pulse oximetry

Pulse oximeters are very commonly used in veterinary practice. They display a pulse rate and a figure representing oxygen saturation. The probe of the pulse oximeter is attached to an unpigmented area of the patient, usually the tongue. It uses red and infrared light to calculate the percentage of haemoglobin that is saturated with oxygen.

Advantages and disadvantages of pulse oximetry

Advantages

- Easy and quick to apply: possibly the quickest of all monitoring aids to set up.
- Adaptable: if the tongue is not available it can often be applied successfully to unpigmented toes, prepuce or vulva (Figure 7.22).
- Individual handheld units are small and light: easily portable through the practice.
- Many models do not need a source of electricity.

Disadvantages

- Does not work well in the presence of peripheral vasoconstriction, e.g. shock or after use of drugs such as medetomidine.
- Can sometimes be difficult to establish probe contact.
- Can be misleading in an anaemic patient. If the patient has low haemoglobin but all the haemoglobin is saturated with oxygen, the pulse oximeter may show a healthy saturation. However, in such a case the amount of oxygen reaching the tissues could still be very low.
- When a patient is breathing 100% oxygen, the pulse oximeter is likely to give a good reading for quite some time, even if ventilation is inadequate. It is when the animal is breathing room air that the pulse oximeter will more quickly detect a problem. Often the pulse oximeter probe is removed at the end of anaesthesia, either as soon as the vaporizer is turned off or when the patient is extubated. In fact it is at this stage that it is most useful. It is after disconnection from the oxygen, and particularly after extubation, that a patient may desaturate. The pulse oximeter is of particular value at this stage.

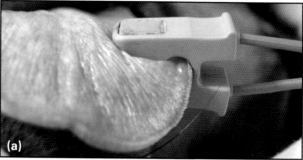

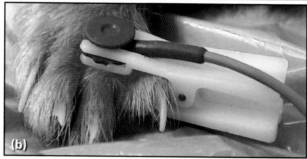

7.22 Sensor of a pulse oximeter. **(a)** On the tongue. **(b)** On a non-pigmented toe. (Reproduced from the *BSAVA Manual of Canine and Feline Anaesthesia and Analgesia, 2nd edition*)

Capnography

A capnograph produces a graphical representation of the carbon dioxide levels throughout the patient's respiratory cycle (a capnogram). It may do this on a screen, a printout or both. As well as a capnogram, it will generally display the respiratory rate, end-tidal carbon dioxide level and sometimes the inspired carbon dioxide level. The carbon dioxide levels may be expressed in mmHg, kPa or as a percentage.

The capnograph takes its measurements using sidestream (Figure 7.23) or mainstream sampling. In sidestream sampling, the gas is sucked off through a narrow tube for analysis in the main unit. This is a slightly less accurate system than mainstream sampling and also causes a delay, so the capnogram may appear out of time with the patient's breathing. Mainstream sampling measures gas directly from the airway and follows exactly the patient's breathing pattern. Mainstream sampling can therefore only be used with intubated patients.

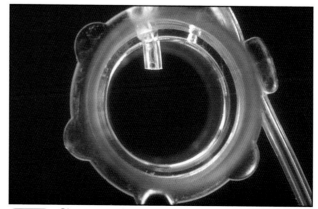

7.23 Close-up of a connector for sampling gas (sidestream capnograph). (Reproduced from the *BSAVA Manual of Canine and Feline Anaesthesia and Analgesia, 2nd edition*)

In a normal capnogram (Figure 7.24) the baseline of the trace should start just as inspiration finishes. It should be touching the baseline, which indicates 0% carbon dioxide. If it does not touch the baseline it indicates that the patient is inspiring carbon dioxide (rebreathing). The trace should rise as the patient starts its expiration and carbon dioxide from the lungs joins the mixture of gases at the sampling point. Towards the end of expiration the trace should level off, climbing more gradually to its highest point, which indicates the end-tidal carbon dioxide level. Then the trace should drop sharply down as the patient starts its inspiration. The trace should return to the baseline (0% carbon dioxide) before the next expiration.

With practice, much can be learnt by studying the traces seen on a capnograph. Rebreathing (Figure 7.25) is easily seen; this may be the result of exhausted soda lime with a rebreathing system or with a non-rebreathing system it is likely to be caused by the fresh gas flow rate being set too low. A leak (Figure 7.26) may occur anywhere in the breathing system but is commonly the result of an inadequately cuffed ET tube. Increased resistance on expiration (Figure 7.27) may be caused by a blocked ET tube or other airway obstruction.

Possibly the most useful function of capnography is the measurement of end-tidal carbon dioxide. Under general anaesthesia a high figure is usually due to hypoventilation and may be an indication that the patient's anaesthetic is too deep. Less commonly, it may be caused by prolonged rebreathing (in which case there would also be a high inspired carbon dioxide level) or by sepsis or malignant hyperthermia. Assuming that the high end-tidal carbon dioxide level is due to hypoventilation, the first response should generally be to turn the vaporizer down and assist ventilation until the carbon dioxide has dropped to an acceptable level.

A low end-tidal carbon dioxide level may be the result of hyperventilation, possibly due to overactive manual ventilation or to the patient's anaesthetic depth being too light. It could also indicate low blood volume or hypothermia. A rapidly falling or absent end-tidal carbon dioxide level, if not caused by technical problems such as disconnection of the patient from the breathing system or breakdown of the capnograph, could indicate respiratory or cardiac arrest.

Advantages and disadvantages of capnography

Advantages

- **Easy to apply, non-invasive equipment.**
- **Provides a great deal of important information, much of which would be difficult to obtain by other means.**
- **A falling end-tidal carbon dioxide level could be a vital early warning sign of respiratory or cardiac arrest.**

Disadvantages

- **Increases equipment dead space from sampling connector.**
- **Increases potential for leaks in the breathing system, including the possibility of increased contamination of the workplace with anaesthetic gases.**
- **Possible spread of infection with reusable sampling lines and connectors.**
- **More expensive and less portable than some other monitoring devices.**

Respiratory gas monitoring

Respiratory gas monitors provide a continuous measurement of the anaesthetic gases in the breathing system, sometimes combined with oxygen and carbon dioxide levels (Figure 7.28). In theory it would be expected that the expired anaesthetic gas measurement should be somewhere close to the MAC.

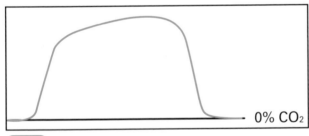

7.24 Capnograph tracing of a normal breath.

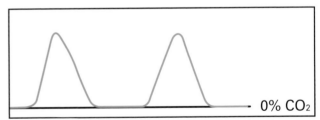

7.26 Capnograph tracing of two breaths showing a leak in the breathing system. Note the rapid fall in carbon dioxide after exhalation.

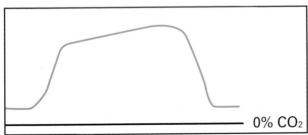

7.25 Capnograph tracing showing rebreathing. Note that the carbon dioxide levels never return to zero (0%).

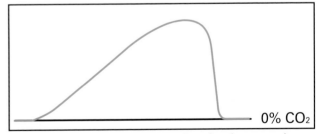

7.27 Capnograph tracing showing increased respiratory resistance. Note the slow rise in carbon dioxide during expiration.

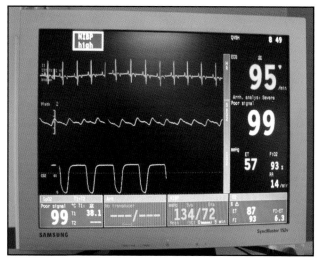

7.28 A monitoring screen displaying respiratory gas concentrations on the left-hand side of the screen.

However, in a balanced anaesthetic, the volatile gas will be only one of the components contributing to anaesthesia, so for example, after a successful and appropriate local anaesthetic nerve block, it is likely to be possible to keep the patient anaesthetized at a figure below the MAC.

Advantages and disadvantages of respiratory gas monitoring

Advantages

- Easy to use and interpret.
- Provides a way of checking the calibration of the vaporizer.
- When using nitrous oxide in a non-rebreathing system, there is a risk (especially at low flows) of developing a hypoxic mix in the system. Respiratory gas monitors that measure oxygen and nitrous oxide levels provide useful information in this situation.
- Useful in a rebreathing system for giving a more accurate picture than the vaporizer provides of the concentration of volatile agent in the system.

Disadvantages

- Cannot be considered to measure the depth of anaesthesia, just the amount of volatile agent in the system. Monitoring of the patient's clinical signs is still necessary.
- Not a particularly inexpensive or portable monitoring device.

Blood gas analysis

This is increasingly popular since small, portable blood gas analysers have come on to the market. Blood gas analysis is used to measure the partial pressures of oxygen and carbon dioxide in the blood. Pulse oximeters and capnographs in their different ways,

use other information (absorption by haemoglobin of infrared light, measurement of gases in the breathing system, respectively) to make an assumption about blood gas partial pressure. They are unable to determine the levels with the accuracy of a monitoring device that measures gases directly from the blood. By measuring pH, it is also possible to assess the acid–base status of the patient, enabling the veterinary surgeon to identify respiratory and metabolic acidosis and alkalosis (see Chapter 6).

A full detailed description of blood gas analysis is outwith the scope of this chapter but as in all areas, understanding grows with familiarity and veterinary nurses should take every opportunity to learn about blood gas analysis in practice and familiarize themselves with normal values (Figure 7.29).

Parameter	Normal values	Decrease	Increase
pH	7.35–7.45	Acidaemia	Alkalaemia
Partial pressure of carbon dioxide in arterial blood (P_aCO_2)	35–45 mmHg	Respiratory component: alkalosis	Respiratory component: acidosis
Plasma bicarbonate (HCO_3^-) concentration	22–26 mmol/l	Metabolic component: acidosis	Metabolic component: alkalosis
Partial pressure of oxygen in arterial blood (P_aO_2)	If oxygen level in inspired gas (F_iO_2) = 21%: 80–100 mmHg (10.7–13.3 kPa)	Hypoxaemia: <60 mmHg (8 kPa)	Due to increased F_iO_2 or increased atmospheric pressure
Saturation of haemoglobin with oxygen (S_aO_2)	95–100%	Hypoxaemia: <90%	

7.29 Normal values from blood gas analysis and interpretation during anaesthesia. (Reproduced from the *BSAVA Manual of Canine and Feline Anaesthesia and Analgesia, 2nd edition*)

Blood sample collection

To assess acid–base status it is acceptable to draw venous blood, so a jugular vein can be used, but for analysis of blood gases, it is necessary to obtain arterial blood. The blood needs to be collected, without air bubbles, in heparinized syringes. Various sites for arterial blood sampling can be employed. Most usually, femoral or dorsal metatarsal arteries are used. However, other sites are available, including radial, lingual and coccygeal arteries. If repeated arterial sampling is to be used it is best to place an arterial catheter, for which the dorsal metatarsal, radial or coccygeal arteries are preferred. After sampling, or after removing an arterial catheter, it is necessary to apply pressure to the site for several minutes.

Advantages and disadvantages of blood gas analysis

Advantages

- High level of accuracy of results.
- Detailed information can be gained.
- Can often be used to measure other parameters such as electrolyte, glucose and lactate levels.

Disadvantages

- More invasive than other forms of monitoring. Poor sampling technique may result in trauma to the sampling area.
- Interpretation is complex and requires considerable knowledge and practice.

Summary

In conclusion, it should be stressed that information gained from monitoring devices should be understood and interpreted in the context of all the observations and impressions that the anaesthetist gathers, not neglecting the evidence of their own senses. The undivided attention of the anaesthetist may well be the most important factor in a safe anaesthetic.

References and further reading

Arbous MS, Grobbee DE, van Kleef JW, *et al.* (2001) Mortality associated with anaesthesia: a qualitative analysis to identify risk factors. *Anaesthesia* **56**, 1141–1153

Brodbelt DC, Blissett KJ, Hammond RA, *et al.* (in press) The risk of death: the confidential enquiry into perioperative small animal fatalities. *Veterinary Anaesthesia and Analgesia*

8

Advanced surgical nursing

Alison Young and Mickey Tivers

This chapter is designed to give information on:

- Theatre personnel and their roles
- Minor surgical procedures – a practical approach to minor surgery
- Advanced surgeries – equipment, general approach, preoperative, intraoperative and postoperative care plans

Introduction

This chapter has been written for veterinary nurses interested in small animal surgery and for those requiring knowledge of more advanced surgical procedures and nursing care plans. It uses knowledge gained from the *BSAVA Manual of Practical Veterinary Nursing* and develops this further with a practical approach to minor surgery in accordance with Schedule 3 of the Veterinary Surgeons Act (1966). The role of the theatre team is discussed, along with more specific duties of theatre nurses.

Theatre management

Successful theatre management is vital for the efficient and effective running of a surgical list in a busy veterinary practice/hospital. Theatre management is usually the responsibility of a veterinary nurse and can provide a defined career path for a qualified, dedicated and experienced nurse. Managing a theatre involves many skills, of which organization is the most important.

Veterinary practice is extremely varied and the theatre team is dependent on the staff, case load and equipment available within the practice. In many circumstances it may be a small team consisting of just a surgeon and a nurse. In busy multidisciplinary hospitals with more than one operating theatre it may be a large team, with veterinary surgeons working alongside surgical assistants, scrubbed nurses, circulating nurses, anaesthetists and anaesthesia nurses or technicians.

The role of the Head Surgical Nurse

Organization of the theatres should be undertaken by a dedicated Head Surgical Nurse or Theatre Manager. Their role should include staffing within the theatres, room/theatre availability and the equipment within these theatres. Although this role may be shared amongst a team of nurses, efficient working requires a dedicated leader. As well as day-to-day management of the running of the theatre team and area, the role may include sourcing equipment and consumables, meeting with suppliers, placing orders, monitoring stock levels, organizing servicing, repairs and maintenance of equipment, as well as teaching newer and less experienced staff.

Hygiene and cleanliness are important issues and all personnel should have a sense of responsibility in maintaining these standards. It is the Head Surgical Nurse who must ensure that this is achieved and maintained. The development of cleaning protocols ensures that no areas or tasks are missed and allows this to be monitored. The Head Surgical Nurse also supervises the general conduct of all personnel entering the theatre area to make sure they are suitably dressed and that theatre protocols are adhered to.

The surgical team

The surgical team can consist of some or all of the following: veterinary surgeons; surgical assistants; scrubbed nurses; circulating nurses; anaesthetists; and anaesthesia nurses or technicians (Figure 8.1).

Use of needle-holders

- **The needle is grasped perpendicular to the needle-holders. In most cases it should be grasped between a half and two-thirds of the way from the point (Figure 8.7).**
- **Appropriately sized needle-holders should be selected for the size of the needle. Fine needle-holders will be damaged if used to hold large needles.**
- **The tip of the needle should not be manipulated by the needle-holders or forceps, as this will blunt it.**
- **Always follow the curve of the needle when passing it through tissue to reduce trauma. The wrist should be rotated to enable the rotation of the needle.**

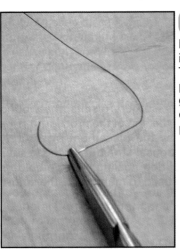

8.7 Needle in position in needle-holders. The needle is held perpendicular and is grasped two-thirds of the way from the point. (© A Young)

Suture material

The choice of suture material will depend on the tissue being sutured (Figure 8.8). When suturing simple skin wounds the following guidelines should be followed:

- Synthetic absorbable suture should be used for ligatures, subcutaneous tissue and when placing subdermal sutures, as they have low tissue reactivity
- Synthetic non-absorbable sutures or skin staples should be used for exposed skin sutures. Such sutures should be removed at an appropriate time (approximately 7–10 days in most cases)
- Suture materials that cause tissue reaction, such as chromic catgut, should be avoided
- The size of suture material used should relate to the inherent strength of the tissue.

Suture patterns

Suture patterns (Figure 8.9) can be divided into interrupted and continuous. The advantages of **interrupted** patterns is that they allow adjustment of tension along the wound and they are potentially more secure as the loss of one suture does not disrupt the whole suture line. The advantages of **continuous** patterns is that they are much quicker to place than interrupted, create a better seal, use less suture material and leave less suture material in the wound. Suture patterns can be **inverting** (turn the edges in), **everting** (turn the edges out) or **appositional** (bring the edges together). In general appositional suture patterns are used when closing skin wounds. Simple interrupted is the most versatile suture pattern and can be used in almost any situation.

Suture material	Characteristics	Uses	Comments
Polyglactin 910 (Vicryl); lactomer 9-1 (Polysorb)	Synthetic Absorbable Multifilament	Subcutaneous, intradermal, muscle, mucous membranes	Easy to handle and minimal tissue reaction
Polydioxanone (PDS); glycomer 631 (Biosyn)	Synthetic Absorbable Monofilament	Subcutaneous, intradermal, muscle, mucous membranes	Very strong with slow rate of absorption Not easy to handle
Poliglecaprone 25 (Monocryl); polyglytone 6211 (Caprosyn)	Synthetic Absorbable Monofilament	Subcutaneous, intradermal	Good handling High initial tensile strength
Chromic catgut	Natural Absorbable Multifilament	Subcutaneous, intradermal, muscle	Causes tissue reaction. Has poor tensile strength, poor knot security when wet and is prone to wicking Synthetic materials generally preferred
Nylon–polyamide (Ethilon, Monosof)	Synthetic Non-absorbable Monofilament	Skin sutures	Generally preferred to multifilament nylon
Multifilament nylon	Synthetic Non-absorbable Multifilament	Skin sutures	Better handling and knot security than monofilament nylon. May increase risk of infection as is braided

8.8 Commonly used suture materials.

Suture pattern	Description	Feature	Uses	Comments
Simple interrupted (SIA)	Individual loops placed at regular intervals across wound (Figure 8.10)	Appositional	Skin, subcutaneous tissue, fascia, gastrointestinal tract and other viscera	Precise suture tension. Easy to apply. Secure anatomical closure
Interrupted intradermal or subcuticular	SIA placed upside-down in dermis and subcutis. Suture does not penetrate epidermis	Appositional	Intradermal skin closure	Does not require removal. Allows more accurate wound closure than continuous pattern. Leaves more suture material in wound than alternative techniques
Cruciate mattress	Two loops placed in same direction. Finished suture forms a cross over the wound	Appositional to everting	Skin; less commonly subcutaneous tissue, fascia, muscle	Stronger closure than SIA. Resists tension. Fast and relatively easy to place
Horizontal mattress	Suture material is passed across wound and then back across parallel to the first pass (Figure 8.11)	Everting	Skin (if tension)	Resists tension
Vertical mattress	Suture material is passed across wound, with entry and exit points reasonably far from the wound edge. Then passed back across the wound in line with the previous pass but closer to the wound edge	Everting	Skin (if tension)	Resists tension
Simple continuous (SCA)	Suture material is passed across wound in a continuous fashion	Appositional	Skin, subcutaneous tissue, fascia, gastrointestinal tract and other viscera	Quicker, good suture economy. Good apposition and tight seal
Ford interlocking	Similar to simple continuous but the suture material is passed through a loop to 'lock' it in place (Figure 8.12)	Appositional	Skin, diaphragm	Similar to simple continuous. Provides additional security. Better tissue apposition
Continuous intradermal or subcuticular (Figure 8.13)	Simple continuous running parallel to skin edge	Appositional	Intradermal skin closure	Does not require removal. Faster than interrupted

8.9   Commonly used suture patterns.

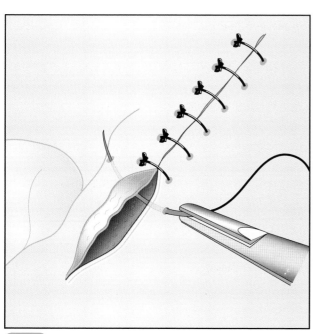

8.10   Simple interrupted skin sutures.

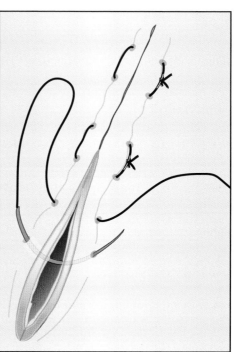

8.11
Horizontal mattress skin sutures.

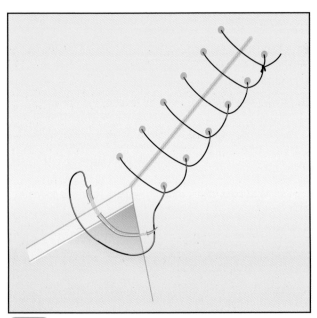

8.12 Ford interlocking suture.

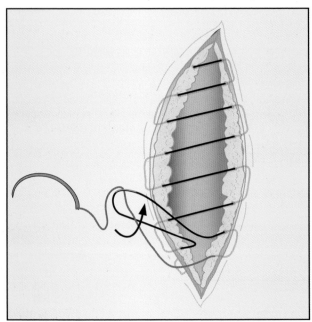

8.13 Continuous intradermal or subcuticular suture.

Suturing a skin wound

Subcutaneous tissue is closed initially to reduce dead space. This is important to reduce the accumulation of fluid postoperatively which otherwise might cause a seroma. Subcutaneous sutures also help to reduce any ongoing haemorrhage. The subcutaneous tissue is closed using simple continuous sutures of synthetic absorbable material such as polyglactin, polydioxanone or poliglecaprone. The tissue is gently apposed with minimal tension.

The skin can be closed over the subcutaneous tissue using a variety of techniques:

■ Skin sutures with a monofilament synthetic non-absorbable material such as nylon are most commonly used. Suture materials that are reactive should be avoided. Monofilament

nylon is preferred to multifilament nylon as there is less risk of infection. A variety of suture patterns are used to close the skin, including simple interrupted, cruciate mattress and Ford interlocking. Simple interrupted sutures (see Figures 8.10 and 8.14) have the advantage of providing good apposition of the skin edges and are more easily removed than continuous or mattress sutures

■ Skin staples are also used commonly in small animal practice. These have the advantage that they are quicker to place and may be useful in very long wounds or unstable patients, but are more expensive

■ Intradermal or subcuticular sutures can also be used to close the skin. This involves placing sutures in the dermis or in the region where the dermis blends with the subcutaneous tissue. A continuous pattern is typically used, although an interrupted pattern is preferred when precise apposition of the edges of the wound is desired. A synthetic absorbable suture material is used in all cases. Intradermal sutures have the advantage that there are no exposed skin sutures and therefore no risk of tracking infection and no sutures to be removed in fractious patients. However, they are slower to place and provide less security than skin sutures. Some surgeons prefer to place an intradermal suture prior to the placement of skin sutures or staples

■ Tissue glue (cyanoacrylate) can also be used for skin closure, particularly in small wounds or incisions.

1. Grasp the needle with needle-holders (see text).
2. Grasp the far edge of the wound with Adson or rat-toothed forceps.
3. Put the point of the needle into the skin approximately 2–3 mm to the side of the far wound edge.
4. Grasp the near edge of the wound with the forceps and pass the needle through the second skin edge. The forceps retain their grip on the wound edge and thus stabilize the needle in the tissue (see A).
5. Grasp the needle-holders with the palm of the hand facing downwards and remove the needle from the tissue. Rotate the wrist to allow the needle to follow its own curve and exit the skin smoothly.
6. Pull the suture material through the skin until approximately 3–4 cm is left protruding from the far side of the wound. Ideally, hold the excess suture material in the non-dominant hand (see B).
7. Tie a square knot with 3–4 throws in total. There should not be any tension in the wound and thus a surgeon's knot is not required (see A,B,C,D).
8. Cut the free ends of the suture material to approximately 1 cm in length to facilitate later removal (see E,F,G).
9. Place subsequent sutures in the same fashion approximately 1 cm apart.

Notes
The wound is sutured from right to left or top to bottom. Nylon suture material of an appropriate size (1.5–3 metric) with a reverse-cutting curved needle is used. Skin sutures should be placed flat on the skin and should not be too tight; this is to allow postsurgical swelling.

8.14 How to place simple interrupted sutures. (© A Young) (continues) ▶

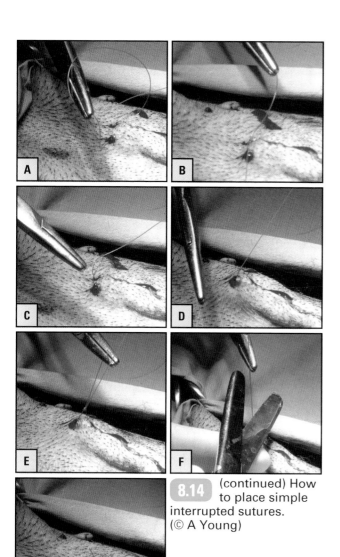

8.14 (continued) How to place simple interrupted sutures. (© A Young)

Antibiotics

Most minor surgical procedures do not require prophylactic antibiotics. Emphasis should be placed on good aseptic technique rather than the indiscriminate use of antibiotic drugs. As a general rule, antibiotics are indicated:

- In surgeries that are expected to last longer then 90 minutes
- Where there is contamination or likely contamination
- When implants are being placed.

If antibiotics are required, they should be administered perioperatively rather than postoperatively. A broad-spectrum antibiotic such as a potentiated penicillin (e.g. amoxicillin/clavulanate) or a second-generation cephalosporin (e.g. cefuroxime) should be given intravenously on induction of anaesthesia and every 2 hours thereafter, for the duration of the procedure, to ensure adequate tissue concentrations during surgery.

Advanced surgeries

With simple surgical procedures the role of the veterinary nurse can be quite limited. More advanced or complicated procedures often require a large team of people and the veterinary nurse's role can be instrumental. With such procedures good teamwork is vital and nurses should be involved in all stages, including: preoperative assessment and preparation; assisting during surgery; and postoperative care. This section aims to outline some of the more advanced surgeries commonly performed, with regards to the specialist equipment used, the general approach to the case and pre-, intra- and postoperative care.

Thoracic surgery

Thoracic procedures include: patent ductus arteriosus (PDA) ligation; lung lobectomy; pericardectomy; diaphragmatic hernia/rupture repair; and thoracoscopy.

Equipment for thoracic surgery

- Oscillating/reciprocating saw for median sternotomy.
- Thoracic retractors, e.g. Finochietto retractors (see Figure 8.17).
- Cardiac set – including long-handled and fine instruments (Metzenbaum scissors, DeBakey forceps, haemostatic forceps). Long instruments are important to enable manipulation of structures within the thorax (Figure 8.15).
- Clamps – Satinsky clamps, ductus clamps, tangential vascular clamps.
- Thoracostomy tubes (chest drains), one-way valves and gate clamps.
- Suction tubing and tips (Poole's suction tip).
- Ligature-passing forceps (e.g. Waterston).
- Surgical stapling equipment (thoracoabdominal (TA) vascular stapler).

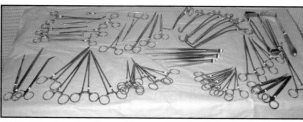

8.15 A selection of instruments for cardiac surgery. (© A Young)

Preoperative considerations

- Thoracic radiography or computed tomography (CT).
- Blood sampling.
- Drainage of any pleural fluid or air.
- Pre-oxygenation prior to anaesthesia.
- Maintenance of patient in sternal recumbency to assist ventilation during patient preparation.
- Placement of vascular access catheters, e.g. arterial and jugular catheters.

Surgical approach

Thoracic surgery is commonly performed through one of two approaches: lateral thoracotomy or median sternotomy. The approach is determined by the surgical procedure being performed.

Lateral thoracotomy

This is the most common approach and allows an excellent view of one side of the thorax. It provides access to all the thoracic organs, although access through any one rib space is limited and a rib resection may be required. A lateral thoracotomy is usually performed between two ribs; the precise rib space used is determined by the surgery to be performed (Figures 8.16 and 8.17).

Procedure	Side of thorax entered	Rib space
Patent ductus arteriosus (PDA) ligation	Left	4th
Pericardectomy	Right	5th
Left cranial lung lobectomy	Left	4th or 5th
Left caudal lung lobectomy	Left	5th or 6th
Right cranial lung lobectomy	Right	4th or 5th
Right middle lung lobectomy	Right	5th
Right caudal lung lobectomy	Right	5th or 6th

8.16   Lateral thoracotomy: side and rib space chosen for different procedures.

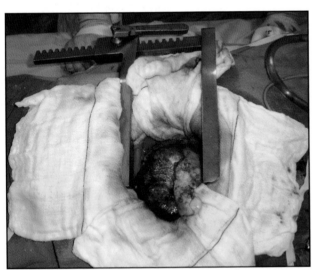

8.17   A right lateral thoracotomy performed for removal of a tumour affecting the right middle lung lobe in a dog. The ribs are being held apart with Finochietto retractors. (© M Tivers)

The skin, subcutaneous tissue and muscles overlying the rib space are incised to reveal the ribs and intercostal muscles lying between. The intercostal muscles are carefully incised to reveal the pleura (membrane surrounding the lungs). The pleura is punctured with care to avoid damaging the lungs. This should be done when the patient is breathing out (in patients that are being ventilated, the ventilation can be briefly interrupted to allow safe entry into the thorax).

Following surgery, sutures of large diameter (3 to 4 metric (2/0 to 1 USP)) synthetic absorbable material are pre-placed around the ribs either side of the incision. Once all of the sutures have been placed they are tied in turn. The muscles, subcutaneous tissue and skin are all closed in a routine fashion. A thoracostomy tube (see below) is placed before the end of surgery and used to empty the chest of air prior to recovery.

Median sternotomy

This approach is used primarily for exploration of the thorax when it might be necessary to access both sides. It is indicated for cases of pyothorax, spontaneous pneumothorax and for combined thoracic and abdominal procedures such as surgical treatment of chylothorax or repair of complicated diaphragmatic ruptures.

The patient is positioned in dorsal recumbency. A midline skin incision is made over the sternum. The muscles are dissected to reveal the sternum. The sternum is cut down the middle with a saw (a reciprocating saw is recommended). The sternum is left intact at one end to assist with postoperative healing.

Following the surgery the sternum is reconstructed using stainless steel wire (4 to 5 metric (1 to 2 USP)) or large-diameter suture material. Careful attention to rigid and accurate closure of the sternum will reduce the amount of discomfort in the postoperative period. The muscles, subcutaneous tissue and skin are all closed in a routine fashion. A thoracostomy tube (see below) is placed before the end of surgery and used to empty the chest of air prior to recovery.

Intraoperative concerns

- Monitoring anaesthesia of a critically ill patient (see Chapter 7).
- Maintenance of adequate body temperature.
- Use of a ventilator.
- Placement of a thoracic drain – this must remain open to the outside until the chest has been closed to prevent a tension pneumothorax being created.

Postoperative considerations

- All patients having thoracic surgery will benefit from oxygen supplementation in recovery.
- Removal of air and blood from the thoracic cavity via the thoracic drain.
- Close monitoring of all cardiovascular parameters during recovery phase, via capnography, pulse oximetry and electrocardiography.
- Analgesia: a multimodal approach is most appropriate using the following: systemic opioids; intrapleural block with local anaesthetic agents; systemic non-steroidal anti-inflammatory drugs (NSAIDs); and, in some cases, epidural or spinal analgesia.
- Adequate analgesia is important as patients in pain may be unable to inspire fully and this may affect oxygenation.
- Sedation and adequate bandaging of the drain may be required to prevent patient interference that could cause considerable morbidity.

Thoracostomy tubes

The placement of a thoracostomy tube (chest drain) is mandatory after most thoracic procedures. Thoracostomy tubes allow the evacuation of the pleural space following surgery, preventing excess fluid or air building up and causing respiratory difficulties. The patient can also be monitored for postoperative haemorrhage by measuring the amount and packed cell volume (PCV) of fluid produced. Thoracostomy tubes also allow local anaesthetic agents to be placed down the tube to provide additional pain relief.

Placement of thoracostomy tubes is much easier during surgery than via a closed technique. Two types of tubes are commonly used: soft silicone tubes; and stiffer polyvinylchloride tubes that have their own stylet (Figure 8.18). Tubes should be placed through a stab incision in the skin over the dorsal thoracic wall, level with the tenth to twelfth ribs. The tube is then tunnelled subcutaneously in a cranioventral direction and enters the thoracic cavity at the level of the seventh to nineth rib space. The tube is sutured in place with a Chinese finger-trap suture.

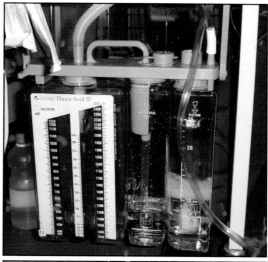

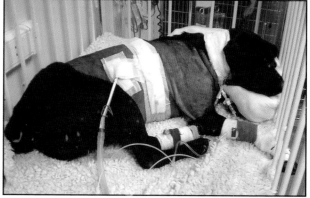

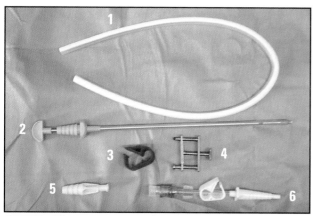

8.18   Thoracostomy tubes and connectors: (1) silicone tube; (2) polyvinylchloride drain with trocar; (3) plastic gate clamp; (4) metal gate clamp; (5) Christmas tree connector; (6) needle-free drain connector. (© A Young)

Postoperative care

Thoracostomy tubes may be drained continuously or intermittently. Continuous drainage requires a very high level of nursing care as the patient must be constantly monitored. The thoracic drain is most commonly connected to a commercially available three-bottle unit (Figure 8.19) and this in turn to a suction device. This method is used if there is a rapid production of air or fluid in the chest cavity that would be life-threatening if not continually drained. It is also used to increase the likelihood of a spontaneous sealing of a pneumothorax.

Intermittent drainage is more common and can be performed by veterinary nurses (Figures 8.20 and 8.21). It is paramount that sterility is maintained during the procedure, as the thoracic drain has the potential to track bacteria into the thorax.

The patient must have the bandage around the chest changed daily – more frequently if soiled. Patients should be supervised as closely as possible to prevent inadvertent removal or damage to the tube, and the use of an Elizabethan collar should be considered.

8.19   Thoraseal unit for continuous drainage. The drain attaches directly to the thoracostomy tube and the gate clamp remains open. (Top photograph: © M Tivers; bottom photograph: © A Young)

Equipment:
- Sterile gloves
- Sterile syringes
- Sterile three-way tap
- Injection caps/bungs
- Alcohol swabs

Procedure
The procedure requires more than one person to be present, as the patient must be suitably restrained.

1. Once the patient is restrained, the person draining the thorax should wear sterile gloves to remove the injection cap on the drain connector.
2. Swab the drain connector with an alcohol wipe before placing a three-way tap and syringe on to the connector.
3. Loosen the gate clamp and open the three-way tap.
4. Gently aspirate the chest.

> ⚠️ **WARNING**
> Extreme care must be taken at this point, as a life-threatening pneumothorax could occur if the patient were to move and the connector become detached.

5. Stop aspiration as soon as any negative pressure is felt.
6. Close the gate clamp and three-way tap and place a new sterile injection cap on the drain connector.

   How to drain a thoracostomy tube.

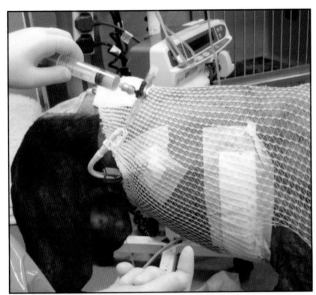

8.21 Thoracostomy tube *in situ* following lateral thoracotomy. Note the dressing covering the surgical incision to the right of the picture. The thoracostomy tube is being drained in an aseptic manner using a three-way tap attached to the tube. (© M Tivers)

Tube removal

For thoracic surgeries in which there was no pre-existing pleural effusion, the thoracostomy tube is often removed within several hours if there is minimal fluid produced. For patients with long-standing pleural space disease, such as spontaneous pneumothorax, pyothorax or chylothorax, the tube may be left in place for longer until the amount of fluid or air has reduced to a minimum. The tube itself will cause a residual volume of fluid to be produced – approximately 2 ml/kg bodyweight per day.

The Chinese finger-trap suture around the tube is removed and the drain is pulled out in one motion. Some surgeons pre-place a purse-string suture at the time of surgery, which can then be tied to close the hole in the skin. The tube stoma is then covered with a small sterile dressing.

Patent ductus arteriosus ligation

PDA is one of the most common congenital heart defects of dogs. In the embryo the ductus arteriosus shunts blood away from the fetal lungs that are not yet in use; it usually closes shortly after birth. A left-to-right shunt, the most common, causes volume overload of the left ventricle that, in time, leads to left-sided congestive heart failure. A palpable cardiac thrill and continuous grade 6/6 murmur, often called a 'machinery murmur', is sometimes present prior to ligation. It is possible to ligate the PDA surgically (see below) or an intravascular coil can be used to occlude it via a catheter placed in the femoral artery, guided by fluoroscopy.

Surgical technique

The PDA is approached through a left lateral thoracotomy at the fourth rib space. The left cranial lung lobe is reflected caudally to allow access to the heart and associated vessels. The ductus arteriosus is identified between the aorta and the pulmonary artery. The ductus is isolated by blunt dissection and two lengths of suture material are passed around the vessel. Silk or a non-absorbable monofilament synthetic suture material such as polypropylene should be used to ligate the ductus. Permanent suture materials are necessary to prevent the ductus from re-opening in the future. The ligature is tied slowly to occlude the ductus. Occlusion of the vessel can cause an increase in blood pressure and a reduction in heart rate (Brahman's reflex). This will usually resolve spontaneously but an anti-cholinergic drug such as atropine is often given to increase the heart rate. Ligation of a PDA is generally associated with an excellent outcome. However, care must be taken to avoid damaging the ductus intraoperatively as this will cause life-threatening haemorrhage.

Patient care and considerations

- These patients are often very young, sometimes only a matter of weeks old, and the care and management of glucose levels and temperature are very important.
- Aseptic management of the thoracic drain may be more difficult in a small struggling patient although typically the chest drain is often removed within a few hours of surgery.
- Initially the drain is aspirated every hour to monitor air and fluid output; this can be reduced when air/fluid is minimal until it is removed.
- Analgesia is very important to ensure these patients are comfortable and they must be monitored closely until awake and responsive.
- As these patients are usually young they often recover rapidly allowing them to be discharged relatively quickly.

Pericardectomy

This procedure is required if a patient has a pericardial effusion, most commonly caused by neoplasia, which may lead to constrictive pericardial disease, or may be performed as part of the surgical management of chylothorax. Pericardial effusion can cause right-sided heart failure with signs including lethargy, weakness, exercise intolerance and collapse and abdominal distension. Pericardiocentesis (drainage of the pericardial fluid via a needle) should be performed prior to surgery to stabilize the patient for general anaesthesia. A pericardectomy can be carried out via a median sternotomy, lateral intercostal thoracotomy or by thoracoscopy.

Surgical technique

In most cases a right lateral thoracotomy through the fifth rib space is performed. A subtotal pericardectomy is performed, ventral to the phrenic nerve. Care is taken not to damage the heart or associated vessels, particularly the vena cava. Pericardectomy also allows inspection of the heart for tumours that could have caused the effusion.

Patient care and considerations

- All patients should be monitored closely until awake and responsive, and returned to a normal temperature as soon as possible.

Portal hypertension

One of the most serious complications of shunt surgery is portal hypertension. Once the shunting vessel has been occluded, the blood flowing down the hepatic portal vein is directed towards the liver. In some patients the liver vasculature is not able to accommodate the sudden increase in blood flow and this causes accumulation of blood in the portal vein, resulting in an increase in venous pressure within the portal circulation (portal hypertension). If left, portal hypertension would cause ascites, intestinal ischaemia and death. Patients are monitored intraoperatively for signs of portal hypertension, including intestinal hypermotility and intestinal and pancreatic cyanosis. Portal blood pressure can be measured through a jejunal catheter (often the same one that was placed for the portovenogram). This allows the blood pressure to be measured before and after ligation and compared, so that a decision can be made on whether the shunt can be fully ligated. If portal pressures are too high, the shunt is partially ligated. A repeat surgery 3 months later usually allows for full ligation of the shunt. Gradual occlusion techniques including ameroid constrictors and cellophane banding are designed to occlude the vessel slowly and thus avoid the risk of portal hypertension as the blood flow to the liver increases gradually.

Patient care and considerations

- Patients that undergo shunt ligation are often young, and small because of their condition. Hepatic function is reduced in these cases. This results in decreased gluconeogenesis, decreased heat production and reduced drug metabolism. These patients are at risk of hypoglycaemia and hypothermia.
- NSAIDs should be avoided and other drugs such as opioids should be given with care. Typically, the dose should not be reduced, but the interval between dosing should be increased.
- These patients should be monitored closely for approximately 3 days postoperatively as there are many potential postoperative complications of shunt ligation. The most concerning of these is portal hypertension (see above): signs include a distended or painful abdomen, haemorrhagic diarrhoea, tachycardia, hypotension and ascites. A tape measure may be used to monitor abdominal girth to assess for abdominal distension due to ascites, although a small amount of ascites is common after shunt ligation.
- Patients should also be monitored for neurological deterioration. In most cases this will be limited to temporary blindness or 'twitchiness' but in other patients it may result in status epilepticus that can be extremely difficult to manage and may lead to death or require euthanasia.

Gastrointestinal surgery

Small intestinal surgery is most commonly required for patients with gastrointestinal obstruction, e.g. foreign bodies (Figure 8.29) or masses. It can also be used as

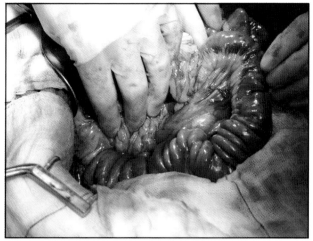

8.29 Exploratory laparotomy in a dog with a linear foreign body. Note how the intestine appears corrugated where it has become 'bunched up' along the foreign body. The foreign body was successfully removed and was an elastic toy! (© M Tivers)

a diagnostic procedure (exploratory laparotomy and intestinal biopsy). Partial thickness gastrointestinal biopsies can be obtained via endoscopy but in some cases this may not be possible or samples may be non-diagnostic. Laparotomy allows full-thickness biopsy at multiple sites along the intestine using a scalpel blade or a skin biopsy punch.

Intestinal foreign bodies are normally removed by making an incision into the intestine (enterotomy) over the foreign body. Linear foreign bodies (such as string or material) may require several enterotomies to remove them.

End-to-end anastomosis, the joining of two pieces of intestine, may be required when a piece of intestine needs to be removed if it has been damaged by a foreign body, intussusception or neoplasia.

Surgical procedure

A routine exploratory laparotomy is performed. Separate instruments should be used when entering the gastrointestinal tract, to prevent contamination of the remainder of the surgical kit. Sometimes this takes the form of a second kit (gastrointestinal kit) which is used in conjunction with a regular kit (Figure 8.30). The first kit is used to open the abdomen and during the exploratory laparotomy. When surgery is performed on the gastrointestinal tract this kit is moved away and the gastrointestinal kit moved in for the 'dirty' procedure. The gastrointestinal tract should be packed off using moist surgical swabs to prevent contamination of the abdominal cavity if gross spillage of intestinal contents occurs. When the surgery is complete the abdomen is lavaged with copious amounts of warmed lavage solution, e.g. normal saline or Hartmann's, which is then removed using suction. The veterinary surgeons then move the gastrointestinal set away, change their gloves and return to using the original kit to close with. This technique of using two kits can also be used when removing a tumour to help prevent spread of neoplastic cells. It may not be possible to have a dedicated gastrointestinal kit but using a few separate instruments is usually sufficient.

Common conditions and surgical treatment:

- Brachycephalic obstructive airway syndrome (BOAS):
    - Elongated soft palate – soft palate resection
    - Everted laryngeal saccules – saccule removal
    - Stenotic nares – rhinoplasty.
- Laryngeal collapse – permanent tracheostomy
- Idiopathic acquired laryngeal paralysis – unilateral arytenoid lateralization ('tie back')
- Temporary tracheostomy.

Equipment for URT surgery

- **Long instruments – Metzenbaum scissors, clamps, forceps.**
- **Tracheostomy tubes (Figure 8.32).**
- **Retractors – Gelpi, Senn.**

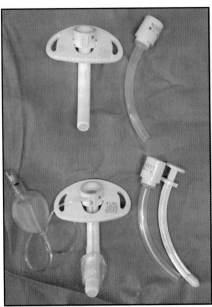

8.32 Tracheostomy tubes. The bottom, cuffed, tube would be used when anaesthetizing or ventilating patients with a tracheostomy tube in place. (© A Young)

Preoperative considerations

- Stabilization of condition – oxygen therapy, body temperature control, administration of corticosteroids.
- Thoracic radiography.
- Emergency tracheostomy.
- Patient sedation to reduce distress.

Intraoperative concerns

- Haemorrhage.
- Swelling.
- Anaesthetic considerations – access to airway.
- Position of veterinary surgeons at operating table – limited access for anaesthetists.

Postoperative considerations

- Anaesthetic recovery – this is the most risky stage as the patient regains control of its airway.
- Analgesia – may cause drowsiness and depress respiration.
- Supplemental oxygen therapy.
- Feeding regimes.

- Position in ward during recovery.
- Avoidance of pressure around the neck.
- Care of tracheostomy tube.

BOAS surgery

Inherited anatomical features mean that it is very common for brachycephalic breeds such as the English Bulldog to require surgery to alleviate URT obstruction. The problem often increases in severity as the dog becomes older. In extreme cases dogs with BOAS can be presented in respiratory distress, especially on hot days, after exercise or long car journeys. Affected dogs may exhibit one or a combination of stenotic nares, overlong soft palate, everted laryngeal saccules and laryngeal collapse. Surgical treatment is designed to correct the underlying problem and should be performed as soon as the problem is identified, as the condition will progress. One or all of the procedures listed above may be carried out on the patient to improve its airway. These patients may be presented in an emergency situation and require immediate treatment to relieve the obstruction via anaesthesia and endotracheal or tracheostomy tube placement.

Surgical technique

The dog's airway is assessed to identify which problems are contributing to the respiratory obstruction. Stenotic nares are enlarged by removing a wedge of tissue, thus enlarging the nostril. The soft palate is assessed; if long, the redundant edge of the soft palate is resected and oversewn. If the laryngeal saccules are everted they are grasped with forceps and resected with scissors. There is no satisfactory surgical treatment for laryngeal collapse. Permanent tracheostomy may be indicated in affected animals to bypass their larynx.

Some surgeons perform a temporary tracheostomy routinely prior to the surgeries outlined above. This is especially true in small breeds. Not only does this provide the animal with a secure airway for recovery but also obviates the need for endotracheal intubation via the mouth and hence reduces interference with the surgical field.

Patient care and considerations

- Postoperatively, patients should be monitored closely, with oxygen therapy close by.
- Patients should remain intubated for as long as possible during recovery and staff should be prepared for an emergency tracheostomy or re-intubation if required.
- Suction machines and catheters should be readily available during recovery.
- Corticosteroids may be given preoperatively to reduce any swelling but if not they may be required postoperatively.
- Patients should be kept calm, cool and rested and not have leads placed around their necks.
- Analgesia is required and may help to keep the patient calm and sedated. Agitated patients may require sedation to calm them down and reduce the risk of respiratory distress.
- Depending on the location of surgery, food may be offered on complete recovery or up to 12–24 hours postoperatively to allow healing and a reduction in swelling.

Unilateral arytenoid lateralization ('tie back')

During normal breathing the larynx opens when the animal breathes in (inspiration), thus enlarging the airway. Laryngeal paralysis is the failure of the larynx (more specifically the arytenoid cartilages) to move during normal inspiration, which leads to obstruction of the airway. It can be congenital, although acquired is more common and affects older, large-breed dogs. Signs of change in bark, progressive inspiratory stridor and exercise intolerance are often noted by the owner. Investigation includes examination of the larynx under a very light plane of anaesthesia. If the larynx does not open during inspiration, a diagnosis of laryngeal paralysis can be made.

Surgical procedure

The dog is placed in right lateral recumbency. A lateral approach is made to the left-hand side of the larynx. Single or multiple sutures are placed through the cartilages of the larynx to hold it in an open position. Sutures are placed between the arytenoid cartilage and the thyroid cartilage and/or the arytenoid cartilage and the cricoid cartilage. This abducts the arytenoid cartilage and holds the larynx in an open position. The patient is extubated prior to recovery and the larynx checked to ensure that it has been fixed in an open position. The patient is then re-intubated and recovered as normal. Surgery is normally performed on one side only; if both sides of the larynx are abducted there is an increased risk of aspiration pneumonia.

Patient care and considerations

- Preoperatively, these patients may be presented in an emergency situation, especially if it is a hot day and the patient has travelled in a hot car or been excessively exercised. Patients in respiratory distress should be sedated and cooled. In some cases patients may require intubation if sedation is ineffective at reducing respiratory distress.
- Postoperatively, these patients must be closely monitored for signs of obstruction due to haemorrhage or swelling.
- Recovery should preferably be in a frequently observed area of a quiet ward to allow constant monitoring. Equipment for emergency intubation, including drugs to induce anaesthesia and small endotracheal tubes, should be close by. A suction machine and oxygen supplementation should also be readily available.
- Sedation postoperatively may be required if the patient continues to bark or gets too stressed or excited. Barking causes sudden outbursts of air, which may pull the sutures through the cartilage. Suture failure may also occur with excessive panting.
- Patients should be kept calm and cool and a harness used to walk them, avoiding leads or collars around the neck. They should not be left unattended for long periods in case they bark or become too excited.
- Food is often withheld for 24 hours post-operatively and then small amounts of a soft sticky food that can be formed into balls can be introduced and fed slowly by hand from a height. This reduces the risk of inhalation of food and hence aspiration pneumonia. Liquid foods, such as milk and gravy, and very soft food should be avoided for at least 6 weeks after surgery.

Temporary tracheostomy

Temporary tracheostomy is performed to bypass the URT for a number of reasons. It is primarily used as an emergency measure in patients in acute respiratory distress due to functional or anatomical airway obstruction (e.g. BOAS, laryngeal mass lesion, laryngeal foreign body, laryngeal paralysis). It can be an elective measure in anticipation of upper airway surgery or extensive oropharyngeal surgery when the endotracheal tube may interfere with surgical access. It may also be used in patients undergoing airway surgery in which excessive swelling or difficulties on recovery are anticipated (bulldogs undergoing BOAS surgery).

Surgery is ideally performed in an anaesthetized patient with endotracheal intubation. It is extremely rare to have to perform a 'slash tracheotomy' in a conscious patient. The patient is placed in dorsal recumbency and the ventral neck is clipped and prepared for surgery. A ventral midline skin incision is made and the muscles of the neck are divided along the midline. A horizontal incision is made between the tracheal rings (between rings four and five). The incision should not be more than 40% of the circumference of the trachea. Long stay sutures are placed around the rings above and below the incision and the tracheostomy tube inserted (Figure 8.33). The stay sutures facilitate replacement of the tube should it accidentally be removed in the conscious patient. The skin incision is closed cranial and caudal to the tube, which is secured with a length of bandage placed around the neck.

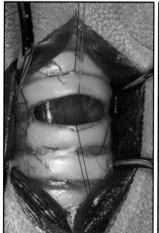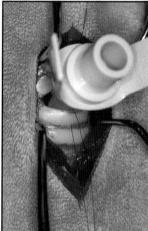

8.33 Tracheostomy tube placement (see text for details). (© SJ Baines)

Patients with tracheostomy tubes need to be monitored at all times and **on no occasion should they be left unattended** as the tube may become blocked with secretions or may fall out, particularly if the patient interferes with it. Small diameter suction tubing can be used to clear mucus or secretions from the tube. Nebulization may be helpful to keep the airway moist and prevent the build up of tenacious secretions. Replacement tubes and suitable sedation or anaesthetic agents should be kept nearby in case the tube needs to be replaced in an emergency. The tube can be removed once the patient is stable and fully recovered from surgery. The wound is left to heal by secondary intention.

Neurosurgery

Neurosurgery is most commonly performed on the spinal cord. Intracranial surgery may also be performed at specialist centres. The postoperative nursing of patients that have undergone neurosurgery can be extremely intensive. Patients may be recumbent for weeks or even months, and considerable time and effort is necessary to nurse them and to ensure a good return to normal function. However, the successful management of these patients can be extremely rewarding.

Procedures include: spinal surgery (hemilaminectomy, dorsal laminectomy, ventral slot); intracranial surgery; and surgery of atlantoaxial subluxation.

Equipment for neurological surgery

- **High-speed air bur.**
- **Retractors – odd-leg Gelpi, Adson-baby, Gosset.**
- **Rongeurs.**
- **Selection of probes, hooks and curettes.**
- **Suction and small flexible suction tip.**
- **Saline lavage solution.**
- **Bone wax and other haemostatic agents.**

Pre-operative considerations

- Analgesia.
- Care on handling, moving and lifting the patient, especially if there is suspicion of spinal fracture or head injury.
- Myelography or magnetic resonance imaging (MRI).
- Urgency of surgery – emergency or elective.
- Urinary retention.

Intraoperative concerns

- Careful positioning of unstable vertebral column.
- Analgesia – surgical procedures are stimulating.
- Ventilation – may be required if high doses of opiates are used, dependent on the location of injury along the spinal cord.

Postoperative considerations

- Analgesia.
- Bladder care and management.
- Fluid therapy.
- Physiotherapy/hydrotherapy.
- No pressure (leads or collars) around the neck.

Spinal surgery

Spinal surgery is indicated for neurological defects as a result of spinal cord compression. This is most commonly due to intervertebral disc disease and less commonly due to neoplasia. Spinal cord surgery is also performed for trauma (spinal fractures), discospondylitis and congenital malformations. The degree of compression corresponds to the severity of the clinical signs. The first clinical sign of spinal cord compression is pain. This progresses to paresis (weakness), paralysis, loss of bladder function and then loss of deep pain sensation. Patients with mild signs (pain and weakness) may respond well to conservative management (rest and anti-inflammatory agents) but surgery is indicated in more severely affected patients or in those that deteriorate. The location of the injury corresponds to the limbs involved: in simple terms, this means that a lesion in the cervical spine will affect the thoracic and pelvic limbs, whereas a lesion in the thoracolumbar spine will affect the pelvic limbs.

Preoperative care and assessment

- Lesion localization is vital in the management of all neurological patients. It is very important in patients with spinal compression to determine the likely area affected and guide further investigation and treatment:
  - A full neurological examination is performed by a veterinary surgeon to determine the severity and location of the spinal cord compression
  - Further imaging is required to determine the precise location of the lesion and the cause. MRI remains the gold standard for imaging the nervous system. However, when this is not available myelography is a good alternative. Myelography involves the injection of a contrast agent around the spinal cord, thus highlighting it on a radiograph
  - In some patients a sample of cerebrospinal fluid may be taken for analysis.
- The timing of surgery is very important and depends on the severity of the lesion:
  - Patients with acute onset of clinical signs or rapid deterioration will benefit from early surgical intervention
  - Although conservative management can be used successfully in dogs with very mild clinical signs, surgery is indicated for patients that are non-ambulatory. In general non-ambulatory patients should have surgery within 24 hours for optimum success
  - Those that have lost deep pain sensation have a much worse prognosis and constitute a surgical emergency. These patients should be operated on as soon as possible
  - Dogs with a more chronic course of disease can be investigated and treated in a more elective fashion.

Surgical procedures

The type of surgery performed will depend on the location of the lesion. Spinal cord compression most commonly results from a disc prolapse ('slipped disc'). In veterinary patients this normally takes one of two forms:

- Type I: Disc extrusion – The disc capsule (annulus fibrosus) ruptures, releasing the calcified

contents (nucleus pulposus) into the spinal canal, which thus compresses the cord. This is most common in chondrodystrophic breeds such as the Dachshund
■ Type II: Disc protrusion – The disc undergoes chronic changes and bulges into the spinal canal, which thus compresses the cord.

The aim of the surgery is to remove the disc material from the spinal canal. Thus the surgeries all aim to produce a 'window' through the bone of the vertebra into the spinal canal. *Hemilaminectomy* is the unilateral removal of the lamina, articular facets and portions of the pedicle of the affected vertebrae in order to reach the spinal cord and remove the disc material that is compressing it; patients are usually positioned in sternal recumbency, and the procedure is commonly performed for disc prolapse in the thoracolumbar (T/L) region (Figure 8.34). *Dorsal laminectomy* is the removal of the dorsal spinous processes and portions of the lamina, articular facets and pedicles of the affected vertebrae; disc prolapses in the lumbosacral (L/S) region are usually treated via this approach. *Ventral slot* surgeries create a window in the ventral aspect of a cervical intervertebral space in order to inspect the ventral spinal canal; they are commonly performed in the cervical spine, with the patient in dorsal recumbency with the neck extended.

Patient care and considerations

■ Analgesia is required peri- and postoperatively. Opioids such as morphine or methadone should be used with NSAIDs, provided that glucocorticoid steroids were not used during the initial treatment.
■ Patients should be handled with care and have cage rest for the first 24–48 hours, followed by limited exercise for the first few days, carrying or using a trolley to take the patient out to urinate/defecate. Paraplegic and quadriplegic patients will need assistance to exercise. For animals with pelvic limb paralysis, a sling placed under the abdomen may be sufficient to facilitate walking (Figure 8.35); larger or quadriplegic dogs may require multiple slings or the use of a hoist to allow them to go outside.
■ Patients should have adequate, soft bedding to prevent pressure sores and skin ulceration.
■ Bladder function may be affected if hindlimb paralysis is present due to nerve compression. Such patients may need to have their bladders emptied by percutaneous compression or may have an indwelling urinary catheter placed. Recumbent patients are at risk of urinary tract infection (UTI) due to urine stasis. An indwelling urinary catheter may be very useful in larger recumbent patients as it will facilitate nursing, but it will also increase the risk of a UTI. Urinary catheters should be connected to a sterile closed collecting system, as this will reduce the risk of ascending infection and facilitate management. Patients should be monitored for signs of UTI, such as change in urine colour or odour, changes on urinalysis, changes in patient's demeanour or pyrexia. If a UTI is suspected, a urine sample should be submitted for culture and sensitivity testing; treatment should be based on the results.
■ It is important to consider the patient's dietary requirements; hand-feeding or tempting to eat and drink may be necessary, especially if recumbent.

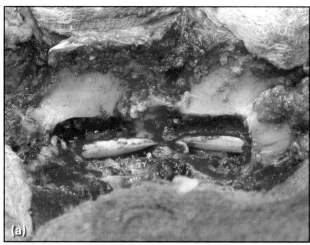

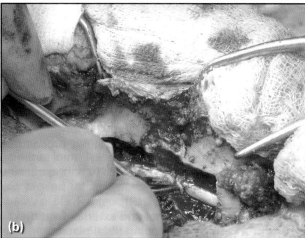

8.34 **(a)** The spinal cord during a hemilaminectomy; note the compression of the cord by disc material. **(b)** The cord after decompression. (© A Young)

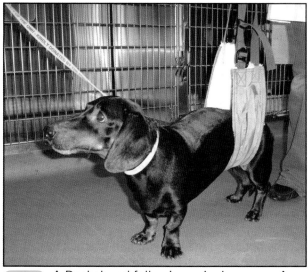

8.35 A Dachshund following spinal surgery. A sling is used to aid walking. (© M Tivers)

Equipment for placing screws through a boneplate

- Drill.
- Plate-bending irons.
- Fracture reduction forceps.
- Drill guide (Figure 8.41).
- Depth gauge (Figure 8.41).
- Tap and tap sleeve (Figure 8.41).
- Selection of screws.
- Screwdriver (Figure 8.41).

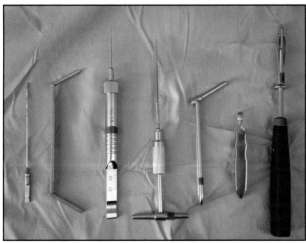

8.41 Left to right, in order of use when placing a screw: drill bit and drill guide; depth gauge; tap and tap sleeve; screw forceps; screwdriver with sleeve. (© A Young)

Placing a boneplate:

1. The plate is contoured to fit the bone across the fracture.
2. The fracture is held in reduction and the plate is held over the fracture site.
3. A hole is drilled in the bone through one of the holes in the plate using a drill guide. Note: if using a DCP then a special guide is used (unless self-tapping screws are used).
4. The depth of the screw hole is measured using a depth gauge.
5. A thread is cut in the bone using a tap and guide.
6. A screw of the appropriate diameter and length is chosen and placed in the screw hole.
7. The procedure is repeated until all of the holes (or sufficient holes) are filled.

External fixation

External skeletal fixation uses a series of pins placed perpendicular to the long-axis(es) of the bone(s). The pins are placed through stab incisions in the skin and then connected by clamps to connecting bars that form a rigid frame. Several systems are available (e.g. Kirschner–Ehmer, Securos, Imex) and in each the clamps and connecting bars come in different sizes to accommodate bones of different sizes. A simple frame will consist of pins and clamps on one side of the leg (uniplanar, unilateral; Figure 8.42). More complicated frames can consist of pins and clamps on

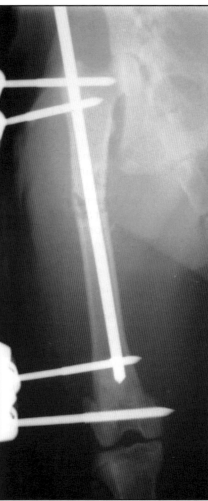

8.42 Cat with a fracture of the right femur following a road traffic accident. The femur has been repaired with an external skeletal fixator and intramedullary pin. The clamps have been covered with pink bandaging material. (© M Tivers)

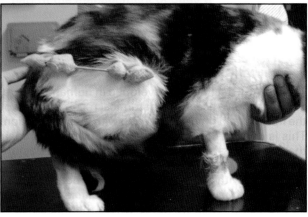

opposite sides of the leg (uniplanar, bilateral) or even on three sides in a triangular arrangement (biplanar, bilateral). Ring fixators or Ilizarov fixators are more complicated frames which use wires under tension and circular frames. These fixators are mainly used for the correction of angular limb deformities.

Epoxy putty or methylmethacrylate may be used instead of clamps in very small patients or for fractures that are in a difficult position, such as metacarpal/metatarsal or mandibular fractures (Figure 8.43).

Although external fixators provide less rigid stabilization of the fracture, they have several advantages over internal fixation:

- The bone heals in a slightly different way, which may result in more rapid healing

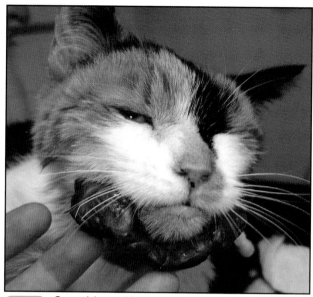

8.43 Cat with multiple mandibular fractures repaired using an external fixator constructed with epoxy putty. (© M Tivers)

- In some cases it is possible to place the fixator without disturbing the fracture site, with less damage to soft tissue structures
- The fixators are very adaptable – pins and clamps can be removed or added as necessary. This means that the fixator can be 'downstaged' as the fracture heals, to allow more weight through the fracture site and encourage further healing
- External fixators are very useful in fractures associated with wounds, as the pins can be placed away from the wounds and thus avoid the risk of infection; the fixator also allows continued access to the wound for management.

Patient care and considerations

- Pre- and postoperatively, adequate analgesia needs to be given; opioids and NSAIDs are often used.
- Radiographs are taken postoperatively to assess fracture reduction and the placement of the implants.
- Patients should have strict cage rest initially, with assistance to take them out to urinate/defecate if appropriate. The kennel should allow room to be comfortable but not so big that the patient can run or jump.
- Soft, comfortable bedding is important as the patient may be recumbent and spend the majority of their time lying on the unaffected side.
- It is important to take care of the whole patient, especially if the fracture is due to trauma. There may be bruising, trauma to other areas of the body, or skin wounds that require treatment in addition to the fracture repair.
- Dogs may have strict lead walks for toilet purposes only. Larger dogs may benefit from sling walking initially.
- In some cases it is important to encourage the patient to use its limb to ensure a good outcome (in particular femoral fractures). This can take the form of gentle physiotherapy and/or gentle

exercise. The patient should start to use the affected limb by 3–5 days postoperatively. If it does not use the limb then it should be re-examined to check for any postoperative complications.
- Patients are typically discharged from the hospital when they are comfortable. They should have instructions for strict rest (cage rest for cats and small dogs).
- Patients should be re-examined 6–8 weeks after surgery, using repeat radiographs to assess fracture healing. This should be repeated until radiographic evidence of fracture healing is seen. The length of time the fracture takes to heal will depend on a variety of factors, including location, severity, method of repair and the age of the patient. Fractures take longer to heal in older patients. Once the fracture has healed satisfactorily the patient can resume full exercise.

Internal fixation

- Internal fixation does not normally require any additional postoperative care.
- Most surgeons do not routinely remove internal implants; however, once the fracture has healed they may be removed if they are causing a problem.

External fixation

- A dressing is usually placed on the limb to reduce any swelling associated with the pins. This is usually changed after 24 hours. The leg should not need to be dressed for longer than 2–3 days.
- Once the surgeon is happy that there is no significant swelling, the ends of the pins and clamps are covered in bandage material to prevent inadvertent injury to the patient, the owner or the owners' furniture!
- It is important to monitor the pin tracts (where the pins enter the skin) for any discharge. A small amount of serous discharge is normal and will form a light scab around the pin tract, which should be left in place. A persistent discharge or an obviously purulent discharge may indicate an infection and would warrant further veterinary attention.

Arthroscopy

This is the use of a rigid endoscope to examine and treat joints. It allows a joint to be examined without the trauma of an arthrotomy and in less surgical time, and is a diagnostic procedure as well as a therapeutic one. Throughout the procedure isotonic fluid such as Hartmann's or saline is constantly flushed through the joint to allow a good view of the joint being examined. Elbows and shoulders are most commonly 'scoped', although stifles, hips and hocks can also be examined. Probes, grasping forceps, curettes and hand burs are used through additional ports into the joint to allow the removal of bone fragments or cartilage. Elbow arthroscopy is commonly performed for the diagnosis and treatment of elbow dysplasia (specifically fragmentation of the coronoid process and less commonly osteochondritis dissecans of the medial humeral condyle and un-united anconeal process). Further details are in Chapter 10 and in the *BSAVA Manual of Canine and Feline Endoscopy and Endosurgery.*

Patient care and considerations

- These are often short procedures and so antibiotic cover is usually not required.
- Opioid analgesia is continued in the immediate postoperative period and patients are usually prescribed a long course of NSAIDs.

Conclusion

This chapter illustrates the vital role a veterinary nurse plays in the treatment and care of surgical patients. Everyone has their role within the team but ultimately it is teamwork that provides a positive outcome for the patient.

A wide range of procedures, which may be seen in a veterinary hospital, have been discussed. Although some are very specialized, veterinary nurses that have achieved or are working towards their surgical diploma will be able to apply their knowledge and skills to each situation. Knowledge of the procedures and equipment will benefit the patient in a number of ways. Surgeries that are organized and run smoothly result in a better outcome than those that are not, and shorter surgery and anaesthesia times can contribute to faster recoveries.

The surgical team also extends to the veterinary nurses working in the ward area for the recovery and rehabilitation phase. Knowledge of the procedure by the ward veterinary nurses is important to understand why and how the patient is responding to treatment that is dependent on the initial surgical procedure.

References and further reading

Anderson D and Smith J (2007) Surgical nursing. In: *BSAVA Textbook of Veterinary Nursing, 4th edn*, ed. DR Lane et al., pp. 590–639. BSAVA Publications, Gloucester

Brockman D and Holt D (2005) *BSAVA Manual of Canine and Feline Head, Neck and Thoracic Surgery.* BSAVA Publications, Gloucester

Coughlan A and Miller A (2006) *BSAVA Manual of Small Animal Fracture Repair and Management.* BSAVA Publications, Gloucester

Denny H and Butterworth S (2000) *A Guide to Canine and Feline Orthopaedic Surgery, 4th edn.* Blackwell Science, Oxford

Fossum T (2002) *Small Animal Surgery, 2nd edn.* Mosby, St Louis

Hoad J (2006) *Minor Veterinary Surgery: A Handbook for Veterinary Nurses.* Butterworth Heinemann/Elsevier, Philadelphia

Houlton JEF, Cook JL, Innes JF and Langley-Hobbs S (2006) *BSAVA Manual of Canine and Feline Musculoskeletal Disorders.* BSAVA Publications, Gloucester

Martin C and Masters J (2007) *Textbook of Veterinary Surgical Nursing.* Butterworth Heinemann/Elsevier, Philadelphia

McHugh D (2007) Theatre practice. In: *BSAVA Textbook of Veterinary Nursing, 4th edn*, ed. DR Lane et al., pp. 561–589. BSAVA Publications, Gloucester

Platt S and Olby N (2004) *BSAVA Manual of Canine and Feline Neurology, 3rd edn.* BSAVA Publications, Gloucester

Scott K and Hotston Moore A (2007) Surgical nursing. In: *BSAVA Manual of Practical Veterinary Nursing*, ed. E Mullineaux and M Jones, pp. 315–370. BSAVA Publications, Gloucester

Slatter D (2003) *Textbook of Small Animal Surgery, 3rd edn.* Mosby, St Louis

Williams J and Moores A (in press) *BSAVA Manual of Canine and Feline Wound Management and Reconstruction, 2nd edn.* BSAVA Publications, Gloucester

Williams J and Niles J (2005) *BSAVA Manual of Canine and Feline Abdominal Surgery.* BSAVA Publications, Gloucester

9

Dentistry

Lisa Milella and Maureen Helm

This chapter is designed to give information on:

- The importance of dental health in dogs and cats
- The role of the veterinary nurse in dental treatment
- The role of the veterinary nurse in client education for oral health

Introduction

Dentistry is one of the most important aspects of veterinary healthcare alongside vaccination and medical care. A high proportion of dogs and cats >3 years old are affected by periodontal disease; routine veterinary dentistry treatment is not only prophylactic but also involves treating existing disease and stopping or slowing down the progression of periodontal disease. In other cases, painful conditions can be alleviated which may not have been noticed by the owner and/or may have been mistaken as a 'normal' ageing process. It is no longer acceptable to ignore these problems or to treat them as minor or secondary problems to be dealt with at the same time as other surgical procedures.

Veterinary oral healthcare needs to be a team effort and neither the veterinary surgeon nor the veterinary nurse alone can take on the role of providing all the dental treatment that the pet will need. The diagnosis of dental disease and surgical treatment are defined as acts of veterinary surgery and so need to be performed by a veterinary surgeon. However, veterinary nurses play a vital role in dentistry in small animal practice. The Royal College of Veterinary Surgeons (RCVS) advises that veterinary nurses are not allowed to perform extractions, but should be able to perform a thorough oral examination, record the findings on a dental chart, take intraoral dental radiographs, perform periodontal therapy (excluding periodontal surgery) and, perhaps the most important role, offer instruction in homecare and ongoing oral hygiene. Although oral surgery, including extraction, is an act of veterinary surgery, it is important that the veterinary nurse understands what the procedures involve, potential complications and the postoperative nursing care that the patient may require following treatment.

Dental terminology

Apical	**Towards the root**
Buccal	**Surface of the tooth towards the cheeks**
Coronal	**Towards the crown**
Distal	**Surface of the tooth away from the front midline**
Interproximal	**Surface between two teeth**
Labial	**Surface of the tooth towards the lips**
Lingual	**Surface of the tooth towards the tongue**
Mesial	**Surface of the tooth towards the front midline**
Occlusal	**Surface of the tooth facing the opposite jaw**
Palatal	**Surface of the tooth towards the palate**

Dental anatomy

Knowledge of the normal anatomy is important to be able to identify and differentiate pathology and any abnormalities occurring in the oral cavity. It also helps with the understanding of the disease processes occurring in the mouth.

Dental formulae

In all species, the number and type of teeth in the mouth can be simply described by the dental formula. In this form, the incisors, canines, premolars and molars are represented by letters (e.g. PM for premolar) and the upper and lower/left and right arcades are represented by numbers (Figure 9.1).

Dog	Deciduous dentition	2 x (I 3/3, C 1/1, PM 3/3) = 28
	Permanent dentition	2 x (I 3/3, C 1/1, PM 4/4, M 2/3) = 42
Cat	Deciduous dentition	2 x (I 3/3, C 1/1, PM 3/2) = 26
	Permanent dentition	2 x (I 3/3, C 1/1, PM 3/2, M 1/1) = 30

9.1 Dental formulae for dogs and cats.

Eruption times

The age at which both deciduous (primary) and permanent teeth erupt is well documented and this knowledge is important in assessing dental development, particularly in young animals. In contrast with other species (notably the horse), the sequence is somewhat variable and cannot be used to age the animal with any reliability. Eruption times in the dog and cat are detailed in Figure 9.2.

Tooth	Tooth eruption (time in weeks)			
	Puppy (deciduous dentition)	Dog (permanent dentition)	Kitten (deciduous dentition)	Cat (permanent dentition)
Incisor	3–6	12–16	2–4	11–16
Canine	3–5	16–24	3–4	16–20
Premolar	4–12	14–24	3–6	16–24
Molar	NA	18–28	NA	16–24

9.2 Eruption times in dogs and cats.

Structure and function

Although the teeth vary in appearance, the anatomical layout is similar for all and is represented in Figure 9.3. Each part of the tooth has particular properties and functions.

Enamel

This is the hardest substance in the body and covers the crown of the tooth. It has no nerve or blood supply. Enamel in dogs and cats is only about 0.5 mm thick. If the enamel is damaged or inadequately formed during development, it may result in faster wear of the tooth and may result in bacterial ingress through the dentinal tubules, resulting in pulp necrosis.

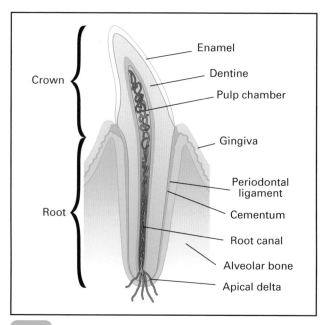

9.3 Incisor tooth structure.

Dentine

The bulk of the tooth is made up of dentine. This has a tubular structure with odontoblastic processes extending the width of the dentine, from the pulp to almost the junction with the enamel. Dentine continues to be produced throughout the life of the animal by the odontoblasts that line the pulp cavity and fill the tubules. If trauma occurs to the tooth, tertiary dentine is laid down faster than secondary dentine is formed after eruption of the tooth, and in a less organized manner to repair the defect and protect the pulp.

Pulp

The pulp cavity is the centre of the tooth containing nerves, blood and lymph vessels, and connective tissue. It is lined by odontoblasts, which produce the dentine. In young animals the cavity is very wide and narrows as the animal ages. The pulp cavity in the crown is referred to as the pulp chamber and in the root, the root canal. The pulp terminates at the apex where the vessels exit/enter the tooth via a delta rather than a single foramen.

Cementum

This is a bone-like structure that covers the root surface. It has no blood supply and acts as part of the attachment structure holding the tooth in place. In most healthy teeth it covers the root up to the junction with the enamel. The cells that produce cementum are called cementocytes. Cementum is capable of repair and resorption and is continually being remodelled.

Periodontal ligament

The periodontal ligament is derived from connective tissue and attaches the cementum to the alveolar bone. The ligament lines the alveolar socket in interwoven strands allowing movement, which gives the tooth a small amount of protection by absorbing some impact when biting down. The periodontal ligament has pain and pressure receptors.

Alveolar bone

This is the bone holding and supporting the teeth. The socket within the bone in which the root is seated is known as the alveolar socket or alveolus.

Gingiva

The gingiva is the specialized oral mucosa that surrounds the tooth. The gingiva can be subdivided into the free gingiva and the attached gingiva. The free gingiva is the edge of the gingiva that is not directly attached to the tooth and separated from the tooth by the gingival sulcus. The gingival sulcus is a 'normal' partial loss of the attachment of the junctional epithelium to the crown. This can be as deep as 3 mm in large dogs. The depth of the sulcus is considered pathological when there is apical migration of the junctional epithelium and attachment to the root. The attached gingiva extends from the free gingival margin to the junction with the alveolar mucosa. The attached gingiva is tightly adhered to the underlying periosteum.

Surrounding structures

There are also some important anatomical structures surrounding the oral cavity (Figure 9.4) to consider when performing dentistry, in order to avoid iatrogenic injury and also to understand the potential involvement of the extraoral tissues in disease processes.

- Orbit: the base of the orbit lies just above the upper molars, and care must be taken to avoid slipping with instruments during extraction of these teeth, which may result in penetration of the eye.
- Nasal cavity: the maxillary incisors, canines and premolars are located in very close proximity to the nasal cavity, and in some areas only a thin layer of bone separates the tooth from the nasal cavity. Care should be taken to avoid accidentally pushing the roots medially into the nasal cavity during extraction or to otherwise damage the bone separating the tooth roots and nasal cavity. In some disease processes the bone may already be destroyed by infection.

- Inferior alveolar canal (mandibular canal): this houses the neurovascular bundle supplying the teeth of the mandible. It runs within the mandible just below the apices of the tooth roots. Care should be taken to avoid damaging the canal during fracture repair, and accidental displacement of tooth roots should be avoided during extraction.
- Foramina: the infraorbital foramen is situated above the mesial root of the third maxillary premolar where the neurovascular bundle exits. The mental foramina are situated below the mandibular incisors, at the apex of the lower canine, and distally below the third premolar. Care must be taken to avoid these structures during dental surgery.

Instrumentation

In order to perform a thorough oral examination and good quality dental work, the correct instruments should be available. A sterile set of instruments should be used for each patient. The instruments must also be cared for properly and sharpened correctly when necessary.

Instruments used for oral examination

The instruments required for an oral examination include (Figure 9.5):

- Periodontal probes
- Dental explorer probes.

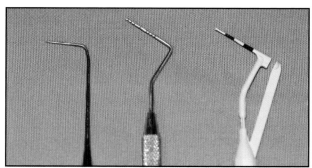

9.5 Instruments used for an oral examination (left to right): explorer probe; periodontal probe; and periodontal teaching probe.

Periodontal probe

The periodontal probe is a blunt-ended instrument with graduations on the tip for measuring. The probe is used to examine the periodontal attachment of the tooth. It is used to measure the depth of periodontal pockets, gingival recession, gingival hyperplasia, bone loss between roots, and can be used to assess mobility of the tooth. Training probes are available that allow the user to gauge the pressure used when probing, so that excessive force or pressure is not used unknowingly. The whole circumference of the tooth should be probed gently to assess loss of attachment without causing damage to the tissues. The probe must be held correctly to allow detailed examination without excessive trauma (Figure 9.6).

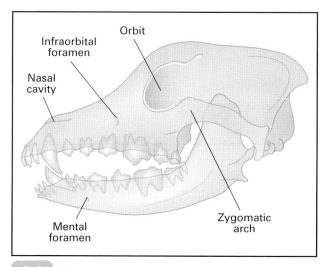

Orbit
Infraorbital foramen
Nasal cavity
Mental foramen
Zygomatic arch

9.4 Skull showing important anatomical features.

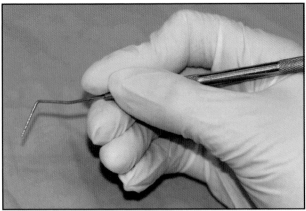

9.6 A modified pen grip is used to hold dental instruments correctly.

Dental explorer probe

This is a sharp pointed instrument. It is used to examine defects in the crown and root, such as caries lesions, resorptive lesions and pulp exposure in fractured teeth. The explorer probe is gently run across a suspicious area of pathology to check if the instrument catches. This may indicate pulp exposure or another crown defect.

Instruments used for periodontal treatment

The instruments required for periodontal treatment include (Figure 9.7):

■ Hand scalers
■ Curettes.

Many different patterns of scalers and curettes are available. The patterns best suited to veterinary dentistry are a sickle-shaped scaler (H6/7) and a Columbia curette (either a 4L/4R or Columbia 13/14).

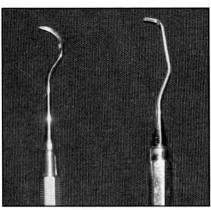

9.7

Hand scaler (left) and curette (right) showing different working tips.

Hand scaler

A hand scaler has a sharp tip and is used to remove supragingival calculus deposits from the surface of the tooth. It should never be used subgingivally as the sharp tip can damage the gingival attachment and periodontal ligament. It is used in a downward motion moving away from the gingival margin toward the occlusal surface of the tooth, removing the calculus by having the sharp edge contacting the surface of the tooth.

Curette

The curette is a modified scaler but has a rounded blunt tip (Figure 9.8) and is used to remove subgingival calculus from periodontal pockets. The curette is gently inserted into the sulcus and then angled to bring the working edge into contact with the surface of the tooth. A pull stroke is then used to dislodge the calculus and bring it out of the sulcus or pocket. The whole area is cleaned by using overlapping strokes.

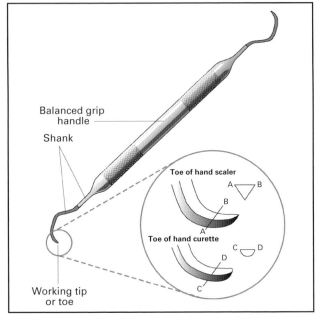

Balanced grip handle

Shank

Toe of hand scaler

Toe of hand curette

Working tip or toe

9.8 Cross-section of a scaler and curette showing the difference in the working tips. (Courtesy of J Robinson)

Instruments used for extraction

The instruments required for extraction include (Figure 9.9):

■ Luxators
■ Elevators (including periosteal elevators)
■ Extraction forceps
■ Small surgical kit.

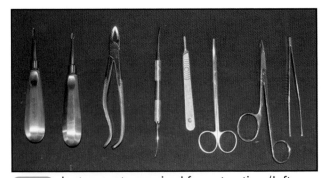

9.9 Instruments required for extraction (left to right): elevators; extraction forceps; periosteal elevator; and a basic surgical kit.

Luxators and elevators

A luxator (Figure 9.10) is a flat-edged cutting instrument used to cut the gingival attachment and periodontal ligament. It is a sharp instrument and must be used with great care to avoid soft tissue injury.

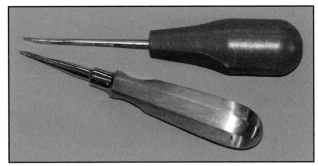

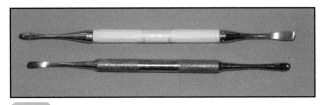 Luxator (top) and elevator (bottom). Note the differences: the luxator is a flatter, sharper instrument, whilst the tip of the elevator is more robust.

An elevator (Figure 9.10) is used after the luxator to break the remaining periodontal ligament attachment. The tip of an elevator is more robust than a luxator and may be modified for a better fit around the root curvature. Winged elevators are also available. The size and concave surface of the instrument should fit the surface of the root. Many patterns are available: Couplands size 1 and 3 are the most utilized elevators in veterinary dentistry. A 1.7 mm elevator, also called a superslim, is required for feline extractions.

Periosteal elevator

This is a sharp instrument (Figure 9.11) used to release the mucosa and attached gingiva with the periosteum from the bone when raising flaps to perform surgical extractions. Different patterns of periosteal elevators are available. The author's [LM] choice is a Goldman–Fox-type periosteal elevator with two different sized ends that can be used with dogs and cats.

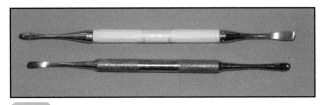

9.11 Goldman–Fox periosteal elevators.

Extraction forceps

Various patterns and sizes are available depending on the tooth requiring extraction. The forceps should make four-point contact with the root of the tooth and be of a suitable size. The best pattern for veterinary dentistry is 76 for dogs and 76N (narrow beaks) for cats.

Small surgical kit

This is required to suture after a surgical extraction. The instruments may vary with personal preference but usually comprise:

- Tissue forceps: DeBakey forceps are ideal as they cause less trauma to the tissue than conventional rat-toothed forceps
- Needle holder: 5 inch Olsen Hagers are a good size and not too bulky for those difficult-to-reach areas
- Scalpel handle

- Scalpel blades (Nos. 15 or 11)
- Metzenbaum scissors
- Suture scissors.

Power tools

Power tools (Figure 9.12) need to be used with great care as, if used incorrectly, they can cause serious damage. There are also operator health and safety considerations when using power tools: a facemask should be worn to avoid inhalation of the aerosol created by power scalers. Safety glasses should also be worn when using scalers to protect the eyes from any calculus, tooth fragments and, when using drills, broken burs that may present a hazard during extraction.

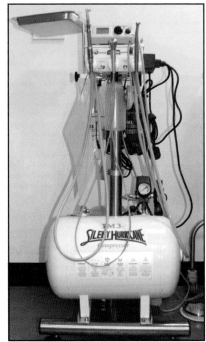

9.12 Compressed air-driven dental unit. The unit has a slow-speed handpiece, water-cooled high-speed handpiece and a three-way air/water syringe. Some machines have fibreoptic handpieces or suction as extra features.

Mechanical scalers

There are two types of ultrasonic scaler available: piezoelectric and magnetostrictive. Scalers work by having a tip that oscillates at an ultrasonic frequency. The vibrations cause the calculus to break up. The vibrating tip produces heat and needs to have a water source to keep it cool. The water coolant should flow to the top of the scaler tip and ensure the whole tip is kept cooled. The water also aids in calculus removal as energy from the tip is transferred to the water causing microscopic bubbles that implode and release energy that helps to dislodge the calculus.

Sonic scalers oscillate at a sonic frequency, which is lower than ultrasonic. These scalers are less effective at removing calculus but generate less heat so reduce the risk of tooth damage from heat.

High-speed handpiece

The high-speed handpiece is also known as the air-turbine. It is used to section teeth and remove alveolar bone to aid with extraction. It is also used in restorative dentistry. The turbine rotates at 350,000–400,000 revolutions per minute. Water is used to cool the bur to avoid thermal damage to tissues from the heat produced, and to prevent the bur from rapidly becoming blunt.

There is a wide selection of bur sizes (Figure 9.13) available to section teeth and remove bone. The most commonly used burs are 701 and 701L tapered fissure burs for sectioning dogs' teeth and a selection of round burs (sizes 1–6) for removing buccal bone. Small round burs (sizes 1 and 2) are suitable for sectioning and removing buccal bone in cats.

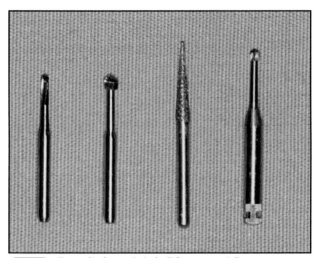

9.13 Burs (left to right): FG tapered fissure; round; diamond; and RA round bur.

Slow-speed handpiece

A straight or contra-angle handpiece is fitted to the slow-speed motor. The straight handpiece is usually used with surgical burs (HP) to remove bone. The contra-angle handpiece may have a latch grip for slow-speed burs (RA) or be a dental polishing handpiece. The cups used for polishing (Figure 9.14) are either latch grip or push-on cups that fit on to a button on the dental polishing handpiece head.

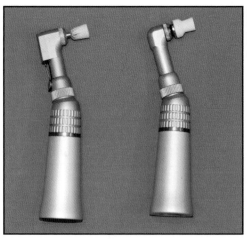

9.14 Polishing cups.

Care of instruments
Sharpening instruments

- All hand instruments with sharp edges should be sharpened after use. Blunt instruments will cause unnecessary damage to the tissue and frustration to the operator. Sharpening does require practice but users must make the effort to learn to do it correctly.

- Before sharpening, instruments should be washed in a suitable cleaning solution to remove any debris, then dried. Dirty instruments should never be sharpened on the stone because the stone is porous and will become contaminated.
- An Arkansas sharpening stone should be used with oil. This is a fine grain natural stone. The stone may be conical or flat, either is suitable.
- To sharpen the instrument, it should be pushed (or pulled) away in gentle strokes through the oil, held at 100–110 degrees, in the same way the instrument would be used to perform the procedure (Figure 9.15).
- Curettes and scalers should be held on a flat angle (i.e. the blade should contact the sharpening stone at a 90 degree angle) with no change as they are pulled along the stone.
- The sharpness should be tested on a test stick (or finger nail); if sharp it should shave off a little sliver.
- After the instrument has been sharpened the residual oil should be wiped off and the instrument sterilized.

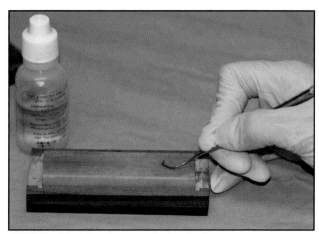

9.15 Sharpening a subgingival curette on an Arkansas stone.

Sterilization

Instruments should be placed in autoclavable bags or instrument trays and autoclaved on the appropriate cycle. The author [MH] personally prefers to cold sterilize instruments with sharp edges (luxators, curettes, scalers and elevators) daily, and once weekly autoclave the instruments in order to maximize the life of the instruments. Probes and the surgical kit should be autoclaved after each procedure.

Sharp tips can be covered with a cork or instrument tips to protect them whilst not in use and to prevent any damage to the tip when stored.

Maintenance and care of power equipment

Power instruments should be washed in a suitable cleaning solution then sterilized as the hand instruments. Care with some solutions for alloy handpieces is needed as they can cause erosion if the instrument is left to soak. The manufacturer's instructions should always be read.

The tip and the whole handpiece of the piezoelectric scaler or the insert tip and magnetostrictive rod can be removed from the handpiece of the magnetostrictive scaler and autoclaved. The tip should be measured for wear against a card available from the manufacturer, and if worn away it should be replaced with a new one. Most ultrasonic scaler tips should be replaced every 6 months if used frequently.

The slow-speed handpiece can also be autoclaved. The handpiece should be dried and oiled (Figure 9.16) before and after autoclaving to maintain the working gears. The high-speed handpiece should be treated in the same way: cleaned, sterilized and oiled. Manufacturers usually supply a blank to fit into the friction grip handpiece so that they are never left without a bur in place except when autoclaving.

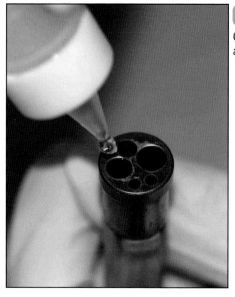

9.16 Oiling the air-turbine.

Dental examination

This is a two-stage procedure: the conscious examination followed by a more thorough examination under general anaesthesia.

Conscious examination

A complete oral examination is not possible in the conscious animal and is limited to a visual inspection only (Figure 9.17). Many animals may have areas of discomfort and may resist examination. Care should be taken when opening the mouth and a gentle technique used. The mouth can be opened by placing one hand over the muzzle and pressing the thumb of the other hand inside the lip, ideally behind the canine teeth to gently hold it open. The forefinger of the other hand can be used to gently lower the mandibular incisors and in doing so, open the mouth. Opening and visualization are helped by raising the head.

Examination under general anaesthesia

The second stage is examination under general anaesthesia (Figures 9.18 and 9.19) where a more thorough examination of the mouth and teeth is possible. The oral soft tissues can be visualized whilst intubating and checked for abnormalities. Further examination of the teeth, including charting can then be carried out.

Area to be examined	What to look for
Extraoral	
Skull: ■ Maxilla ■ Mandible ■ Cranium ■ Temporomandibular joint (TMJ)	Symmetry Protruberences Areas of discomfort
Muscles: ■ Temporal ■ Masseter	Symmetry Pain Muscle wastage
Lymph nodes: ■ Mandibular ■ Retropharyngeal ■ Cervical	Size
Salivary glands: ■ Parotid ■ Mandibular ■ Zygomatic (not usually palpable)	Pain Swelling
Occlusion: ■ Maxilla and mandible lengths	Relationship of each jaw quadrant to each other
Intraoral	
Occlusion	Relationship of the teeth to each other (see Figure 9.26a)
Alveolar mucosa and gingiva	Inflammation Ulceration Oral masses Colour Draining sinuses
Teeth	Fractured teeth (see Figure 9.28) Discoloured teeth Missing/extra teeth (see Figures 9.22 and 9.26c) Resorptive lesions (see Figure 9.29a)

9.17 Conscious oral examination.

Oral soft tissues	Tongue Hard palate Soft palate Tonsils Pharynx Larynx Salivary duct openings
Tooth unit	Gingival attachment Periodontal attachment Tooth

9.18 Examination under general anaesthesia.

Examination	What to assess	Findings	Disease present	Abbreviation used on dental chart
Gingiva	Inflammation and bleeding	Slight reddening	Gingivitis	G1
		Red and swollen and bleeds on probing		G2
		Swollen/ulcerated gingiva/bleeding		G3
	Margin (level of the gingiva relative to the cementoenamel junction of the tooth)	Increased	Hyperplasia Inflammation (see above) Gingival mass	GH
		Decreased (see Figure 9.27bcde)	Periodontitis	GR (mm)
Periodontal support	Periodontal probing depth	Increased (see Figure 9.27g)	True pocket False pocket (as a result of gingival hyperplasia)	PPD (mm)
	Furcation	Area in between roots can be felt with probe	Periodontitis	F1
		Probe passes about 1 mm horizontally	Periodontitis	F2
		Probe passes horizontally between the roots (see Figure 9.27c)	Periodontitis	F3
	Mobility	Tooth moves in one direction	Periodontitis Root fracture	M1
		Tooth moves more than 1 mm		M2
		Tooth moves vertically and horizontally		M3
Crown	Absent	Tooth/root present on radiograph	Unerupted tooth (see Figure 9.22b) Root remnant	Circle crown RR
		Absent on radiograph	Missing tooth	Circle whole tooth
	Fracture	Uncomplicated	No evidence of pulp exposure	UCF
		Complicated (see Figure 9.28a)	Pulp is exposed	CCF
	Worn teeth	Explorer catches	Pulp is exposed	AB PE
		Smooth brown discoloration, no catch on probing	Tertiary dentine	AB
	Discoloured	Purple/pink/grey crown	Pulpitis Pulp necrosis	Colour area on crown
		Brown discoloration on occlusal surface	Stain Caries lesion (see Figure 9.28c)	CA or stain
	Enamel dysplasia	Defect on crown where enamel missing	Enamel hypoplasia Enamel hypocalcification	ED
	Resorptive lesion	Defect on crown or root surface; explorer catches (see Figure 9.29)		RL
Position	Tooth out of normal position/alignment	Rotated teeth Abnormal jaw length	Malocclusion	Arrow on chart

9.19 Dental examination criteria for each tooth.

All abnormal findings need to be recorded on a dental chart (Figure 9.20), which can then be referred to at the time of treatment, at discharge to discuss the treatment performed with the owner, or at following dental procedures to compare dental status. The chart is a diagrammatic representation of the dentition. Most charts make use of the modified Triadan system (Floyd, 1991) (Figure 9.21) where each tooth is allocated a three digit number. The first number denotes the quadrant of the mouth and whether the tooth is permanent or deciduous. The second and third digits denote the tooth itself. In dogs the teeth are numbered consecutively from the midline whereas in cats, some numbers are skipped as not all teeth are present. Canine teeth are always numbered 04 and molars are always 09. To complete the examination, intraoral radiographs should be taken where necessary.

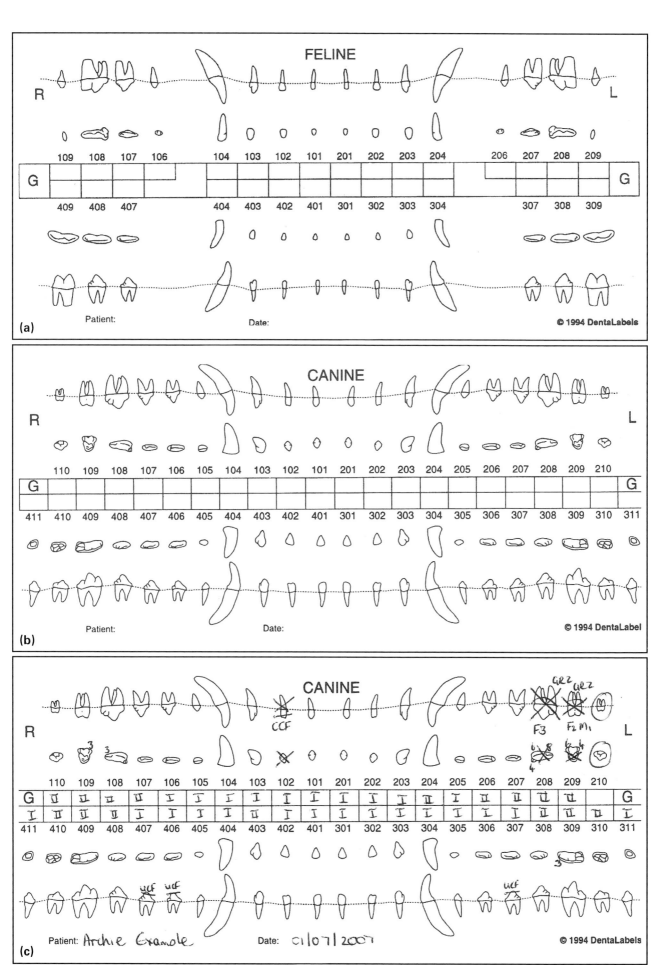

9.20 (a) Feline dental chart. (b) Canine dental chart. (c) An example of a completed canine dental chart. (© DentaLabels, J Robinson)

Permanent dentition	
Right upper = 1	Left upper = 2
Right lower = 4	Left lower = 3
Deciduous dentition	
Right upper = 5	Left upper = 6
Right lower = 8	Left lower = 7

9.21 Quadrant numbering in the modified Triadan system.

Dental radiography

Dental radiography is one of the most important tools available to aid in the diagnosis and treatment of dental disease. The bulk of the tooth can only be visualized by means of radiography and much pathology can be missed without its use. In some cases a lesion can be recognized clinically but the full extent of the pathology can only be evaluated with the use of radiography (Figure 9.22).

Equipment

X-ray machine

A standard veterinary X-ray machine can be used for taking dental radiographs but it has limitations. Usually the X-ray machine is not in the same room where the dental procedures are to be carried out, which means moving the patient around the clinic. The tube head is usually rigidly mounted, making positioning and adjustments in collimation and angulation difficult. Dental X-ray units have a moveable head and the collimation is confined by the cone. The cone also controls the film–focal distance. The kilovoltage (kV) and milliamperage (mA) are fixed, the timer being the only adjustable control. Wall-mounted or mobile machines are available.

Intraoral film

Intraoral or dental films should be used for taking dental radiographs. Intraoral films do not have intensifying screens and thus need a high exposure. Dental film is available as speed D (ultra) and speed E (ektra). Speed D is the equivalent of other non-screen film but speed E is rated at twice the speed of D, requiring half the exposure, but with a small loss of quality.

Films are available in different sizes but the three most commonly used in veterinary dentistry are:

- Occlusal film (5 cm x 7 cm) or size 4
- Adult periapical (3 cm x 4 cm) or size 2
- Child periapical (2 cm x 3.5 cm) or size 1.

Each film packet has individual wrapping to protect the film from light and moisture (Figure 9.23). The film inside the packet is wrapped in a black paper envelope. There is a lead foil backing which is positioned opposite the side exposed to the X-ray beam to protect against secondary radiation and reduce the effect of scatter.

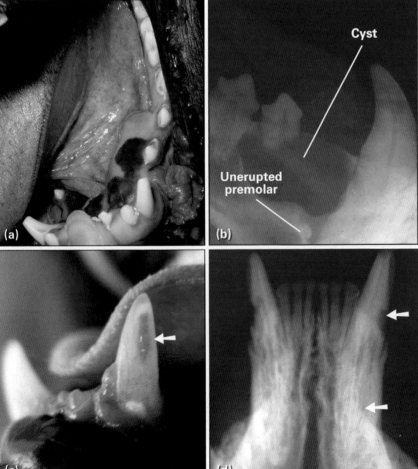

(a)
(b) Cyst / Unerupted premolar
(c)
(d)

9.22 (a) Missing first mandibular premolar. (b) Intraoral radiograph showing an unerupted premolar (radiodense area surrounded by a radiolucent halo) and the formation of a dentigerous cyst (radiolucent area) as a result. (c) Resorptive lesion (arrowed) affecting the crown of 304. (d) The true extent of the resorptive process can only be assessed by intraoral radiography. The tooth shows no normal root anatomy: no periodontal ligament, dentine or root canal (bottom arrow) can be identified. The area of crown resorption (top arrow) is seen clinically. The right canine tooth is also undergoing resorption.

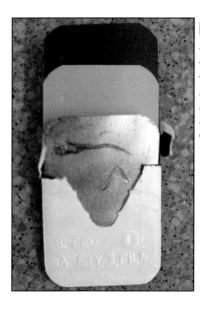

9.23 Dental film. An open film packet showing the paper covering the film, the film and the foil backing, all enclosed within a water-resistant envelope.

Self-contained films are also available in size 2 (periapical). The envelope contains the film with a separate compartment containing combined developer and fixer. These films are relatively expensive but useful when radiographs are only taken occasionally. The exposed films unfortunately do not keep unless they are fixed for longer than the period suggested by the manufacturers as they discolour with age.

A dimple can be found on the corner of the film. The convex surface always faces towards the X-ray beam and so identifies the front for viewing. It also serves as an orientation marker and helps determine the left- from the right-side of the patient.

Processing

Films can be processed in a darkroom using cups containing the processing chemicals or in a chair-side developer light-protected box. Some automatic processors will take dental film or separate automatic processors are available for dental film. The automatic processors deliver a fully fixed and dried film within 5 minutes. Ease of use and convenience are advantages but the cost and time to develop the films remain disadvantages. A chair-side light box system is convenient to use and the films can be developed in the dental procedures room. Rapid processing chemicals are available, resulting in a processed film within a minute. The box is designed with a special top that prevents light from entering and causing fogging of the film. Clips are also available. Each film is opened, a clip attached to the corner, and then submerged in the developer for 15 seconds, washed, then fixed for 30 seconds, and finally thoroughly washed under running water and hung up to dry.

The films are too small to label individually but they can be mounted in special mounts or stored in small envelopes with the client, patient and treatment details.

Techniques

Intraoral techniques produce radiographs without superimposition of the contralateral side of the head, which occurs if an extraoral technique is used. To obtain the best results:

- The appropriate size film, allowing the best possible positioning, should be used
- The film should be positioned inside the mouth as close to and as near parallel as possible to the structures to be radiographed without bending the film. This minimizes the risk of distortion
- A paper towel, foam or cotton-wool should be placed behind the film to wedge it and maintain its position.

Parallel technique

- The animal is placed in lateral recumbency with the side to be radiographed uppermost.
- The film is placed parallel to the tooth. This is only possible in the mouth when the film can be placed intraorally parallel to the teeth (i.e. for the mandibular posterior teeth caudal to the caudal limit of the mandibular symphysis).
- The intraoral film is placed lingual to the premolar or molar with the dimple facing towards the teeth. The film should be gently pushed ventrally to get the lower edge of the film as close to the ventral border of the mandible as possible.
- The X-ray beam is positioned perpendicular to the film.

Bisecting-angle technique

- When taking radiographs of teeth other than the mandibular premolars and molars, it is not anatomically possible to position the film parallel to the tooth root.
- The film should be placed as close to parallel as possible (Figure 9.24a).
- If the X-ray beam is directed perpendicular to the film, the image will be foreshortened (Figure 9.24b). If the X-ray beam is directed perpendicular to the long-axis of the tooth, the image will be elongated (Figure 9.24c).
- To avoid these problems, an imaginary line is drawn half way between the plane of the film and a plane through the long-axis of the tooth. This is known as the bisecting-angle (Figure 9.25). The X-ray beam is then directed perpendicular to this line.

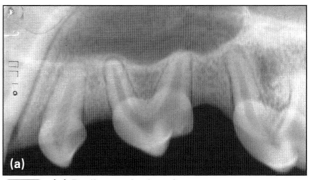

(a)

9.24 (a) Radiograph showing an accurate representation of the teeth, proving that the dental film was correctly positioned. (continues) ▶

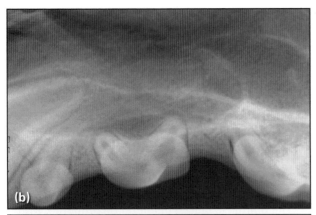

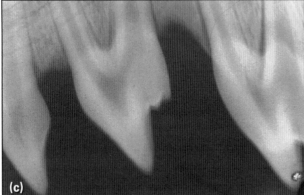

9.24   (continued) **(b)** Foreshortened image: the X-ray beam was directed perpendicular to the film. **(c)** Elongated image: the X-ray beam was directed perpendicular to the long-axis of the tooth.

Common dental pathology

For a more complete explanation of dental and oral conditions, the reader is referred to the *BSAVA Manual of Canine and Feline Dentistry, 3rd edition*.

Anatomical and developmental disease

The anatomical and developmental dental diseases affecting dogs and cats include:

- Malocclusions (Figure 9.26a)
- Missing and/or extra teeth
- Enamel defects (Figure 9.26b)
- Persistent deciduous teeth (Figure 9.26c).

Not all anatomical or developmental diseases require treatment. Some malocclusions may be functional and not cause any soft tissue or dental trauma (for example, brachycephalic dog breeds such as Boxers). Malocclusions that result in trauma will require treatment (for example, base narrow canine teeth). Persistent deciduous teeth and extra teeth may predispose the animal to periodontitis, as do teeth severely affected by enamel dysplasia. Teeth with enamel defects should also be radiographed to ascertain whether the pulp has become necrotic or has any root pathology. Missing teeth may be truly missing or unerupted, and can be distinguished with the help of radiography. If unerupted, the tooth may require treatment.

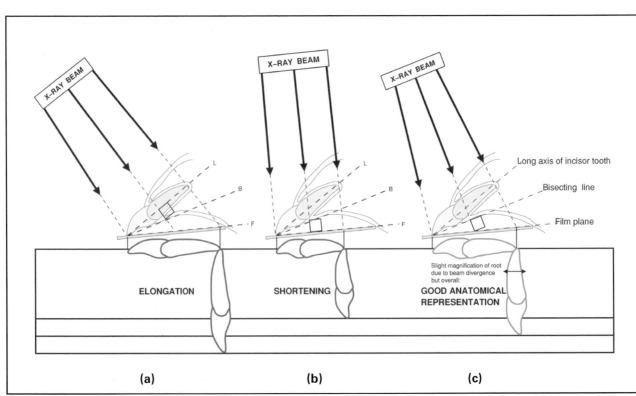

9.25   **(a)** Incident beam perpendicular to the tooth results in elongation of the image. **(b)** Incident beam perpendicular to the film results in foreshortening of the image. **(c)** Incident beam perpendicular to the bisecting line results in a life-size image. (© D Crossley)

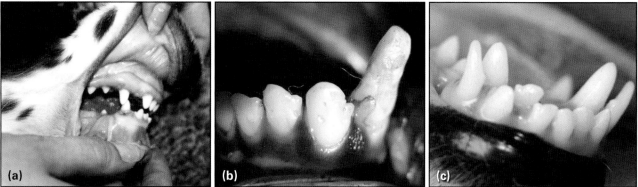

9.26 **(a)** Malocclusion: the lower canine is occluding distally and palatally to the correct position, causing trauma to the palate. This malocclusion needs treatment as the bite is not functional or comfortable. **(b)** Enamel dysplasia affecting the canine and incisors. Normal enamel should be smooth and not pitted or discoloured. **(c)** Persistent deciduous teeth, resulting in a malocclusion.

Periodontal disease

Periodontal disease (i.e. gum disease, periodontitis) (Figure 9.27) is by far the most common disease affecting pet cats and dogs. Bacteria are normal inhabitants of the mouth and can be found on the mucous membranes, tongue and in saliva. Periodontal disease is caused by plaque. Plaque can be described as a microbial community found on the tooth surface embedded in a matrix of polymers of bacterial and salivary origin. A film of proteins and glycoproteins is adsorbed rapidly to a clean tooth surface. Plaque formation involves the interaction between bacterial colonizers and this film (acquired enamel pellicle).

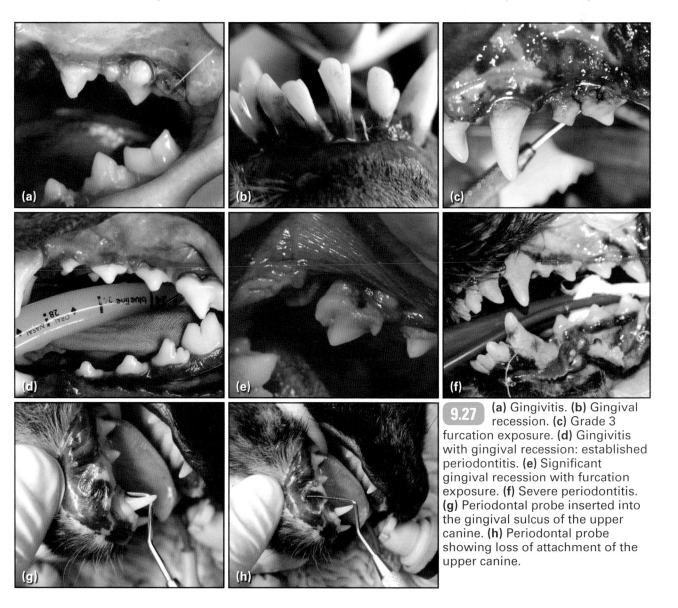

9.27 **(a)** Gingivitis. **(b)** Gingival recession. **(c)** Grade 3 furcation exposure. **(d)** Gingivitis with gingival recession: established periodontitis. **(e)** Significant gingival recession with furcation exposure. **(f)** Severe periodontitis. **(g)** Periodontal probe inserted into the gingival sulcus of the upper canine. **(h)** Periodontal probe showing loss of attachment of the upper canine.

Plaque is soft, sticky, yellowish white in colour and not always visible on the tooth surface. Plaque accumulation at the base of the crown results in inflammation of the gingiva that can progress to periodontitis if left untreated. Gingivitis is inflammation of the gingiva and is reversible. There is no periodontal attachment loss at this stage. Periodontitis is inflammation and loss of the supporting structures of the tooth. This condition is irreversible but may be controlled with vigilant homecare and regular professional dental treatment including extractions. Calculus or tartar is mineralized plaque. In itself calculus is not harmful but it is porous and rough and harbours plaque. Calculus can only be removed by scaling the teeth.

Periodontal disease can be diagnosed by assessing loss of attachment using a periodontal probe.

Endodontic disease

Endodontic diseases (diseases of the pulp) include:

- Fractured teeth (Figure 9.28ab)
- Worn teeth with or without pulp exposure
- Caries lesions (tooth decay) (Figure 9.28c)
- Non-vital teeth.

If the pulp is affected in any disease process the tooth will require treatment, as the condition is not only painful but also results in infection and the development of pathology associated with the tooth root. Treatment options are extraction or root canal treatment. Root canal treatment is only suitable for teeth that are periodontally healthy, and that have no root fractures or vertical fractures.

Feline odontoclastic resorptive lesions

As many as 29% of cats in the general population are affected by feline odontoclastic resorptive lesions (FORLs) (Figure 9.29). There is no known aetiology and the current treatment remains extraction of the affected teeth. With this disease odontoclasts progressively resorb tooth substance. Two types of resorptive lesions are seen: type 1, where there is resorption of the tooth but no replacement of bone or cementum on the root surface; and type 2, where the tooth roots undergo resorption and are replaced with bone, resulting in spot ankylosis (loss of the periodontal ligament resulting in fusion) of the tooth with the alveolar bone. The two types can only be distinguished by radiography.

Dental treatment

Anaesthetic considerations

A full oral and dental examination must be performed under general anaesthesia. The full extent of the pathology and the treatment required can only then be assessed.

- A cuffed endotracheal tube should always be placed during dental surgery in dogs to prevent aspiration of water, blood and dental debris (calculus, tooth remnants, bone) that can result in inhalation pneumonia, which is a very serious complication. In cats the use

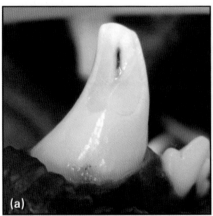
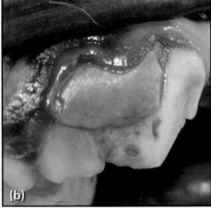
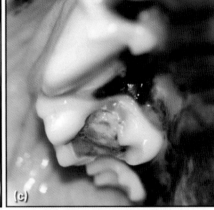

9.28   (a) Complicated crown fracture with a visible necrotic pulp (black spot). (b) Slab fracture of the carnassial tooth, exposing the pulp and extending subgingivally. (c) Upper molar affected by caries.

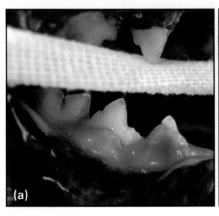
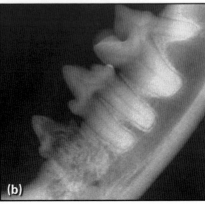

9.29   (a) Lower premolar affected by a FORL. The gingiva has grown over the defect in the crown of the tooth. (b) Radiograph of the affected tooth showing resorption of the roots and crown.

of a cuffed endotracheal tube is controversial and some people prefer to use a snugly fitting plain endotracheal tube, but a water-tight seal has to be a high priority in dental patients and may not be achieved with the use of uncuffed tubes. A cuffed endotracheal tube is therefore recommended for dental procedures in cats but should be used with extreme caution. The cuff should only be sufficiently inflated to achieve a seal. The endotracheal tube should also be tied as far back along the tube as possible to avoid movement of the tube during anaesthesia. In dogs it is recommended that the tube is tied to the muzzle or mandible and not behind the ears to help prevent movement of the tube.

- A throat pack should also be used for extra airway protection and changed if/when it becomes saturated. It is advisable to tie the throat pack to the endotracheal tube so that its removal is guaranteed and it is never accidentally left in place during recovery.
- Animals may be under general anaesthesia for a considerable time during dental procedures. Appropriate anaesthetic monitoring should be arranged and intravenous fluid therapy used when indicated.
- Many patients requiring advanced dental treatment are senior patients and should be placed on intravenous fluids prior to surgery.
- Dental patients getting excessively wet will develop hypothermia. The mouth is open and patients lose heat via the mouth. Water is constantly used during dental procedures and may cool the patient further. Hypothermia should be avoided by checking the body temperature at least every 15 minutes. Heat pads, circulating hot air blankets and other heat insulation methods should be used.
- Adequate pain control is necessary and anaesthetic regimes should be based upon the treatment required. Pre-emptive analgesia should always be administered at the discretion of the veterinary surgeon as even procedures such as subgingival scaling have been shown to

cause pain and discomfort to the patient. Local analgesia and regional nerve blocks should be considered when extensive surgery (oral tumour resection or full-mouth extractions) is planned.

Periodontal treatment

Periodontal treatment consists of two main areas: professional periodontal therapy and maintenance of oral hygiene. The steps involved in performing periodontal therapy (Figure 9.30) are:

1. Examine and record findings on a dental chart.
2. Rinse the mouth with a chlorhexidine mouthwash before starting any scaling.
3. Supragingival scaling: remove gross calculus using calculus forceps, taking care not to damage the gingiva. Use an ultrasonic (or sonic) scaler to remove any residual calculus above the gingival margin. Use a gentle stroking movement across the surface of the tooth with the side of the tip. Using the tip of the instrument causes gouging of the tooth surface. A sharp sickle-shaped hand scaler can also be used.
4. Subgingival scaling: remove calculus below the gingival margin. Only specialized mechanical instruments can be used below the gingival margin, with care, so usually hand curettes are used in practice.
5. Polishing: remove any remaining subgingival plaque with polishing aids. Polishing is usually performed using a soft rubber cup and a mildly abrasive paste rotating slowly on a slow-speed handpiece. The handpiece should be running very slowly to prevent excessive heat damage to the tooth. The polishing cup should be flared under the free gingiva to remove any plaque in the gingival sulcus. Excessive pressure will result in too much friction and produce heat that may cause pulp inflammation.
6. Sulcular lavage: remove any free-floating debris from the gingival sulcus. A diluted chlorhexidine gluconate solution can be used.
7. Extractions as necessary.

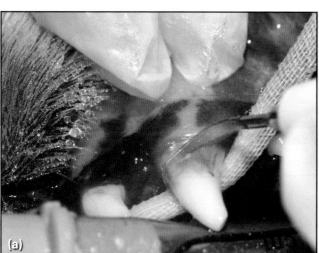
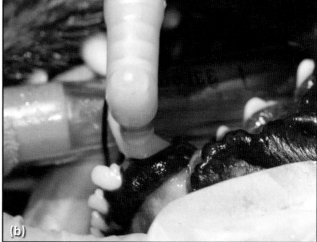

9.30 **(a)** Removing supragingival calculus using an ultrasonic scaler with a fine tip. The fine water spray generated by the machine helps cool the tip and dislodge calculus. **(b)** Polishing helps smooth the tooth surface and remove any remaining plaque. The cup can be flared by applying gentle pressure to clean subgingivally.

Extraction

Extractions are considered to be major oral surgery and an act of veterinary surgery, and so the RCVS advises that veterinary nurses are not allowed to perform them. The indications for tooth extraction are given in Figure 9.31.

Severe periodontal disease (mobility, furcation exposure, periodontal probing depths)
Complicated crown fracture (pulp exposed)
Worn tooth with pulp exposure
Crown root fracture
Odontoclastic resorptive lesion
Caries lesion
Non-vital tooth
Persistent deciduous teeth
Teeth involved in a jaw fracture
Unerupted teeth causing pathology
Teeth causing malocclusions
Supernumerary teeth
Chronic gingivostomatitis

9.31 Indications for tooth extraction.

Equipment

The following equipment is required for extractions:

- Luxators: size 3 mm and 4 mm, straight and curved
- Elevators: Couplands sizes 1 and 3, and a superslim for cats
- Goldman–Fox periosteal elevator
- Scalpel handle and blades
- Extraction forceps: pattern 76 for dogs and 76N for cats
- Selection of round and tapered fissure burs
- Soft tissue protector
- Surgical kit for closure of oral flaps.

Techniques

There are two techniques used for extractions: open (surgical) and closed (non-surgical). The choice of technique depends on operator preference, tooth morphology and disease present. The technique used may also depend on the findings of preoperative radiographs, which are always recommended prior to an extraction.

Surgical or open technique

This technique (Figure 9.32) should always be used for extraction of canine teeth, for retrieval of root remnants and if any abnormal tooth morphology exists. It may also be the surgeon's preference to use a surgical technique if multiple adjacent teeth need to be extracted.

- Releasing incisions are made mesially and distally to the tooth to be extracted.
- A mucoperiosteal flap is raised using a periosteal elevator.
- The overlying buccal bone can be removed using a round bur on a high-speed handpiece with water-cooling.
- Grooves can be made along the mesial and distal aspects of the root to create space for placement of a dental elevator. An elevator of an appropriate size is then placed in the groove and gently rotated to tear the periodontal ligament fibres.
- The tooth is extracted using forceps or fingers once movement has been created. The edges of the socket are then smoothed using a bur, bone file or rongeurs.
- The flap is then replaced and sutured without tension using a fine monofilament absorbable suture material.

There are significant complications associated with dental extraction, which the veterinary nurse should be aware of; these are detailed in Figure 9.33.

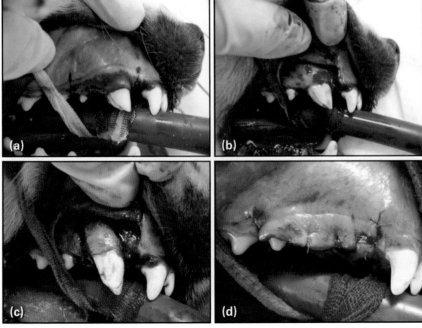

9.32 Surgical extraction of a canine tooth. **(a)** Vertical releasing incisions are made mesially and distally to the tooth. **(b)** A mucoperiosteal flap is raised. **(c)** Grooves are made along the mesial and distal aspects of the tooth root to facilitate placement of the dental elevators. The grooves are connected across the buccal surface of the root. **(d)** Following extraction of the tooth, the flap is replaced and sutured using a simple interrupted suture pattern.

Complication	Cause and avoidance
Tooth fracture (crown/root/both)	Incorrect technique – careful use with elevators and luxators Extraction forceps should not be used before the tooth is adequately loosened
Oronasal communication	May be due to infection or iatrogenic damage – avoid excessive force during extraction
Jaw fracture	Preoperative radiographs should be taken to assess bone loss in advanced periodontal disease Incorrect technique (placement of luxators and elevators, especially associated with the lower canine) must be avoided
Haemorrhage	Accidental damage to neurovascular bundle during surgery Haemorrhage may occur as a result of a root fracture Pre-existing disease (identified before surgery if possible)
Displaced root fragments	Avoid downward force in cats as the root fragment may be displaced into the mandibular canal Avoid excessive force on the palatal root of the upper carnassial in dogs to avoid pushing the root into the nasal turbinates
Thermal bone damage	Adequate cooling of high-speed bur when used
Emphysema	Incorrect use of the high-speed handpiece. Avoid blowing air into soft tissue or bone
Soft tissue injuries (gingiva, tongue, frenulum, lip, eye)	Use spatulas to avoid accidental damage when using the high-speed bur Controlled force when using elevators and avoid slippage by correct holding of instrument and stabilization of the patient's head
Wound breakdown	Avoid tension when suturing in the mouth. Periosteal releasing incisions can be made on the surface of mucoperiosteal flaps to release tension, or increase the size of the flap by increasing the releasing incisions to relieve tension. Careful flap planning prior to extraction is necessary

9.33 Complications of extractions.

Non-surgical or closed technique

This technique is used for all single-rooted teeth or teeth that have been sectioned into individual roots.

- The gingival attachment is cut around the whole circumference of the tooth using a No.11 scalpel blade or a sharp luxator.
- Either a luxator or elevator of appropriate size is then inserted into the periodontal ligament space to cut the periodontal ligament fibres.
- Once a space is created between the tooth and the bone, an elevator is used to work circumferentially around the tooth applying apical and rotational pressure at an acute angle to the tooth root. Pressure should be applied

for 10 seconds at a time to break down the periodontal ligament fibres. It is important that the tooth is not levered.
- Once the tooth is mobile it can be delivered from the socket using either fingers or extraction forceps. It is important to use extraction forceps correctly to avoid root fracture. The forceps should be applied as low down the root as possible. The forceps are initially used in a slight rotational manner to break down any remaining fibres and, when the tooth is loose, the tooth can gently be pulled from the socket.

To section teeth into individual roots a tapered fissure bur on a high-speed handpiece with water-cooling is used. A small diameter (010 or 012) bur should be used. The furcation needs to be identified and, as a general rule, it lies below the main cusp of the crown. Once the furcation has been identified the tooth can be sectioned from the furcation towards the cusp, from the buccal to lingual/palatal aspect of the tooth. Care should be taken not to damage the gingiva at the furcation. To check that the tooth has been adequately sectioned, an elevator should be placed between the two sections of the tooth and gently rotated: both parts of the crown should move independently.

Advanced dental treatment

Root canal treatment

Strategic teeth (canines and carnassials, and incisors in some working dogs) with complicated crown fractures can be referred for restoration by root canal treatment (Figure 9.34). The tooth must be periodontally sound and the fracture should not extend subgingivally. The pulp is removed using a combination of flushing and filing, and once clean the empty pulp chamber and root canal are obturated and sealed. The fracture site is then restored.

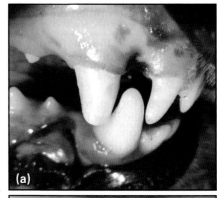
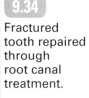
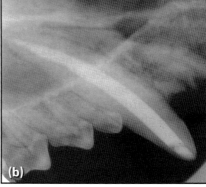

9.34 Fractured tooth repaired through root canal treatment.

accepting of new things and it is easier to introduce oral hygiene into their daily routine. Puppy parties provide the opportunity for veterinary nurses to talk about oral care and point out the benefits of tooth brushing. This should be made a fun experience, so toys with toothpaste applied to them should be used to get the pet used to the taste. Leaflets explaining how to introduce tooth brushing should be given out and owners invited back for an individual consultation to go through tooth brushing more thoroughly and reinforce the importance of oral care. Initially puppies should become accustomed to having their mouths held, gums rubbed and teeth examined, but a toothbrush should only be introduced once all the permanent teeth have finished erupting. When the permanent teeth are erupting, the gingiva may be inflamed and sensitive, and some deciduous teeth may be mobile. If a toothbrush is used too early it may cause discomfort to the puppy and cause the animal to become head shy or avoid further dental care. It is also important that pets have their mouths checked at 6 months of age to assess eruption and check for any malocclusion problems.

Senior pet clinics

Most senior patients will have dental disease of varying stages. Senior pet clinics provide the opportunity to show the owner with their own pet what is happening, using pictures to help explain the diseases present and what treatment may need to be performed. It is important to explain the systemic consequences of the disease to the owner and discuss the fact that their pet may be in pain, even if it is still eating. Pets will often chew on one side of the mouth and very seldom lose their appetite completely. Old dogs may have fractured teeth requiring treatment. The owners should be warned about the high incidence of oral tumours. As veterinary nurses are unable to diagnose disease, if they have any concerns about the mouth they should advise the owner to book an appointment for a consultation with the veterinary surgeon to discuss any treatment required.

In the clinics the possibility of introducing home-care and how this will improve the animal's health and quality of life can be discussed. Pictures and leaflets should be provided for owners to read at home. A follow-up telephone call can help after they have had a chance to read and digest the information that has been given out. Some owners will feel guilty and possibly react defensively. Quite often with a previous pet, dental care or dental problems will have never been mentioned or even noticed. The client should be reassured and time taken to explain that veterinary dentistry is important for their pet's overall health and welfare.

References and further reading

Floyd MR (1991) The Modified Triadan System: nomenclature for veterinary dentistry. *The Journal of Veterinary Dentistry* **8(4)**, 18–19

Gorrel C (2004) *Veterinary Dentistry for the General Practitioner.* WB Saunders, Edinburgh

Gorrel C and Derbyshire S (2005) *Veterinary Dentistry for the Nurse and Technician.* Elsevier, Butterworth Heinemann, Oxford

Holmstrom SE (2005) *Veterinary Clinics of North America: Small Animal Practice.* WB Saunders, Philadelphia

Mulligan T, Aller M and Williams CA (1998) *Atlas of Canine and Feline Dental Radiography.* Veterinary Learning Systems, USA

Tutt C, Deeprose J and Crossley D (2007) *BSAVA Manual of Canine and Feline Dentistry, 3rd edition.* BSAVA Publications, Gloucester

Wiggs RB and Lobprise HB (1997) *Veterinary Dentistry Principles and Practice.* Lippincott-Raven, Philadelphia

10

Endoscopy

Emma Barty and Philip Lhermette

This chapter is designed to give information on:

- The principles of flexible and rigid endoscopy – instrument selection, care and maintenance
- Tracheobronchoscopy
- Gastrointestinal endoscopy
- Protoscopy and colonoscopy
- Rhinoscopy
- Urethrocystoscopy
- Laparoscopy
- Thoracoscopy
- Arthroscopy

Introduction

The word endoscopy literally means to 'look inside', and instruments have been available for many years to enable physicians to peer into various body cavities and take diagnostic samples. More sophisticated instrumentation has now greatly increased the scope and usefulness of these techniques to include interventional surgery. As equipment costs come down, endoscopy is being integrated into many veterinary practices as a routine procedure.

Principles of flexible and rigid endoscopy

The flexible endoscope

Instrument construction

Most flexible endoscopes consist of an umbilicus, a handpiece and an insertion tube.

Umbilicus

The umbilicus plugs into the light source and usually has connections for irrigation and suction (Figure 10.1). There is also a pressure compensation valve, which is used for pressure testing the endoscope. A pressure compensation cap is provided for use during air shipment or gas sterilization. This cap opens the

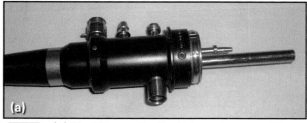

10.1 **(a)** Umbilicus of a flexible endoscope. The probes on the right connect to the light source for provision of light and insufflation. The side connectors are for attaching the wash bottle and suction, and for cleaning. (continues) ▶

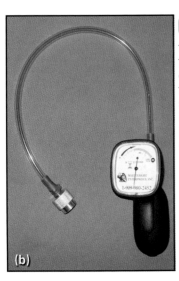

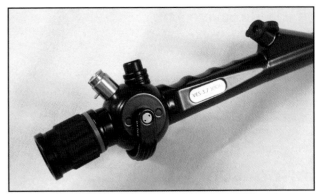

10.1 (continued) **(b)** Leak tester that can be attached to the endoscope before cleaning to check the integrity of the seals. Entry of fluid into the endoscope is a potentially catastrophic event.

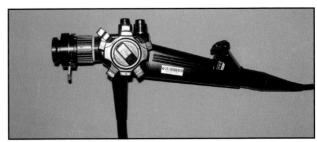

10.2 Handpiece of a gastroscope. This shows two rings, which allow four-way deflection of the tip, together with an instrument channel, and buttons for insufflation/irrigation and suction.

inner workings of the endoscope to the air and great care must be taken not to allow any fluid to enter the endoscope as this will cause irreparable damage.

The umbilicus contains non-coherent light guide fibres that continue through the handpiece and down to a lens at the tip of the insertion tube. These fibres are fragile and can be damaged by excessive torsion. Care should be taken not to twist or coil the umbilicus excessively or to knock it against a hard surface, as this will damage fibres and reduce illumination. Fibres retain a 'memory' if stored in a coiled position and are more prone to breakage when straightened. For this reason flexible endoscopes are always stored hanging with the umbilicus and insertion tube in a straight position. This also facilitates drainage from the channels.

Handpiece

Gastroscope

The handpiece of a gastroscope (Figure 10.2) is designed to be held in the left hand, allowing the index finger and middle fingers to operate the suction and irrigation/insufflation buttons, respectively. The irrigation/insufflation button has a hole in the top, through which air is pumped continuously. Covering the hole with the middle finger diverts the air down the irrigation/insufflation channel to insufflate the bowel or stomach and provide a space in which to work. Pressing the button down all the way stops the air and pumps water down the irrigation channel to wash the video lens at the tip when it becomes obscured by mucus or debris. The suction button is used to remove air from the stomach or bowel or to drain fluid. The inner wheel controls the up and down movement of the tip and can be operated with the left thumb or right hand as required. Anticlockwise rotation will give maximum deflection of 180–210 degrees to allow examination of the cardia of the stomach (J manoeuvre). A small friction brake is also available to maintain the position of the tip, e.g. during biopsy. The outer wheel controls left and right movement of the tip and is operated in a similar fashion. A friction brake is also available on this control.

At the top of the insertion tube is the instrument channel port, fitted with a removable rubber cap. Flexible biopsy forceps, grasping forceps, cytology brushes or lavage tubing can be introduced here, and must be

designed for the appropriate length and diameter of the instrument channel. Instruments should be inserted and withdrawn through the tip of the insertion tube only when it is straight. Failure to do this may damage the rubber lining of the flexible tip, allowing fluids to enter the inner workings of the endoscope which can cause irreparable or very costly damage.

Bronchoscope

The handpiece of a bronchoscope (Figure 10.3) is typically simpler, with a lever providing up and down movement in place of the control wheels. The bronchoscope may not have an umbilicus at all, in which case there will be connectors for a separate light guide cable, suction and pressure compensation valve on the handpiece itself. There is also a button to control suction and an instrument channel as on the gastroscope.

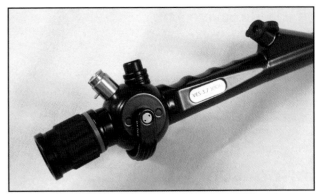

10.3 Handpiece of a bronchoscope. There is a single control to allow two-way deflection of the tip.

Insertion tube

The insertion tube contains the light guide fibre bundle and the various channels for suction, irrigation and instrumentation. It also contains guidewires for manipulating the flexible tip and either a coherent fibre bundle (fibreoptic endoscope) or wires to a CCD (charged couple device or digital camera) chip (videoendoscope) at the tip to convey the image to the operator. The flexible tip contains an imaging lens and a lens that provides illumination from the light source (Figure 10.4). There are also openings of the channels for suction/instrumentation and irrigation. The irrigation channel terminates in a small flange, which deflects water over the surface of the imaging lens to clean it during procedures.

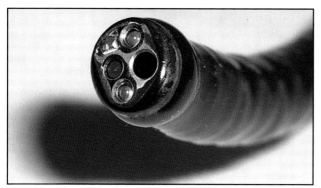

10.4 Tip of the insertion tube of a gastroscope. There is a single lens for image collection, two lenses for illumination, a large combined channel for instruments/suction and a smaller channel for insufflation/irrigation.

Instrument selection

No single endoscope is suitable for all procedures in small animal practice. It is therefore important to understand the specific clinical requirements of the practice, including the types of patient most commonly seen, and then to understand enough about endoscope design and function to find an instrument to match them.

Flexible endoscopes commonly used in veterinary medicine can be divided into two main types: gastroscopes and bronchoscopes. These are generally available as either videoendoscopes or fibreoptic endoscopes, and each has its own particular characteristics (Figure 10.5).

Fibreoptic endoscopes transmit the image from the tip to the eyepiece via a bundle of glass fibres. These fibres are arranged spatially in the same order throughout the bundle from one end to the other, so that a true image is seen at the eyepiece. This is termed a coherent light fibre bundle, and results in a pixellated image rather like magnified newsprint, which is viewed directly through the eyepiece or, via an attached camera, on a monitor.

A videoendoscope has no eyepiece, the image being transmitted electronically from a CCD video chip at the tip of the insertion tube directly to a video monitor. This gives a vastly superior image with no pixellation but at much greater cost, since each endoscope essentially incorporates its own camera system.

Both fibreoptic and videoendoscopes contain glass fibre bundles to carry light from the light source to the tip. Glass fibres are delicate and easily damaged by severe bending or rough handling, and this can reduce the amount of illumination provided, and in the case of a fibreoptic endoscope, cause black spots to appear in the image corresponding to individual broken fibres.

Given the variation in size of veterinary patients, no single gastroscope is ideal for all. An insertion tube diameter of 7–8 mm will be suitable for cats and small to medium-sized dogs, and can double as a bronchoscope for larger dogs. In larger dogs an insertion tube diameter of 9–10 mm will provide a larger image, better illumination and a larger instrument channel, allowing the use of more robust instruments and larger biopsy forceps, which provide bigger and more diagnostic samples. Endoscopes much larger than this are not suitable for small animal use as they will not pass through the pylorus.

The length of insertion tube is also important. Many human gastroscopes are 100 cm long, which is adequate for small dogs, but larger dogs will require an insertion tube of 130–150 cm in order to reach the duodenum or caecum.

Most bronchoscopes are fibreoptic, since it is difficult and expensive to produce CCD video chips small enough to fit the tip of the insertion tube. An outer diameter of 3.5–5 mm is ideal for all adult dogs and cats, and a tip deflection of 180 degrees in one direction will allow retroflexion over the soft palate to examine the caudal nares.

The ability to sterilize the endoscope adequately between patients is paramount, and for this reason it is essential to ensure that the endoscope is fully immersible to allow adequate cleaning and disinfection. Some older second-hand endoscopes are not fully immersible and should be avoided.

The rigid endoscope
Instrument construction

The rigid endoscope is inherently simpler than the flexible endoscope, and is essentially a hollow steel tube that contains solid glass rod lenses, with an oculus or eyepiece at one end and a light guide post to which a flexible light guide cable is attached.

Property	Gastroscope	Bronchoscope
Tip deflection	Four-way	Two-way
Field of view	At least 180 degrees in one direction	At least 180 degrees in one direction
Controls	Two wheels to control tip movement left/right and up/down	One lever to control up/down
Channels	Separate instrument/suction and insufflation/irrigation channels Biopsy/instrument channel of at least 2 mm, preferably 2.8 mm	Usually one instrument/suction/irrigation channel Biopsy/instrument channel of at least 1.8 mm
Working length	At least 100 cm, preferably 130–150 cm	At least 80 cm
Outer insertion tube diameter	7.9–10 mm	3–5 mm

10.5 Characteristics of gastroscopes and bronchoscopes.

Light is transmitted to the tip via a circular array of light guide fibres that surrounds the imaging lens. This simple construction provides high-quality illumination and an extremely high-quality magnified image that can be viewed directly through the eyepiece or, more commonly, via an attached camera system on a video monitor.

Rigid endoscopes come in a variety of lengths and diameters, and are also available with varying angles of view. Zero-degree endoscopes provide a view straight ahead, like a conventional telescope, and are the simplest to learn to use. A 30-degree endoscope provides a view ahead at an angle of 30 degrees to the long axis (Figure 10.6). The advantage of this is that by rotating the endoscope around its long axis the field of view can be increased. This can be extremely useful, especially in a confined space, such as a joint, the nose or the trigone of the bladder. Endoscopes <4 mm in diameter are extremely fragile and are always used in a protective sheath or cannula.

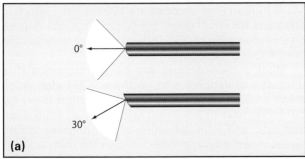
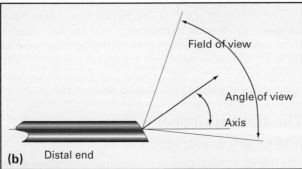

10.6 Fields of view for angled rigid endoscopes. (a) The most commonly used veterinary endoscopes are 0 and 30 degrees. (b) Relation between angle of view and field of view in a rigid endoscope.

Instrument selection

The selection of a rigid endoscope will depend upon the procedure undertaken. The most commonly used and versatile rigid endoscope is 2.7 mm in diameter with a 30 degrees viewing angle and 18 cm in length. This endoscope is used for urethrocystoscopy, rhinoscopy and arthroscopy, and can also be used for laparoscopy and thoracoscopy in cats and small dogs. For laparoscopy and thoracoscopy, especially in medium to large dogs, a 5 mm 0 degrees endoscope is generally used, although a 5 mm 30 degrees endoscope can be useful for thoracoscopy. For arthroscopy it is sometimes useful to have a 1.9 mm or 2.4 mm 30 degrees endoscope, and these can also be useful for urethrocystoscopy in the queen.

Ancillary equipment

A variety of ancillary equipment (Figure 10.7) is necessary for both flexible and rigid endoscopy and in most cases can be used for both:

- Light source – preferably xenon or metal halide as these produce a brighter and whiter light, but halogen may be sufficient
- Suction/irrigation
- Camera system (or video processor if using a videoendoscope)
- Monitor – preferably a medical monitor
- Insufflator – separate carbon dioxide insufflator for laparoscopy or integrated into light source for flexible endoscopy
- Electrosurgery unit.

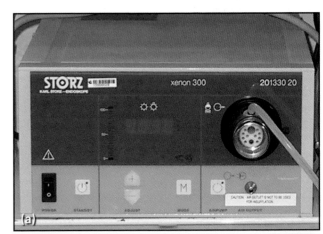

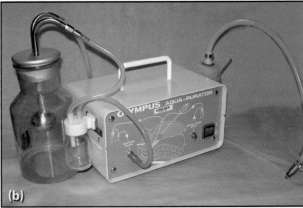

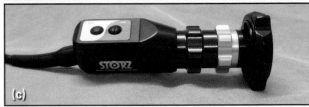

10.7 Ancillary equipment. (a) Light source. This example is adaptable for both rigid and flexible endoscopy (the adaptor for flexible endoscopy is in place). (b) Combined suction/irrigation device. The large bottle on the left is for collection of aspirated fluids and the smaller bottle on the left is a fluid trap to protect the suction pump. The bottle on the right is the wash bottle for irrigation. (c) Camera head for attachment to the eyepiece of a rigid endoscope. Adaptors are available for connection to flexible endoscopes. (continues) ▶

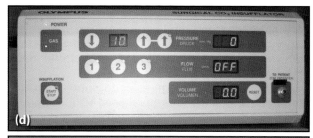

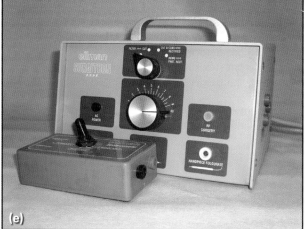

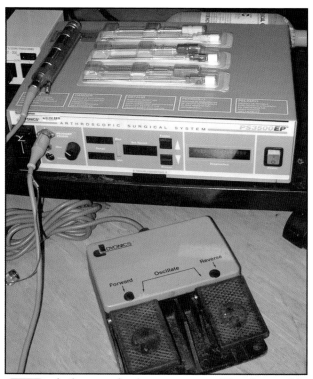

10.7 (continued) Ancillary equipment.
(d) Automatic carbon dioxide insufflator.
There are controls for selected intracavitory pressure and maximum gas flow rate, and displays for actual intracavitory pressure, instantaneous gas flow and total volume used during the procedure. The gas cylinder connector is not shown. **(e)** Electrosurgery unit suitable for connection to instruments for open or endoscopic surgery.

Some other useful, though not essential, additions are:

- Image capture device – video and still image (VHS or digital)
- Arthroscopic shaver system
- Diode laser system.

An arthroscopic shaver (Figure 10.8) is a hand-held rotating blade system incorporating suction and is used for debriding tissue in joints and can also be useful in the nose. It is particularly useful, indeed almost essential, in the stifle joint, where the peripatellar fat pad obscures visualization and must be removed before the joint can be explored. It is also useful for debriding cartilage following removal of osteochondrosis dissecans (OCD) lesions.

A diode laser system (Figure 10.9) is extremely useful for endoscopic surgery, since the laser light is delivered by means of a flexible quartz fibre which can be passed through the instrument channel of a flexible endoscope or rigid endoscope sheath. Since diode laser light is absorbed by pigment (haemoglobin), it can be used in a fluid medium such as in the bladder or in the nose under saline irrigation and can therefore be used for tumour ablation and haemostasis. Other lasers in common use, such as carbon dioxide lasers, do not work in a fluid medium and the operative arm cannot be passed through an endoscope, restricting their use to open surgery.

10.8 Arthroscopic shaver system. The disposable handpieces are seen on the top of the equipment and the foot pedal is in front of it.

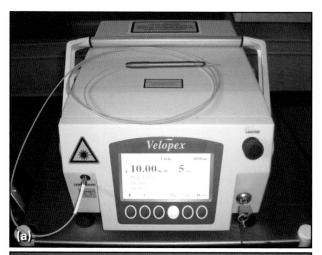

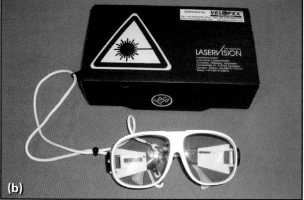

10.9 **(a)** Diode laser with coiled laser fibre attached. A handpiece is shown which can be removed when the fibre is used endoscopically. The aiming laser (not the surgical laser) is illuminated at the tip. **(b)** Specialized eye protection such as these goggles must be worn whenever the laser is in use.

WARNING
Suitable eye protection must be worn by all personnel whenever the laser is in use.

The veterinary nurse should be familiar with the operation of all the ancillary equipment in use. Invariably the endoscopist will require images to be captured during the procedure, or changes to insufflation rates and electrosurgical settings. Cameras must be white-balanced before use in order to give a true colour rendition.

Instrumentation

Flexible endoscopy

Instrumentation for flexible endoscopy (Figure 10.10) must be matched to the size and length of the instrument channel for the individual endoscope. A basic set of accessories should include:

- Cleaning brush
- Biopsy forceps – preferably oval serrated fenestrated cups to give the largest and highest quality samples
- Grasping forceps – plain, serrated and toothed
- Polypectomy snare for polyps and some foreign bodies
- Three- or four-pronged grasping forceps
- Basket forceps for foreign bodies
- Sterile irrigation/bronchoalveolar lavage tubing.

It is also useful to have a range of balloon dilators for oesophageal strictures.

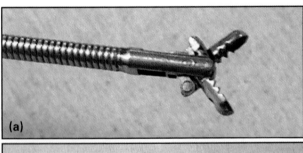

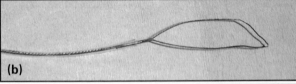

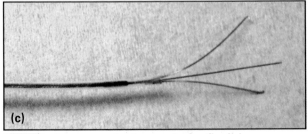

10.10 Accessory instruments for flexible endoscopy. **(a)** The tips of a pair of serrated flexible biopsy forceps. **(b)** Polypectomy snare used to encircle the base of a polypoid mass or to retrieve foreign bodies. **(c)** Three-pronged grasping forceps used to retrieve foreign bodies.

Rigid endoscopy

For rigid endoscopy the instrumentation will largely depend on the procedures undertaken. A more comprehensive list is included later under each procedure.

For the 2.7 mm 30 degrees endoscope the instrumentation will usually be purchased with the endoscope and matched with it:

- 14.5 Fr cystoscopy sheath (Figure 10.11) with two irrigation/insufflation ports and a 5 Fr instrumentation channel
- 7 Fr 40 cm flexible biopsy forceps
- 7 Fr 40 cm flexible grasping forceps
- 7 Fr 40 cm flexible scissors.

This set up can be used for rhinoscopy, urethro-cystoscopy and otoscopy.

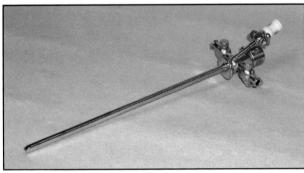

10.11 Cystoscopy sheath for a rigid endoscope, with two irrigation/insufflation ports and an instrumentation channel.

Laparoscopy and thoracoscopy

In cats and small dogs, additional requirements are:

- 3 mm protection sheath
- 3.5 mm laparoscopy cannula and sharp trocar (or Endotip® cannula).

Additional instruments for laparoscopy and thoracoscopy (Figure 10.12) are usually of a standard 5 mm diameter, and are used with 6 mm diameter cannulae. Cannulae of 11 mm are sometimes used with 10 mm instruments or for specific procedures that require a slightly larger incision. Clip-on reducers are available to allow use of 5 mm instruments with these cannulae. Instruments include:

- 6 mm laparoscopy cannulae with sharp trocars or Ternamian Endotip® cannulae
- 11 mm laparoscopy cannula with sharp trocar
- 11 mm/6 mm reducer
- 6 mm flexible thoracoscopy cannulae with blunt trocars
- Palpation probe
- 5 mm biopsy forceps, cup type
- 5 mm Babcock's grasping forceps
- 5 mm serrated grasping forceps
- 5 mm curved scissors
- 5 mm haemostatic clip appliers
- Commercially available pre-tied loop ligatures on a knot pusher.

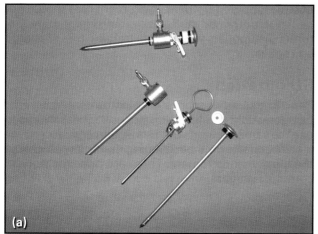

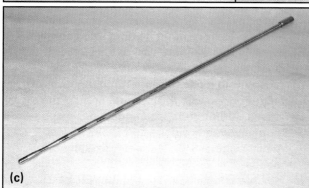

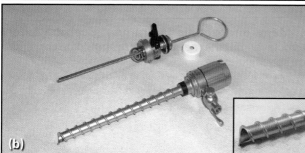

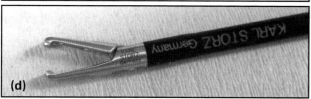

10.12 Additional instruments for laparoscopy and thoracoscopy. **(a)** Reusable laparoscopic cannula with sharp trocar (assembled above; disassembled below). **(b)** Ternamian Endotip® cannula. The threaded cannula allows controlled insertion and retains the cannula in the body wall during the procedure. The insert shows tip detail. **(c)** Palpation probe. Note the blunt tip (left) and graduations to allow assessment of lesion size and depth. **(d)** Babcock forceps (5 mm), such as might be used to grasp the ovary or stomach wall.

A vast range of instruments is available for specific laparoscopic and thoracoscopic endosurgical procedures, including needle-holders, staplers and bipolar electrosurgical instruments for sealing and resecting tissue.

For laparoscopy an insufflator is required in order to create a space in which to work. The gas commonly used is carbon dioxide as it is non-flammable and

easily absorbed, thereby reducing the risk of gas embolism. New and second-hand carbon dioxide insufflators are easily available, but it is important to ensure that an electronic insufflator is used, as this will automatically monitor and maintain intraperitoneal pressure at a preset level. Manual insufflators are also available but, as they require a dedicated operator to monitor and adjust the gas flow constantly, are generally not suitable for routine use.

An electrosurgery unit is extremely useful for maintaining haemostasis. Many laparoscopic instruments are insulated and have a monopolar electrosurgery connector on the handle to enable them to be used for haemostasis. If a machine for open surgery is already available, leads and adaptors can usually be provided for endoscopic instruments. This enables one machine to be used for open procedures as well as endoscopic surgery. A bipolar facility is useful. Specialist endosurgical units like the Ligasure® (Tyco/Valleylabs) or Harmonic Scalpel® (Ethicon) are available and greatly facilitate endosurgical dissection, but at a cost prohibitive to most general practitioners.

Arthroscopy

Additional accessories (Figure 10.13) include:

- A high-flow arthroscopy sheath designed for the endoscope used
- A selection of probes
- Arthroscopic grasping forceps
- A range of instrument cannulae (2.3–3.5 mm diameter) with switching sticks to facilitate instrument introduction and switching
- Hand milling drills
- Arthroscopic curettes
- Arthroscopic knives
- Infusion pressure jacket or an electronic arthroscopic infusion pump for pressurized saline (Hartmann's) irrigation.

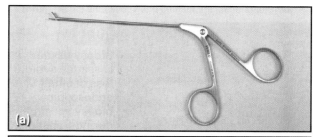

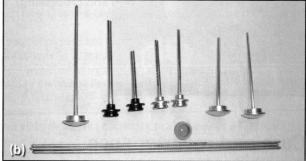

10.13 Additional instruments for arthroscopy. **(a)** Arthroscopic forceps, such as might be used to grasp cartilage flaps or bone fragments. **(b)** Arthroscopic cannulae (centre) with trocars (left and right), a spare seal and switching sticks (bottom). (continues) ▶

require a plentiful supply of warmed (to 37°C) sterile saline solution. Saline infusions containing glucose are not suitable for use in rhinoscopy, as they may provide a favourable environment for microorganisms.

Specific requirements:

- Light source
- Camera system
- 3.5–9 mm flexible endoscope
- Mouth gag
- 2.7 mm 18 cm 30 degrees endoscope
- 14.5 Fr cystoscopy sheath with 5 Fr instrument channel
- 7 Fr 40 cm biopsy forceps
- 7 Fr 40 cm grasping forceps
- 3 mm rigid biopsy forceps
- Biopsy tissue cassettes
- Giving set
- Normal saline (at least 1 litre)
- Gridded table.

The key to successful rhinoscopy is aggressive saline irrigation, as nasal mucosa bleeds readily, especially in the presence of inflammation. A gridded table is ideal, but if not available a deep tray covered with a grid will make an acceptable substitute.

> ⚠️ **WARNING**
> The nose is highly vascular and continuous irrigation with very cold saline can significantly affect core body temperature in smaller patients. Careful monitoring of body temperature is essential, especially in prolonged procedures.

The patient is positioned in sternal recumbency, with the table angled so the head is lower than the rest of the body, and a rolled up towel under the chin. With a mouth gag inserted, a flexible bronchoscope or small gastroscope is inserted into the mouth and retroflexed over the soft palate to view the pharynx and choana. Biopsy and swab samples are taken as required.

- The cuff on the endotracheal tube should be checked carefully to ensure a good seal. The lungs should be manually inflated and listened to in order to determine if any gas is escaping around the tube.
- A sterile gauze pack should be placed over the larynx, leaving the free edge of the soft palate clear for fluid to drain into the mouth.
- A litre bag of saline on a high drip stand should be attached to the irrigation post of the cystoscope sheath using a standard giving set. The controls should be opened on the giving set, such that fluid flow is controlled using the tap on the cystoscope port.

The cystoscope is lubricated with a sterile water-based gel and inserted into the nostril. Saline irrigation is turned on and the dorsal, middle and ventral meatus are examined in turn. In most cats and dogs, the ventral meatus can be explored back to the pharynx and the openings of the Eustachian tubes (Figure 10.21).

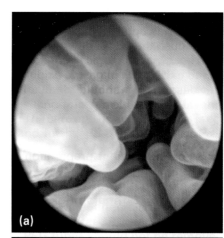

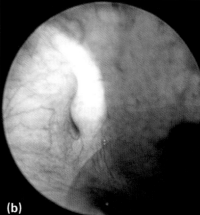

10.21
Rigid rhinoscopy. **(a)** Normal turbinates in the ventral meatus of a dog during saline irrigation. **(b)** Pharyngeal opening of the Eustachian tube (the slit to the left of the image) in a dog. (Reproduced from the *BSAVA Manual of Canine and Feline Endoscopy and Endosurgery*)

Multiple biopsy samples can be taken. They need to be sufficiently deep, as inflammatory mucosal proliferation may overlie more sinister pathology. Taking serial samples at the same site is helpful. Placing 3 mm or larger biopsy forceps alongside the endoscope enables larger samples to be obtained. Small samples are removed from the forceps and placed in a biopsy tissue cassette (see above). Larger samples can be teased off with a needle and placed directly in a formalin pot. Care should be taken that biopsy sites are noted and the subsequent samples labelled with their origin.

Postoperative care

- Premedication with acepromazine will reduce blood pressure and help limit haemorrhage. Postoperative acepromazine may also be considered if haemorrhage is severe.
- The patient should be maintained under anaesthesia until haemorrhage has ceased.
- Throat packing should be removed and the pharynx and oral cavity cleared but extubation should be left until the last minute to ensure adequate laryngeal reflexes.
- A quiet and slow recovery should be allowed. Hospitalization overnight should be considered – raised blood pressure on greeting owners may result in recrudescence of haemorrhage.
- Haemorrhage can be profuse but stops in 10 minutes, assuming there are no underlying coagulopathies. If bleeding persists, adrenaline flushes or cold compresses may be used.

■ Premedication with analgesics is advised, and pain is managed aggressively postoperatively.

■ Antibiotics are used as appropriate.

Urethrocystoscopy (in the bitch and queen)

Urethrocystoscopy is the gold standard for examination of the lower urinary tract. Flexible endoscopes or a laparoscopic approach must be used in male dogs and tom cats.

In bitches and queens, the equipment used is the same as for rhinoscopy (see above), with an additional giving set attached to an access port on the cystoscope to drain urine from the bladder into a suitable receptacle on the floor. A wet table or grid and tray are required to collect saline irrigant. A smaller endoscope (1.9–2.4 mm) with examination sheath may be required in queens and very small bitches. In very large dogs a 4 mm cystourethroscope is used.

The patient is positioned in sternal or lateral recumbency, with the vulva near the edge of the table. The authors prefer sternal recumbency with a rolled up towel under the pelvis and sandbags or positioning cradles for support, as required. The vulva and perineum are cleaned with chlorhexidine scrub and the tail elevated out of the way. An endoscope in a lubricated cystoscopy sheath is placed in the dorsal commissure of the vulva, avoiding the clitoral fossa, and the lips of the vulva are gripped by the left hand of the veterinary surgeon to form a seal around the shaft of the cystoscope. Saline flow is commenced and the vestibule can be seen to inflate, revealing the vaginal os and urethral orifice below (Figure 10.22).

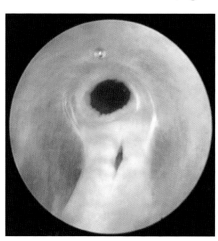

10.22

Endoscopic image of the vestibule of a bitch, showing the vaginal os dorsally and urethral opening below. Infusion of saline has distended the tissues, making the anatomy accessible.

The endoscope is advanced to examine the vagina, then retracted and redirected ventrally into the urethra. The urethra is examined for ectopic ureters or pathological changes as the endoscope advances. On entering the bladder, fluid flow is stopped and the bladder examined for obvious pathology. The effluent port is then opened to drain the urine, and the bladder is partially refilled with saline to improve visibility. The bladder and ureters can then be examined in detail. It is important not to overinflate the bladder, as this can cause damage and also makes examination and biopsy more difficult. The endoscope is withdrawn to the trigone and rotated through 360 degrees (keeping the camera stationary) to view the whole circumference of the trigone. In large dogs, if using a 2.7 mm endoscope,

it is often helpful for the veterinary nurse to manipulate the bladder externally to bring the proximal wall into view. Biopsy samples are taken using flexible biopsy forceps through the instrument channel. The samples are removed in saline and filtered through a biopsy tissue cassette before being stored in formalin.

A diode laser may be used to resect paramesonephric remnants or ablate bladder polyps or transitional cell carcinomas. Protective glasses should be worn at all times during laser use, and non-essential staff should not be permitted in the operating area.

> ⚠️ **WARNING**
> **Instilling a large volume of cold saline into the core of the body can result in hypothermia. The use of tepid saline and/or heated pads, and careful monitoring of body temperature is advised.**

Periurethral injections for urethral sphincter mechanism incompetence

A non-invasive treatment for urethral sphincter mechanism incompetence (USMI) involves the injection of a bulking substance, such as collagen, submucosally into the urethral wall just inside the proximal urethra about 1 cm from the trigone. Injection is usually done at three equidistant points using a 30 cm 23-gauge needle through the instrument channel of the cystoscopy sheath (Figure 10.23).

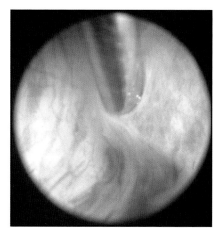

10.23

Treatment of urethral sphincter mechanism incompetence. Injecting bulking agent into the urethral wall using a 23-gauge needle. Note the magnification afforded by the endoscope.

■ Once the needle has been positioned by the veterinary surgeon, a syringe containing the bulking agent is attached to the hub by the veterinary nurse.

■ The solution is usually made up in saline and glycerine for added viscosity.

■ It is important to make a firm attachment and hold the needle hub firmly, since forcing a moderately viscous solution down a narrow-gauge needle requires considerable pressure, and if the syringe and needle separate the bulking agent will be lost.

■ The use of a small extension set with locking hubs on the needle and syringe should be considered.

■ Approximately 1–2 ml is injected at each site to form a bleb that partially occludes the urethral lumen.

In most cases resolution of signs is instant but will not be permanent. The bulking agent will eventually be resorbed, with return of clinical signs in 6–18 months. The procedure may then be repeated.

Postoperative care

■ In some cases, especially where there is urethral damage or pathology, a Foley catheter may be placed for a few days postoperatively to facilitate micturition without excessive straining. This should be capped and attached to a closed drainage system and precautions taken to prevent interference with the catheter by the patient.
■ Postoperative pain relief is advised for all patients, and should be managed aggressively following prolonged procedures such as laser resection of masses.
■ Infection is rarely a problem, due to the flushing effect of copious amounts of saline, but short-term antibiotic cover may be given.

Laparoscopy

Laparoscopy has many potential advantages over conventional open surgery:

■ Smaller incisions cause less postoperative pain and need a shorter recovery period
■ Excellent optics give the surgeon a well illuminated magnified view of the whole abdomen from a small access site
■ Reduced manipulation of tissues leads to reduced postoperative inflammation and adhesions
■ Smaller skin wounds and the absence of a large open wound during surgery reduce the incidence of postoperative infection
■ Biopsy samples can be taken under direct visual control, from several sites at once, with minimal trauma.

Specific requirements:

■ Camera system and monitor
■ Xenon, metal halide or halogen light source
■ Electronic carbon dioxide insufflator
■ Veress needle (Figure 10.24)
■ Sterile insufflation tubing
■ 5.0 mm 29 cm Hopkins 0 degrees endoscope
■ 6 mm laparoscopic cannula with sharp trocar (x3) (or Ternamian tip cannulae)
■ 11 mm laparoscopic cannula with sharp trocar
■ 10/5 mm reducing valve
■ 5 mm endoscopic biopsy forceps (cup and/or punch type)
■ 5 mm endoscopic grasping forceps
■ 5 mm endoscopic Babcock forceps
■ 5 mm palpation probe with centimetre markings
■ Sterile de-ionized water for rinsing instruments
■ Standard laparotomy surgical kit.

The peritoneal cavity is a *potential* space. In life, serosal surfaces are in contact with each other, so a space must be created in order to be able to visualize areas of interest. To do this the abdomen is insufflated with carbon dioxide using an electronic

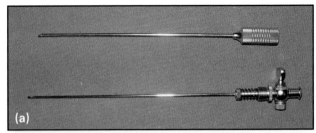
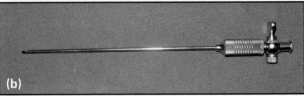

10.24 Veress needle. **(a)** Disassembled, with the outer sharp cannula above and the inner spring-loaded blunt needle below. **(b)** Assembled. Insufflation tubing is attached to the tap on the right.

insufflator (see Figure 10.7d). The gas is delivered into the abdomen via a Veress needle, a hollow needle containing a blunt trocar to minimize trauma on insertion (Figure 10.24). Most insufflators can be set to several gas flow rates. Initial flow rate must be slow (1 l/min) to allow the cardiovascular system to adjust to increased intra-abdominal pressure. Gas pressure in the abdomen presses on the diaphragm, reducing diaphragmatic movements and reducing thoracic and pulmonary volume, thereby reducing tidal volume. Pressure on the caudal vena cava also reduces venous return to the heart. If the increase in pressure is slow and a maximum pressure of 15 mmHg is used (12 mmHg in cats), then these changes are minimal and the circulation quickly adapts so that the changes become insignificant in the healthy patient. Patients with pre-existing cardiovascular or respiratory disease should be monitored extremely closely and minimal intra-abdominal pressures used. Pulse oximetry should always be used. Capnography and electrocardiography are useful additions.

If necessary the anaesthetist should be prepared to instigate positive pressure ventilation.

Once the abdomen is insufflated, the veterinary surgeon will insert the first cannula and introduce the endoscope into the abdomen. Local anaesthetic is often used at port sites to further reduce postoperative discomfort. The peritoneal cavity is examined for any iatrogenic damage or haemorrhage before inserting the operating cannula. The number and position of the cannulae (ports) will depend on the procedure being performed and the site of interest in the abdomen. Biopsy of the liver, kidney or pancreas will generally require two ports, whereas operative surgery will require at least three.

Most laparoscopic procedures are performed with the patient in dorsal recumbency, although left lateral recumbency is preferred by some for liver biopsy, and dorsolateral positions are required for endoscopic-guided needle biopsy of the kidneys. In any case, a tilting table is very useful as the patient may be manipulated during the procedure to move the internal organs out of the veterinary surgeon's field of view.

- A wide surgical clip is used and the abdomen prepared and draped as for open surgery.
- If complications occur, the veterinary surgeon should always be prepared to convert to an open surgical procedure immediately. A suitable surgical laparotomy kit should be available.

Following the procedure, the abdomen is checked for haemorrhage from any surgical sites, deflated, and the ports removed. Ports of 5 mm diameter usually only require skin closure; 10 mm ports are closed in two layers. In almost all cases, no preventive measures (such as a Elizabethan collar) are required, but it is important to assess the character of each animal, as persistent licking around port sites will lead to dermatitis and potential infection. Analgesics and antibiotics are administered as required.

Biopsy

Liver biopsy is performed under direct observation, allowing abnormal areas to be selected. Following insertion of the camera port, an operating port can be inserted under direct visualization from within the abdominal cavity to prevent iatrogenic damage. Instruments are always inserted under direct observation and followed down to the site of interest. A blunt palpation probe is inserted first and the liver examined in detail (Figure 10.25a). This is then replaced with cupped biopsy forceps and several samples taken. Haemorrhage is usually minimal and easily controlled (Figure 10.25b). The biopsy samples must be carefully teased off the jaws of the forceps with a hypodermic needle and placed directly in formalin. These samples are too large to place in biopsy tissue cassettes and attempting to do so will cause crush artefacts.

Pancreatic biopsy is performed in a similar manner, ideally using punch-type biopsy forceps and avoiding the central duct area.

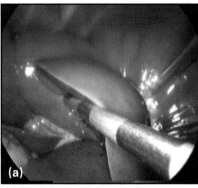
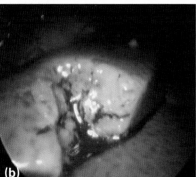

10.25 Liver biopsy. **(a)** Examining the liver of a dog using a palpation probe to separate the lobes and assess the texture. The liver in this patient is pale and brown. **(b)** Immediately following biopsy with cup forceps. Haemorrhage is usually minimal, as in this case. (Reproduced from the *BSAVA Manual of Canine and Feline Endoscopy and Endosurgery*)

Kidney biopsy is performed with the patient in dorsolateral recumbency. Samples are usually taken from the right kidney in bilateral disease, since this kidney is more fixed in position and the approach avoids the spleen on the left side. A camera and operating port are inserted around the midline and a palpation probe is inserted in the operating port. A 14–16 gauge spring-loaded biopsy needle is inserted percutaneously under direct visual guidance over the caudal pole of the kidney and directed into the parenchyma at an angle (Figure 10.26). The biopsy needle is fired and withdrawn and the palpation probe applied to the resulting wound to control haemorrhage. The sample is then removed from the biopsy needle and placed in formalin solution. Again, great care must be taken in teasing the sample from the needle to avoid artefactual damage.

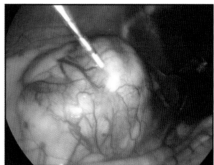

10.26 Kidney biopsy. The spring-loaded needle is passed into the cortex and away from the hilus.

Operative surgery

Operative surgery usually requires three ports and, although it can sometimes be performed by a single veterinary surgeon, it is helpful to have an assistant or veterinary nurse to operate the endoscope whilst the veterinary surgeon manipulates the instruments to perform the operation. It is essential that the veterinary nurse has adequate experience in manipulating the endoscope before assisting in live surgery. Laparoscopy involves manipulations within a three-dimensional environment, viewed on a two-dimensional screen. Perception of depth is lost and can be partially corrected for by skilful use of the endoscope. Moving close to the site of interest aids intricate manipulation and depth perception, whilst moving away from the focal point of interest broadens the view and helps when directing instruments into the abdomen and down to the operative site. The endoscope must be moved under the direction of the veterinary surgeon to follow closely the operative procedure without damage to surrounding structures. From time to time the view may be obscured by misting or contamination of the tip with body fluids. Gently wiping the tip on a serosal surface is usually sufficient to clear the view, but it may be necessary to remove the endoscope and clean it with a moistened swab.

PRACTICAL TIP

A laparoscopy trainer can easily be made using a small lightproof cardboard or plastic box with a few small holes cut into it for insertion of ports.

Ovariohysterectomy/ovariectomy

Laparoscopic ovariohysterectomy requires three ports. These are usually placed in the midline: cranial to the umbilicus; caudal to the umbilicus; and just cranial to the pelvic brim. With the ports in place, and the endoscope placed in the central port, the patient is rotated 45 degrees to one side and tilted into a head-down position to allow the viscera to fall away from the body wall and reveal the uterus (Figure 10.27a) and ovary on that side. Babcock forceps are placed in the caudal port and the ovary grasped and elevated. A bipolar cautery/cutting device is then placed through the cranial port and the ovarian ligament is transected. It is important that the cutting/cauterizing tip of the cautery device is kept within central view of the endoscope at all times. The ovary is then dropped over the bladder and the patient rotated on to the other side. The contralateral ovary is dissected in the same manner and is then withdrawn to the mouth of the cannula. The cannula, forceps and ovary are then withdrawn from the abdomen together. The remainder of the uterus and the remaining ovary are exteriorized and the cervix is ligated and transected as normal (Figure 10.27b). The operative ports are removed and closed with a single absorbable suture and skin adhesive.

Ovariectomy is widely performed in Europe and increasingly elsewhere. A two-port approach is used, cranial and caudal to the umbilicus. The ovary is grasped and elevated to the abdominal wall. An ovariectomy hook is introduced percutaneously to hook around the ovary and hold it in place. The grasping forceps can then be replaced with bipolar cutting forceps and the ovary is dissected free of the pedicle and uterus. The ovary is then grasped once more, the hook removed, and the ovary exteriorized either through the port or following removal of the port if required. The procedure is then repeated on the other side. This procedure requires a wide clip up the side of the abdominal wall to accommodate insertion of the ovariectomy hook.

Removal of a cryptorchid testicle

An endoscope port is placed near the umbilicus and an 11 mm port is placed lateral to the rectus abdominis muscle about halfway between the umbilicus and the pubis on the affected side. The testicle is easily located and grasped and is elevated to the mouth of the cannula. The cannula and testicle are then removed from the abdomen together (Figure 10.28). The vas deferens and spermatic vessels are then ligated and the testicle removed in routine fashion.

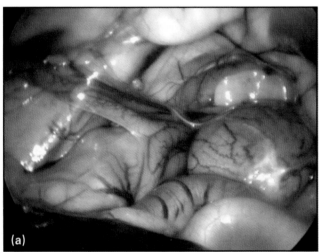
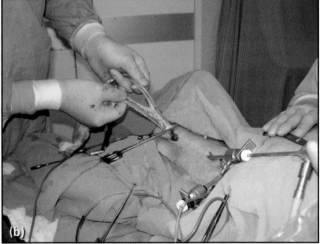
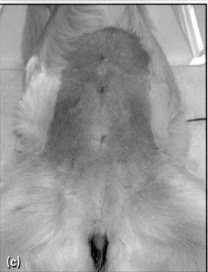

10.27 Laparoscopic ovariohysterectomy in a bitch. **(a)** View of the uterus; the bladder is to the right and the bifurcation is seen immediately cranial to this. **(b)** The uterus exteriorized following transection of the ovarian pedicles and broad ligament. The endoscope is seen in a cannula, close to the umbilicus, on the right of the picture. **(c)** Abdomen after laparoscopic spay, showing the three portal sites: cranial to the umbilicus; caudal to the umbilicus; and slightly cranial to the pubis. For ovariectomy only the two most cranial ports are required. (Reproduced from the *BSAVA Manual of Canine and Feline Endoscopy and Endosurgery*)

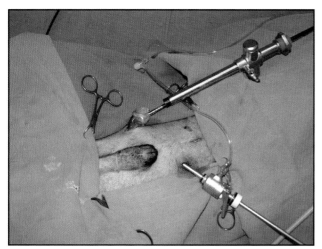

10.28 Laparoscopic removal of a cryptorchid testicle from a dog. The testicle has been retrieved through an enlarged instrument portal. The endoscope is in a portal to the left of the prepuce. Light from the endoscope is seen transilluminating the instrument portal. (Reproduced from the *BSAVA Manual of Canine and Feline Endoscopy and Endosurgery*)

Laparoscopic gastropexy

Following insufflation the primary camera port is introduced, to the right of the midline about 7–10 cm caudal to the umbilicus. A second port, preferably 10 mm with a 5 mm reducer to accommodate the instruments, is introduced under direct visualization, on the right side approximately 5 cm lateral to the umbilicus and 3–4 cm caudal to the last rib. A suitable section of stomach near the pyloric antrum is selected and grasped with Babcock forceps. The forceps are withdrawn to bring the stomach up to the mouth of the cannula, and the forceps, cannula and attached stomach wall are withdrawn, as one, through the trocar incision in the abdominal wall. In most cases the abdominal incision at the port entry site will need to be enlarged to about 3–5 cm with a No.15 blade to enable adequate exposure. Stay sutures are placed in the gastric wall and a 3 cm incision is made into the muscularis of the gastric wall, without penetrating the gastric lumen. The edges of this incision are sutured to the muscular abdominal wall with a simple continuous pattern of 2 metric (3/0 USP) monofilament absorbable suture material. The subcutaneous tissue and skin are then closed in a routine fashion. The gastropexy site is viewed through the endoscope before desufflating the abdomen and removing the endoscope and cannula. Port closure is routine.

Laparoscopic-assisted cystoscopy

Male dogs and cats, and patients with large cystic calculi are not amenable to rigid urethrocystoscopy. In these cases a laparoscopic-assisted approach is preferred. The enormous magnification afforded by the endoscope provides excellent visualization and enables the veterinary surgeon to remove even the smallest stones.

Prior to surgery a Foley catheter is placed in the bladder and the bladder drained and flushed with saline. The abdomen is insufflated and a camera port established at the umbilicus. An 11 mm operative port

is established over the bladder and the cranial pole of the bladder is grasped with Babcock forceps and brought up to the mouth of the cannula. The cannula is then removed, bringing the bladder wall into the abdominal incision, where it is held in place with stay sutures. The abdomen is desufflated. The bladder is then incised and the endoscope placed into the bladder directly. The bladder is examined and the urethra can be followed as far as the pelvic flexure (Figure 10.29). Instruments are placed alongside the endoscope to take biopsy samples, remove stones or resect masses. Following surgery the endoscope is removed and the bladder wall sutured and returned to the abdomen. Closure is routine.

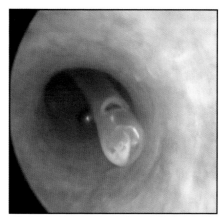

10.29 Laparoscopic-assisted cystoscopy in a dog. View from inside the bladder of the urethra at the pelvic flexure; a polyurethrane urethral catheter is seen extending into the bladder. (Reproduced from the *BSAVA Manual of Canine and Feline Endoscopy and Endosurgery*)

Postoperative care

- Recovery from laparoscopy is usually excellent compared with open surgery.
- Pain relief should always be given for at least the first 24 hours and thereafter as required.
- Wounds should be checked routinely after 3 days.

Thoracoscopy

Thoracic surgery has historically been associated with difficult surgical access, prolonged recovery and severe postoperative pain. Rigid thoracoscopy provides the veterinary surgeon with excellent access. There is minimal postoperative discomfort and patients generally show dramatically improved recovery times compared with open surgery.

Preoperative considerations

Any entry into the thorax will result in pulmonary collapse requiring *positive pressure ventilation*. This can be provided manually, using bag compressions, or mechanically with a mechanical ventilator.

- Care must be taken to adjust the tidal volume to an appropriate value for the individual patient.
- Manual compressions can be timed to assist the veterinary surgeon by keeping inflated lung out of the visual field at crucial times, but can be tiring if the procedure is lengthy.

- Single lung intubation is sometimes used, but requires specialist equipment. It has the advantage of freeing the veterinary surgeon's field of view almost completely.
- Careful monitoring is essential to ensure adequate oxygenation; pulse oximetry and capnography should be employed.

Patient position and port sites will vary according to the procedure. Lateral or ventral recumbency will be required to access the coronary vasculature or dorsal thorax for thoracic duct ligation. However, many diagnostic procedures, as well as pericardectomy, are done from a ventral approach with the patient in dorsal recumbency. This gives access to both sides of the chest and, because the lungs fall dorsally under gravity, exposes the ventral surfaces of the heart and lungs and much of the mediastinum.

- A wide clip must be employed over the whole of both lateral walls of the chest and extending back 8 cm caudal to the xiphisternum. This enables port placements on either side of the chest as required.
- As in laparoscopy, the team must be prepared to convert to open surgery at any time, and a full thoracotomy kit should be readily available.

Diagnostic thoracoscopy

Specific requirements:

- Camera and monitor
- Xenon or halogen light source
- Veress needle
- Sterile insufflation tubing
- 5.0 mm 29 cm Hopkins 0 degrees endoscope
- Flexible 5 mm disposable thoracic cannulae with blunt obturators
- 11 mm laparoscopic cannula with sharp trocar
- 5 mm endoscopic biopsy forceps (cup and/or punch type)
- 5 mm endoscopic grasping forceps
- 5 mm endoscopic scissors
- 5 mm endoscopic haemostats
- Palpation probe with cm markings
- Sterile de-ionized water
- Thoracic drainage kit
- Standard thoracotomy surgical kit.

With the patient in dorsal recumbency, a Veress needle is inserted through a stab incision just lateral to the sternum at about the eighth or ninth intercostal space to create a pneumothorax. Positive pressure ventilation should be started immediately.

> **WARNING**
> **Care must be taken by the veterinary nurse to time intermittent positive pressure ventilation (IPPV) inflations so that the veterinary surgeon is not in danger of damaging the lung whilst placing the port. Good communication between the veterinary surgeon and veterinary nurse is imperative.**

Initial port placement is just lateral to the xiphisternum. The port is placed through the diaphragm into the ipsilateral hemithorax. In most patients a 5 mm endoscope will enable examination as far forward as the thoracic inlet. The endoscope is then passed through the mediastinum into the contralateral hemithorax to complete the examination. Additional ports can be inserted under direct visualization near a point of interest in order to take biopsy samples or resect masses, etc. The valve assembly is always removed if laparoscopic cannulae are used, as a gas-tight seal is not required and can lead to a tension pneumothorax.

Thoracoscopic pericardectomy

The paraxiphoid approach described above is used. Since this is a surgical procedure requiring the veterinary surgeon to use two instruments, the assistance of a camera/endoscope operator is required. The same principles apply as described above for laparoscopy.

Additional operative ports are placed just dorsal to the costochondral junctions at the sixth and tenth intercostal space on the right side, or at the nineth intercostal space on each side. The caudal mediastinum is resected from the sternum, with close attention to haemostasis, to provide access to the whole of the ventral surface of the heart. The pericardium is then grasped at the apex with forceps, elevated, and incised with scissors. A pericardial window can then be carefully removed and withdrawn through one of the ports.

Closure

Following thoracoscopy a chest drain is introduced to provide drainage and resolution of the pneumothorax (see Chapter 8).

Arthroscopy

Joint surgery invariably causes a degree of trauma that can result in arthritic changes later in life. Surgical access also requires resection and/or retraction of ligaments and soft tissues around the joint, resulting in considerable postoperative discomfort, and even then access is often poor. Arthroscopy provides a minimally invasive method of examining joints in greater detail than is possible by open means, and surgical procedures can often be carried out at the same time, reducing perioperative pain and allowing the patient to regain use of the joint in the shortest possible time.

The most commonly used arthroscopes in veterinary surgery are the 2.7 mm 30 degrees endoscope, the 2.4 mm 30 degrees endoscope and the 1.9 mm 30 degrees endoscope. These small endoscopes are very easily damaged by torsion or flexion and are always used in a protective sheath to minimize the risk of this occurring. The 2.7 mm endoscope is used in the stifle and shoulder of medium and large dogs and can even be used in the elbows of large dogs. The 2.4 mm endoscope is best suited to elbows and hocks in medium to large dogs. In smaller dogs and cats the 1.9 mm endoscope is used.

Specific requirements:

- Camera and monitor
- Xenon or halogen light source

- 1.9 mm, 2.4 mm or 2.7 mm 30 degree endoscope
- Appropriately sized arthroscope sheath and blunt obturator
- Right angle probes
- Arthroscopic cannulae (with obturator and switching sticks)
- Large grasping forceps
- Milling drill
- 5-0 curette
- Banana knife
- Sickle knife
- Hartmann's solution (lactated Ringer's) (at least 1 litre)
- Giving set
- Infusion pump or pressure cuff for saline bag
- 18-gauge 40 mm needle
- 20-gauge 25 mm needle
- Electric arthroscopy shaver system (for stifle) (see Figure 10.8)
- Radiosurgery system (for stifle).

Elbow joint

The elbow joint is a common site of lameness in the dog, and radiographs are often difficult to interpret. Arthroscopy is the gold standard for examination of the joint and for removal of fragmented coronoid processes (FCP) (Figure 10.30) or treatment of osteochondrosis lesions.

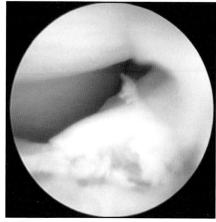

10.30 Elbow arthroscopy: fragmented coronoid process in a dog. Note the disrupted articular cartilage of the coronoid process in the lower half of the image, compared with the intact cartilage of the humeral condyle in the upper part.

- The joint should be shaved and prepared as for open surgery with a wide clip all round the limb above and below the elbow.
- Draping should allow for manipulation and mobility of the limb during surgery.
- Waterproof drapes prevent strikethrough and maintain surgical sterility.
- The patient is positioned in lateral recumbency with the affected limb down and a sandbag placed under the elbow joint to act as a fulcrum (Figure 10.31).

Three ports are generally used: an egress port; a camera port; and an instrument port. The egress port is established first, either with a bespoke cannula or,

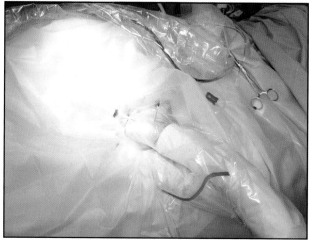

10.31 Elbow arthroscopy: dog positioned in semidorsal recumbency and draped for a medial approach to the left elbow. Saline has been injected to distend the joint (the syringe on the left) and a needle has been placed cranial to this to establish the access for the arthroscope.

more commonly, with an 18-gauge 40 mm needle. This is placed in the caudomedial joint capsule cranial to the anconeal process. A 10 ml syringe is attached and the joint is distended with lactated Ringer's solution. The camera port is established next. The joint space is widened by internal rotation and flexion of the joint over a fulcrum (an appropriately sized sandbag) and the arthroscope sheath with blunt obturator is introduced just distal to the medial epicondyle. The obturator is removed and replaced with the endoscope, and the fluid bag is attached to the inlet port of the arthroscope sheath. Following inspection of the joint an instrument portal is established in the craniomedial part of the joint. Different sized ports can be inserted to suit the instrumentation. Switching sticks are used to maintain access to the joint whilst repositioning ports.

The joint is inspected and probed for lesions. Fragments of bone or cartilage are removed via the instrument port and the underlying bone debrided to form a good bed for cartilage regrowth. The joint is flushed to remove any cartilage particles or bone fragments. Saline flow is turned off and the joint is infused with bupivacaine to reduce postoperative discomfort. Ports are removed. The wounds are closed with a single non-absorbable stitch or skin adhesive.

Shoulder joint

Lameness of the shoulder is commonly due to OCD lesions (Figure 10.32) or soft tissue injury. OCD lesions can be treated arthroscopically and the joint assessed for soft tissue injuries that would not be visible with radiography or computed tomography (CT).

- The patient is positioned in lateral recumbency with the affected leg uppermost.
- The joint is clipped as for open surgery.
- The leg is draped in a hanging limb preparation to provide a wide freedom of movement during the procedure. Lateral drapes may be used if preferred, but provide less manoeuvrability.

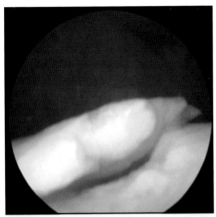

10.32 Shoulder arthroscopy: osteochondrosis dissecans in a dog. A large fragment of articular cartilage is seen, separated from the underlying humeral head (below) by an obvious cleft.

An egress port is established with an 18-gauge 40 mm needle placed in the cranial joint space, and 10–12 ml of lactated Ringer's solution is injected. The arthroscope with blunt obturator is then inserted directly distal to the acromial process of the scapula. The obturator is removed and replaced with the endoscope and the fluid bag is attached to the inlet port of the arthroscope sheath. Following inspection of the joint an instrument portal is established approximately 2 cm caudal and slightly distal to the acromium. This is the optimum position for debridement and removal of OCD lesions of the humeral head. Different sized ports can be inserted to suit the instrumentation. Switching sticks are used to maintain access to the joint whilst repositioning ports.

The joint is inspected and probed for lesions. Fragments of cartilage are removed via the instrument port and the underlying bone debrided to form a good bed for cartilage regrowth. The joint is flushed to remove any cartilage particles or bone fragments. Saline flow is turned off and the joint is infused with bupivacaine to reduce postoperative discomfort. Ports are removed. The wounds are closed with a single non-absorbable stitch or skin adhesive.

Tarsal joint

The tarsal joint (hock) is very small and requires the use of a 1.9 mm or 2.4 mm endoscope. Even so, arthroscopy can be challenging as arthritic changes progress.

- The patient is clipped and prepared as for open arthrotomy.
- A hanging limb preparation is recommended to give maximum manoeuvrability during surgery.
- The patient is positioned according to the site of interest. For dorsal lesions, dorsal recumbency is selected and for plantar lesions ventral recumbency with the hindlegs extended is best.

The site of the lesion will ideally have been identified radiographically prior to surgery, and will dictate the exact position of the portals. Two or three portals are required depending on the procedure. As the joint is very small, the egress port sometimes doubles as an instrument portal. A dorsolateral egress portal is established and 3–6 ml of lactated Ringer's solution is injected. A plantarolateral camera port and a plantaromedial instrument port are established next. Joint closure is routine.

Stifle joint

The stifle joint is a common site of injury in medium to large dogs, with cruciate ligament and meniscal injury topping the list of conditions seen. The stifle presents a challenge to the arthroscopist, as access to the joint is hampered by the patellar fat pad, and synovial proliferation and hyperaemia often lead to intra-articular haemorrhage that can obscure the view. It is therefore necessary to have a motorized shaver and radiosurgery equipment available. A large diameter fenestrated outflow cannula is also required since smaller portals can easily become blocked by synovium.

Arthroscopic cruciate surgery is in its infancy and it is more usual to perform an arthroscopic examination of the joint to assess for meniscal damage prior to a traditional open stabilization technique. If the damage is limited to the menisci, these can be treated arthroscopically without further resort to open surgery.

- The leg is clipped and prepared as for open arthrotomy.
- The patient is placed in dorsal recumbency with the affected leg over the end of the table.
- The opposite leg is tied laterally so that the affected leg is upright and hanging straight.
- The limb is draped for open surgery, as this is often performed following arthroscopic assessment.

A craniolateral port, just lateral to the tibial crest is established first. With the leg in extension, a blunt switching stick is inserted into the first portal and guided through the joint, under the patella until it exits the skin just medial to the quadriceps tendon. The outflow cannula is slid over the switching stick and into the joint. The switching stick is then removed and the egress cannula repositioned in the medial joint compartment. The arthroscope cannula with blunt obturator is then introduced into the first craniolateral port site and advanced under the patella into the midline proximal joint pouch. The obturator is replaced by the endoscope and inflow is established from the pressure bag or infusion pump. The joint is flushed to obtain a clear view. The proximal joint, trochlear ridge and medial and lateral joint compartments are explored. A craniomedial port is then established directly opposite the primary camera port. A motorized shaver is introduced to remove the fat pad, and haemorrhage is controlled by radiosurgery or electrocautery. Once the fat pad and synovial proliferation have been removed the cruciate and menisci can be examined and treated. Joint closure is routine.

Postoperative care

- Opiate analgesics are given routinely postoperatively in conjunction with non-steroidal anti-inflammatory drugs (NSAIDs) which are continued for 5–7 days.

- A cold pack is applied to the joint during recovery, for a period of 15 minutes, to relieve pain and swelling. Two applications (15 minutes on and 10 minutes off) are applied daily for 48–72 hours until the surgical swelling is absent.
- Heat therapy is then applied as a moist heat pack or warm towel (test against your own elbow for 30 seconds first); 10-minute applications are followed by gentle passive flexion and extension of the joint, starting with small movements and increasing slowly, for 1–2 minutes. The animal must be observed closely for any discomfort, and the range of motion used adjusted accordingly. It is sensible initially to have a second person to restrain the animal while physiotherapy is being provided (see Chapter 4).
- Exercise is limited for 4 weeks after surgery to on-lead exercise only. Walking in high grass or shallow water forces the dog to pick up the feet and increases the range of movement of the joints. If possible, consider referring the dog for postoperative hydrotherapy at an appropriate centre once skin wounds have healed, as this will provide the most comprehensive method of postoperative rehabilitation (see Chapter 4).
- From 4 to 8 weeks, exercise is gradually increased to normal levels.

References and further reading

Lapish J and Van Ryssen B (2006) Arthroscopic equipment. In: *BSAVA Manual of Canine and Feline Musculoskeletal Disorders,* ed. JEF Houlton *et al.,* pp. 177–183. BSAVA Publications, Gloucester

Lhermette P and Sobel D (2008) *BSAVA Manual of Canine and Feline Endoscopy and Endosurgery.* BSAVA Publications, Gloucester

Van Ryssen B (2006) Principles of arthroscopy. In: *BSAVA Manual of Canine and Feline Musculoskeletal Disorders,* ed. JEF Houlton *et al.,* pp. 184–192. BSAVA Publications, Gloucester

11

Advanced imaging

Lindsay Crane and Esther Barrett

This chapter is designed to give information on:

- Advanced radiographic positioning
- Advanced contrast radiography
- Digital radiography
- Fluoroscopy
- Ultrasonography
- Computed tomography
- Magnetic resonance imaging
- Scintigraphy

Advanced radiographic positioning

Patient positioning for routine radiographic examinations is comprehensively described in the *BSAVA Manual of Practical Veterinary Nursing*. For some routine radiographic examinations of cats and dogs there are several alternative positioning techniques, and a number are described in Figure 11.1. The indications and patient positioning for a selection of more specialized radiographic examinations is also described. These views are not part of a routine radiographic examination, but should be used at the specific request of the veterinary surgeon when trying to answer a specific question about the condition being investigated. These advanced radiographic positioning techniques are also described in Figure 11.1.

Area to be radiographed	Beam centring	Positioning and collimation	Comments
Spine			
Left 45° ventral–right dorsal oblique (Lt45°V–RtDO) view Right 45° ventral–left dorsal oblique (Rt45°V–LtDO) view 45°	Palpate the spine and centre on the area of interest as for a ventrodorsal spinal radiograph	Place the patient in dorsal recumbency and then rotate 45° laterally. Support the patient in this position with foam wedges and sandbags. The side of the spinal column closer to the cassette will be highlighted ventrally and should be labelled accordingly with a L/R marker placed on the ventral aspect of the animal. Repeat the radiograph with the animal rotated to the opposite side	Oblique views of the spine are useful to assess the obliquely positioned intervertebral foramina in the cervical spine, and for a fuller evaluation of suspected lesions noted on myelography. Together with the lateral and ventrodorsal views, the oblique views will help to identify which side of the spinal cord is affected

11.1 Positioning techniques for advanced radiography. General anaesthesia is required to facilitate the positioning described. All images must be appropriately labelled with a L/R marker. (continues)

Area to be radiographed	Beam centring	Positioning and collimation	Comments
Feline tympanic bulla			
Rostral 10° ventral–caudodorsal oblique (R10°V–CdDO) view	Centre in the midline over the pharynx, just caudal to the ramus of the mandible	Place the cat in dorsal recumbency supported in a trough. Secure forelimbs caudally with sandbags. Flex the head so that the hard palate is positioned 10° beyond the vertical and support in position using a foam wedge	This view enables visualization of the tympanic bullae whilst keeping the mouth closed. It is a useful alternative to the open-mouth rostrocaudal (RCd) view, especially in cats. It is important to make sure the head and body are kept in a straight line. Make sure the anaesthetic circuit is adequately supported while performing this view
Temporomandibular joint (TMJ)			
Left lateral 20° rostral–right lateral caudal oblique (Lt20°R–RtCdO) (closed mouth) view Right lateral 20° rostral–left lateral caudal oblique (Rt20°R–LtCdO) (closed mouth) view	Centre on the caudoventral border of the uppermost zygomatic arch at the level of the external ear canal	Place the patient in lateral recumbency with the side under examination closer to the cassette. Place head in true lateral recumbency, with the hard palate positioned perpendicular to the cassette. Elevate the nose between 10° and 30° to the cassette with a triangular foam wedge: ■ Dolichocephalic breeds = 10° ■ Mesaticephalic breeds = 15° ■ Brachycephalic breeds = 20–30° Collimate to include the area of interest	This view allows the TMJ to be visualized without superimposition of other structures. By raising the patient's nose, the TMJ adjacent to the cassette is highlighted rostrally and should be labelled L or R as appropriate. When investigating jaw-locking or TMJ pain, these views should be repeated with the mouth open
Pelvis			
Dorsal acetabular rim (DAR) view	Palpate the lumbosacral region and centre in the midline	Place the patient in sternal recumbency. A trough may be useful, especially for a narrow-chested animal. Extend the hindlimbs cranially so that they lie along the side of the body. Using a tie, bind the femurs to the caudal abdomen, keeping them parallel with and close to the torso. This should rotate the pelvis under the caudal abdomen so that its long-axis is perpendicular to the cassette, with the animal effectively sitting on the tuber ischii. The stifles should be flexed to 90°. Small pads placed under each hock will help with positioning of the hindlimbs. Collimate to include the ilial wings and greater trochanters laterally	The DAR view is used to look at the cranial and dorsal areas of the acetabular region of the pelvis. The DAR region is the main weight-bearing area of the hip and may show evidence of degenerative change before this can be seen on a standard ventrodorsal pelvic radiograph

11.1 (continued) Positioning techniques for advanced radiography. General anaesthesia is required to facilitate the positioning described. All images must be appropriately labelled with a L/R marker. (continues) ▶

Area to be radiographed	Beam centring	Positioning and collimation	Comments
PennHIP views (extended limb, distraction and compression views) This is described for information only. The view requires manual restraint of the patient and is therefore not used in the UK 	Centre as for a ventrodorsal pelvic radiograph	Place the patient in dorsal recumbency and support symmetrically with sandbags or a trough. A standard extended limb ventrodorsal pelvic view is taken. For the compressed view, the hips are flexed to 90° and the femurs manually pushed down to seat the femoral heads fully within the acetabulum. For the distracted view, a special frame is placed between the femurs. The femurs are then held tightly against the frame, placing a lateral force on to the femoral heads; increase to demonstrate any joint laxity	This procedure has been named after The University of Pennsylvania Hip Improvement Program (PennHIP), which is similar to the BVA hip score scheme. The procedure comprises a set of 3 pelvic radiographs: a standard ventrodorsal extended leg view and compressed and distracted views to assess joint laxity. The Distraction Index (DI) is the measurement of joint laxity and is calculated by comparing the position of the femoral head centre in the compressed and distracted views 0.0 DI = Fully congruent 1.0 DI = Luxation Hips with a DI <0.3 rarely develop secondary osteoarthritis **This procedure is not performed in the UK as it requires manual restraint**
Pelvic inlet view: ventro20°cranial–dorsocaudal (V20°Cr–DCd) view Pelvic outlet view: ventro20°caudal–dorsocranial (V20°Cd–DCr) view 	Centre as for a normal ventrodorsal pelvis view	Place the patient in dorsal recumbency and support with sandbags or a trough. The X-ray tube is tilted 20° cranially for the pelvic inlet view and 20° caudally for the pelvic outlet view	These views are performed to assess the cranial and caudal openings of the pelvis. This can provide additional information in the assessment of the post-traumatic pelvis
Limbs			
Carpus Dorsopalmar (DPa) laterally and medially stressed views 	Centre in the midline at the level of the antebrachio-carpal joint	Place the patient in sternal recumbency with the head supported on a foam pad to reduce rotation. Extend the forelimb under investigation cranially and secure it, using foam wedges and sandbags to prevent rotation **Medial distraction:** Place adhesive tape or a tie around the distal radius/ulna proximal to the carpus (without obscuring any of the carpal bones). Secure the tape medially (a sandbag may be useful). Place a second piece of tape around the foot and distract the distal limb laterally and secure it in the same way. Collimate to include the distal third of the radius/ulna and the foot **Lateral distraction:** Repeat as for the medial distraction view but reverse the tapes	These stressed views are used when collateral joint instability is suspected. They can also be used to highlight suspected carpal fractures but care must be taken not to cause additional fracture displacement. It is important to include the foot as this will help to visualize the degree of laxity in the joint. Markers should be used at the level of each tape to identify the direction of forces used to stress the joint

11.1 (continued) Positioning techniques for advanced radiography. General anaesthesia is required to facilitate the positioning described. All images must be appropriately labelled with a L/R marker. (continues)

Area to be radiographed	Beam centring	Positioning and collimation	Comments
Mediolateral extended (ML extended) view Mediolateral flexed (ML flexed) view 	Centre at the level of the antebrachio-carpal joint	Place the patient in lateral recumbency with the limb under investigation adjacent to the cassette. The other limb should be secured caudally using a tie. Using the adhesive tapes or ties proximal and distal to the carpal joint, the carpus should be secured in maximum extension for the extended view, and in maximum flexion for the flexed view. Collimate to include the distal third of the radius/ulna and the foot	Including the foot helps to visualize the degree of laxity in the joint
Tarsus			
Plantarodorsal (PID) laterally/ medially stressed views 	Centre in the midline at the level of the tibiotarsal joint	Place the patient in sternal recumbency with the head supported on a foam pad. Place padding under the hindlimb not under investigation. This helps to rotate the pelvis so that the limb of interest can be fully extended caudally. Apply adhesive tapes or ties proximal and distal to the tarsal joint, distracting the proximal limb medially and the distal limb laterally. Collimate to include the distal third of the tibia and the foot. Reverse the tapes to distract the joint medially	Markers should be used at the level of each tape to identify the direction of forces used to stress the joint
Mediolateral extended (ML extended) view Mediolateral flexed (ML flexed) view 	Centre at the level of the tibiotarsal joint	Place the patient in lateral recumbency with the limb under investigation adjacent to the cassette. The other limb should be secured out of the way using a tie. Apply the adhesive tape or a tie proximal and distal to the tarsal joint and secure the joint in maximum extension or in maximum flexion as required. Collimate to include the distal third of the tibia and the foot	Including the foot helps to visualize the degree of laxity in the joint

11.1 (continued) Positioning techniques for advanced radiography. General anaesthesia is required to facilitate the positioning described. All images must be appropriately labelled with a L/R marker. (continues) ▶

Area to be radiographed	Beam centring	Positioning and collimation	Comments
Dorsoplantar (DPI) flexed skyline view	Centre in the midline at the level of the tibiotarsal joint	Place the animal in dorsal recumbency, using sandbags to keep it straight. Place a foam pad between the stifles and secure with adhesive tape so that they are level and parallel. Place the tarsi on top of a pad/block (10–25 cm in height depending on the size of patient), again using a foam pad to keep them separated and parallel. Flex the tarsocrural joint so that the digits are extended 15° beyond the vertical. A cassette is placed under the tarsi, on top of the supporting block. Collimate to include the area of interest	This view is used to examine the distal tibia without superimposition of the calcaneus
Shoulder Cranioproximal–craniodistal oblique (CrPr–CrDiO) flexed skyline view	Centre over the bicipital groove between the greater and lesser tuberosities of the humerus	Place the patient in sternal recumbency, with the head supported on a foam pad and rotated away from the shoulder to be radiographed. The sternum should also be rotated slightly away from the shoulder. Pads placed under the opposite forelimb may help with positioning. The limb under investigation needs to be fully flexed and the carpus brought caudally so that it is under the shoulder, with the foot placed slightly medially. The elbow needs to be held close to the body, which will help to keep the humerus straight. The cassette needs to be positioned into the crease of the elbow, held in position between the humerus and radius. Collimate to include the area of interest	This view is useful in the investigation of mineralized opacities seen on a mediolateral view, and helps to determine whether such opacities lie within the bicipital groove. It is also useful for showing any new bone formation within the groove
Elbow Craniolateral–caudomedial oblique (Cr15°L–CdMO) view	Centre as for a craniocaudal elbow view	Place the patient in sternal recumbency, with the head supported on a foam pad and rotated away from the elbow to be radiographed. The limb under investigation should be extended cranially. It is important to ensure that the shoulder, elbow and foot are in a straight line. Placing a pad in the opposite axilla helps to slightly rotate the trunk and straighten the limb. Support the thorax with a large sandbag to prevent too much rotation. A small pad behind the olecranon helps to keep the elbow extended. Rotate the limb medially (pronate) by 15° and secure with sandbags. Collimate to include the distal third of the humerus, proximal third of the radius/ulna and the lateral skin borders	This view of the elbow is useful for radiographic evaluation of the medial coronoid process of the ulna in cases of possible coronoid disease, and for further investigation of the medial humeral condyle in cases of possible osteochondrosis. It may also help in the identification of incomplete ossification of the humeral condyles. It is difficult to rotate the limb more than 15° for this view
Craniomedial–caudolateral oblique (Cr45°M–CdLO) view	Centre as for a craniocaudal elbow view	Position the animal as for the Cr15°L–CdMO view, but rotate the limb laterally (supinate) by 45°. Collimate as above	This view is useful for investigating the lateral humeral condyle in cases of suspected incomplete ossification of the humeral condyles

11.1 (continued) Positioning techniques for advanced radiography. General anaesthesia is required to facilitate the positioning described. All images must be appropriately labelled with a L/R marker. (continues)

Area to be radiographed	Beam centring	Positioning and collimation	Comments
Stifle Caudocranial (CdCr) horizontal beam view	Palpate the lateral and medial femoral epicondyles and centre just distally on the femorotibial joint	The hindlimb under investigation should be uppermost and fully extended, using foam pads to keep it parallel to the X-ray table. Palpate the femoral condyles to make sure that there is no rotation of the limb and the patella is in the midline. Using a tie, secure the limb in extension. Place a cassette vertically positioned against the cranial edge of the stifle. The cassette will need to be pushed against the abdomen and held in position with a pad/sandbags. A horizontal X-ray beam is then centred at the level of the stifle. Collimate to include to the distal third of the femur, proximal third of the tibia and skin margins NB. as the cassette is resting on the abdomen it is important that the exposure is made during the respiratory pause to avoid the cassette moving with respiration	It is easier to keep the stifle straight for a caudocranial horizontal beam view than for a similar view with the animal positioned in dorsal or sternal recumbency. However, the use of a horizontal beam increases the risk of radiation exposure. Horizontal beam radiography must only be carried out where this is permitted by the local rules and due attention must be paid to radiation safety

11.1 (continued) Positioning techniques for advanced radiography. General anaesthesia is required to facilitate the positioning described. All images must be appropriately labelled with a L/R marker.

Advanced contrast radiography

Contrast media are used in veterinary radiography to enable the visualization and differentiation of body tissues which would otherwise be indistinguishable from each other. Positive contrast media is more radiopaque than the surrounding structures, whilst negative contrast media is more radiolucent than the surrounding structures. An introduction to the different types of contrast media, as well as their use in gastrointestinal, urogenital and myelographic studies is given in the *BSAVA Manual of Practical Veterinary Nursing*. The increased availability of endoscopy and ultrasonography in general veterinary practice has, in some cases, reduced the need for radiographic contrast studies. However, in many cases, the information provided by these contrast studies is complementary to that provided by ultrasonography and endoscopy, and helps to build up a better overall understanding of the disease process being investigated. The following section describes some of the more advanced contrast radiographic procedures currently being used in veterinary practice.

Shoulder arthrography

Shoulder arthrography is most commonly used in dogs and is helpful in the radiographic assessment of the shoulder joint. This relatively simple procedure should be carried out with the patient under general anaesthesia. Before commencing the contrast study, routine craniocaudal and mediolateral views of the shoulder should be taken to evaluate the joint. There are three types of shoulder arthrography that can be performed:

- *Positive contrast studies* using sterile, water-soluble iodinated contrast media. Non-ionic contrast media is preferable to ionic media as it tends to be less irritant and remains visible in the joint space for longer
- *Negative contrast studies* using room air
- *Double contrast studies* using a combination of both. Care must be taken to avoid small air bubbles forming within the positive contrast media and confusing the image.

Positive contrast arthrography is the most frequently performed technique and is discussed below. For further information on negative and double contrast arthrography the reader is referred to the *BSAVA Manual of Canine and Feline Musculoskeletal Imaging*.

Indications

Shoulder arthrography is used to allow visualization of the articular surfaces of the proximal humerus and distal scapula, the shoulder joint space and its different pouches, the synovial membrane, and the biceps tendon. It is especially useful in identifying defects and cartilage flaps affecting the caudal articular surface of the humeral head in dogs suffering from shoulder osteochondrosis (OC). These changes to the articular surface are often not recognized with plain radiography.

Equipment

The following equipment is required:

- Clippers
- Surgical scrub supplies
- Sterile gloves
- Low osmolar water-soluble iodinated contrast media diluted to 100 mg I/ml with sterile water
- 10 ml syringe
- 20–22 gauge 25 mm needles.

Technique

The dog should be positioned on the X-ray table with the shoulder of interest uppermost and the area surgically prepared. The contrast media should be drawn up and diluted to 100 mg I/ml in an aseptic manner. A 20–22 gauge 25 mm needle should be positioned approximately 1 cm distal to the acromion and inserted distally, medially and caudally into the joint space (Figure 11.2). Correct needle placement is confirmed by aspiration of joint fluid.

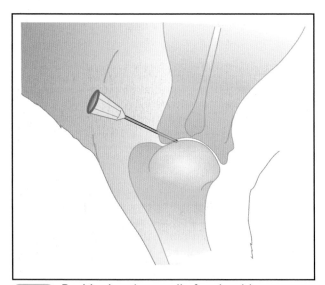

11.2 Positioning the needle for shoulder arthrography.

A total of 2–7 ml of contrast media should then be injected. Lower volumes are needed for evaluation of the joint space alone, whilst higher volumes are needed to fill the biceps tendon sheath. Following injection, the needle is immediately withdrawn, pressure is applied to the injection site and the shoulder manipulated to distribute the contrast media evenly throughout the joint space. The dog is then turned over so that the shoulder of interest is adjacent to the X-ray table. Once the contrast media has been injected, it is important to take the required radiographs relatively quickly as the contrast media will be re-absorbed within 10–15 minutes. As a minimum, standard mediolateral and craniocaudal

views should be taken. In some cases, especially when assessing the biceps tendon sheath, a cranioproximal–caudodistal (skyline) view may also be required.

Potential complications

The possible problems encountered when using this technique include:

- Too little or too much contrast media used
- Small air bubbles introduced whilst injecting (these can look like small joint mice)
- Injection of contrast media into soft tissues outside the shoulder joint space
- Leakage of contrast media into the periarticular structures.

Angiography

The term angiography refers to the use of contrast media to highlight the vascular system. It is performed by injecting a bolus of low osmolar water-soluble iodinated contrast media into the blood stream. Angiographic techniques currently used in veterinary medicine include portovenography, angiocardiography and peripheral angiography. The most commonly used of these techniques is portovenography.

Portovenography

Portovenography is used to visualize the flow of blood through the hepatic portal system and is generally considered to be the gold standard for diagnosis of portosystemic shunts (PSSs). PSSs occur where blood from the hepatic portal vein is shunted directly into the venous system, usually the caudal vena cava, without first being filtered and metabolized by the liver. The condition results in both metabolic and neurological abnormalities, with patients typically presenting with a history of poor growth and sometimes seizures. (See Chapter 8 for further information about the investigation of a patient with suspected PSS.)

Ultrasonography of the hepatic portal system is useful in the diagnosis of PSS, and has the advantage of being non-invasive and possible to carry out in the conscious patient. Ultrasonography also allows the detection of uroliths in the bladder; urate calculi are a common finding in patients with PSS, which can be missed on plain radiographs as they may be radiolucent. Where facilities are available, scintigraphy is also very useful in the diagnosis of PSS. Routine survey radiographs should also be part of the initial workup and will help to identify the size of the liver (typically small in a patient with PSS), kidneys (sometimes enlarged with PSS) and may allow the detection of bladder calculi.

Indications

Portovenography is used to identify the presence and location of a shunting vessel(s) between the hepatic portal and systemic venous systems. It also allows the veterinary surgeon to establish whether a shunt is intrahepatic or extrahepatic, and whether there are one or more shunting vessels. Figure 11.3 summarizes the more common types of PSS that may be identified. Following occlusion of the shunting vessel(s), portovenography also allows an assessment to be made of blood flow through the normal portal vasculature.

Type of PSS	Comments
Congenital	Typically a single (occasionally double) shunting vessel. In large breeds of dog they are usually intrahepatic, whilst in small breeds and cats they are usually extrahepatic. Commonly affected breeds include Irish Wolfhounds, Maltese dogs, Yorkshire Terriers and Persian cats
Acquired	These are typically composed of multiple shunting vessels and are seen in patients suffering from chronic portal hypertension. Although older animals are more commonly affected, acquired shunts are seen in younger patients secondary to arterioportal fistulae or congenital portal vein atresia
Single	One (occasionally double) shunting vessel
Multiple	Many shunting vessels
Intrahepatic	The shunting vessel(s) is located within the liver
Extrahepatic	The shunting vessel(s) is located outside the liver

11.3 Types of PSS that may be identified with portovenography.

Equipment

The following equipment is required:

- Sterile small animal surgical kit, including sterile swabs
- Suture material for wound closure
- Low osmolar water-soluble iodinated contrast media 300 mg I/ml
- 2–10 ml syringe (depending on the size of the patient)
- 18–22 gauge intravenous catheter
- Extension set
- Three-way tap or T-connection
- 0.9% saline solution to flush catheter
- Sterile bowls for saline and contrast media
- X-ray machine
- X-ray cassettes
- X-ray cassette holder (to position under the patient)
- Lead protective clothing
- Personal dosimeters.

Technique

Portovenography is carried out under sterile surgical conditions with the patient under general anaesthesia. Before the patient is placed on the operating table, the X-ray cassette holder, covered with a sterile drape, should be positioned so that it will be underneath the patient. The holder can be made of any radiolucent material and needs to be large enough to accommodate the cassette (and grid if necessary). Use of the holder allows the cassette to be removed and replaced whilst maintaining sterility and without moving the patient. It is advisable to take preoperative radiographs once the patient is positioned on the operating table so that positioning and exposure settings can be assessed.

The operating veterinary surgeon performs a laparotomy. A large mesenteric vein is selected and catheterized using an 18–22 gauge sterile intravenous catheter. Once the catheter has been secured in position and flushed, the animal is positioned in lateral recumbency and water-soluble iodinated contrast medium is injected at a dose rate of 1 ml/kg bodyweight. A lateral radiograph of the cranial abdomen and caudal thorax (centred on the liver) is taken at the time of contrast medium injection. In the normal animal, the contrast medium should pass into the hepatic portal vein which then branches throughout the liver, resulting in a general contrast enhancement of the liver parenchyma. When an abnormal shunting vessel(s) is present, this will be outlined by the contrast medium (Figure 11.4), resulting in poor or non-opacification of the normal hepatic portal system. In order to localize the shunting vessels more accurately, the animal can be repositioned in dorsal recumbency, the contrast medium injection repeated and a ventrodorsal radiograph taken. Once the shunting vessel has been identified, the veterinary surgeon may wish to temporarily occlude it, forcing blood to flow into the hepatic portal system. The contrast medium injection is repeated to outline this portal vasculature, allowing the surgeon to assess how well developed it is. All personnel present in the operating theatre at the time of radiography should be wearing protective lead clothing and personal dosimeters.

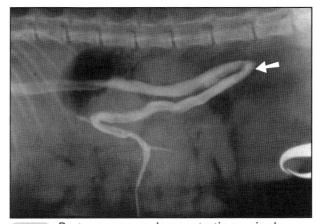

11.4 Portovenogram demonstrating a single congenital extrahepatic shunting vessel (arrowed) in a cat. (Courtesy of F Barr)

A C-arm is a mobile fluoroscopy unit (see below) which may be used for real-time imaging of the flow of contrast medium from the catheterized mesenteric vessel. The use of a C-arm has several advantages: watching the contrast medium flow in real-time often makes it easier to identify any shunting vessels; the image is detected by the C-arm itself with no need to reposition the animal to accommodate an X-ray cassette; and the image is produced instantly, avoiding the delay caused by the processing of standard X-ray film. However, the equipment required is expensive and typically only available in specialist referral centres.

fur with contrast medium as this could confuse interpretation of the images. Orthogonal radiographs should be taken to help identify the position and extent of the tract(s).

Potential complications

The possible problems encountered when using this technique include:

- Difficulty visualizing the total extent of the sinus tract/fistula
- Purulent debris and air bubbles masking the appearance of foreign bodies
- Leakage of contrast medium.

Ultrasonography is also a useful tool when investigating sinus tracts, especially when looking for foreign bodies. However, as ultrasonography often provides limited information about the direction and extent of the tract, sinography should be considered a useful and complementary imaging technique.

Dacryocystorhinography

Dacryocystorhinography involves the use of water-soluble iodinated contrast media to evaluate the nasolacrimal duct system. Situated in the medial canthus of each eye are the lacrimal puncta. These are small openings into which drain the tears produced to lubricate and protect the conjunctiva. The tears drain into the lacrimal duct, via the lacrimal sac, and into the nasolacrimal duct, finally emptying into the nares.

Indications

Dacryocystorhinography is indicated in the investigation of a suspected nasal/paranasal mass or foreign body that may cause obstruction of the lacrimal system. It is also useful in the investigation of abnormal overflow of tears (epiphora), especially in cases where the ophthalmological examination appears normal.

Equipment

The following equipment is required:

- Swabs
- Sterile gloves
- 0.9% sodium chloride solution
- Low osmolar water-soluble iodinated contrast medium diluted to 150 mg I/ml with sterile water
- 5 ml syringe and needles
- Lacrimal catheter
- Otoscope (to help visualize the nasal puncta if retrograde flush is required).

Technique

This procedure should be performed with the patient under general anaesthesia. Lateral and dorsoventral survey radiographs of the skull should be taken to look for any relevant bony changes or radiopaque foreign bodies. For the contrast study, the patient is placed in lateral recumbency with the side of interest uppermost. A lacrimal catheter is inserted into the tear duct. The nasolacrimal system should be flushed with saline to clear any purulent discharge that may be present before injecting the contrast medium. If a

foreign body is suspected, retrograde flushing with saline is advised to avoid lodging the foreign body further into the duct. However, visualizing the distal duct puncta in the nares is difficult in all but large breeds of dogs. Once the duct has been flushed, 1–1.5 ml of contrast medium should be injected, using digital pressure applied to the distal end of the duct (i.e. at the nares) to minimize contrast medium leakage. During contrast medium injection, it is also advisable to hold a swab over the lacrimal punctum to collect any leaking contrast medium at this site. The radiograph should be taken immediately on completion of the contrast medium injection, taking due precautions to ensure the radiation safety of the personnel involved. A prefilled extension set attached to the lacrimal catheter allows the radiograph to be exposed during the injection, with the person carrying out the injection wearing full lead protective clothing and standing as far away from the animal as possible.

Potential complications

The possible problems encountered when using this technique include:

- Contrast medium leakage
- Difficulty advancing the lacrimal catheter and injecting the contrast medium.

Lymphangiography

Lymphangiography involves the injection of contrast medium into the lymphatic system, either directly via catheterization of a lymphatic duct, or indirectly by injection into a lymph node or by subcutaneous injection into the tissues drained by a local lymph node in the area of interest. A series of radiographs is then taken to monitor the passage of the contrast medium through the lymphatic system (Figure 11.9).

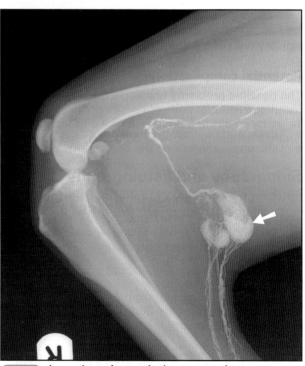

11.9 Lymphangiograph demonstrating an enlarged popliteal lymph node (arrowed) in a crossbred dog.

Indications

Indications for lymphangiography include the investigation of lymphoedema (the collection of fluid within the interstitial space associated with an interruption to normal lymphatic drainage), chylothorax and suspected primary or secondary neoplasia of the lymphatic system.

Equipment

The following equipment is required:

- Sterile small animal surgical kit including sterile swabs
- Suture material for wound closure
- Sterile gloves
- 25–27 gauge lymphatic cannulation needle
- Low osmolar water-soluble iodinated contrast media – for direct lymphangiography a total dose of 100 mg I/kg diluted in 0.25 ml/kg sterile saline has been recommended
- Sterile syringe and needles
- Extension set to attach to the cannula
- Vegetable dye (e.g. methylene blue) to highlight lymphatic drainage.

Technique

Before lymphangiography is carried out, survey radiographs should be taken. These radiographs should be assessed for any findings that will explain the reason for the presenting condition (e.g. neoplasia, trauma, sites of infection). The survey radiographs will also help to ensure that patient positioning and exposure settings are appropriate.

Direct lymphangiography

This should be carried out with the patient under general anaesthesia. The site should be aseptically prepared. A dye (usually methylene blue) is injected into the tissues distal to the area of interest, which is then taken up by the lymphatic vessels. Surgical exposure of the area of interest allows identification of the highlighted vessels, which can then be catheterized, and contrast medium injected directly. A series of radiographs is taken to document the passage of contrast medium through the lymphatic vessels.

Indirect lympangiography

This can be carried out with the patient under sedation. No surgical exposure is needed. A lymph node is identified distal to the lymphatic vessels of interest. Contrast medium is injected either directly into this lymph node, or into the surrounding tissues drained by that lymph node. A series of radiographs need to be taken to record the progress of contrast medium absorption and passage through the lymphatic system.

Potential complications

The possible problems encountered when using this technique include:

- Contamination of the area of interest by contrast medium leakage
- Interpretation of the images can be challenging as there are many vessels that can take up the contrast medium.

Digital radiography

The use of digital radiography is now standard in human hospitals and is becoming more widespread in veterinary practice. With digital radiography X-rays are generated and passed into the patient, interacting with the tissues in the same way as conventional radiography. The difference is the way in which the X-ray photons which pass through the patient are detected. In conventional radiography, the X-ray photons are detected using film (± intensifying screens) where they produce a latent image. The film is then chemically processed in order to produce a visible image (for more information see the *BSAVA Manual of Practical Veterinary Nursing*). In digital radiography, two alternative digital systems are currently used for detecting and recording the X-ray photons: computed radiography and direct digital radiography.

Computed radiography

Computed radiography replaces the conventional film–screen combination with a phosphor-based imaging plate. When X-ray photons strike the imaging plate, instead of producing a latent image on film, the plate temporarily stores the image as a pattern of excited electrons. The plate is then processed by a computed reader (Figure 11.10) which uses a laser beam to impart energy to the electrons, allowing them to 'release' the image as flashes of light which are digitally detected. A second laser is used to erase any traces of the image from the plate, which is then ready for re-use. The reading process typically takes somewhere between 1 and 3 minutes. The processed image is then displayed on a dedicated viewing monitor.

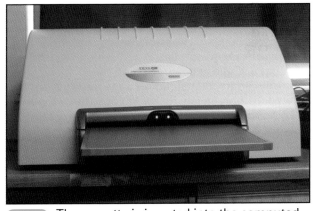

11.10 The cassette is inserted into the computed reader. The reader will extract the imaging plate from the cassette, scan and then erase the image and reload the cassette ready for re-use.

Direct digital radiography

Direct digital radiography replaces the film–screen combination with an X-ray sensitive panel which, in small animal radiography, is usually permanently attached to the X-ray table. The most popular technology uses flat panels (Figure 11.11) made of either selenium or silicon. The X-ray photons passing through the patient are detected by this panel and instantly (within 4–10 seconds) displayed as an image on the viewing monitor. Using this system, the size of the image that can be detected will be limited

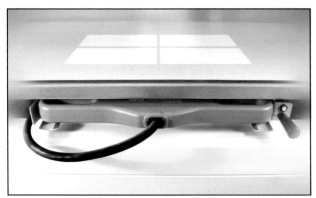

11.11 A flat panel positioned in the Bucky tray of an X-ray table. The wire attaches the panel to the computer, transferring the image information almost instantaneously on to the computer screen. (Courtesy of BCF Technology Ltd)

by the area of the panel. Direct digital radiography is considerably more expensive than computed radiography: its main advantage is the increased speed of image processing.

Both systems of digital radiography share similar advantages and disadvantages. It is important to appreciate that the image quality achieved with digital radiography is generally comparable with that achieved with conventional radiography.

Advantages

The advantages of digital radiography include:

■ Conventional X-ray film has a relatively narrow latitude, meaning that it is limited in the range of exposures which can be displayed as perceptibly different on the image. An important advantage of digital radiography is that it has a much wider latitude, making it possible to achieve good images of both soft tissue and skeletal structures using a single exposure setting
■ Within limits, digital radiography systems are able to compensate for overexposure. In theory this should result in fewer repeated films due to exposure errors, and therefore a reduced risk of staff exposure to radiation
■ Using digital radiography, all image processing is carried out by a dedicated computer. In theory such a system is cheaper to run as there are no costs associated with providing X-ray film, processing chemicals or maintaining the X-ray processor
■ The instant image production achieved with direct digital radiography saves a considerable amount of processing time. The processing time needed for computed radiography is comparable with the time taken by an automatic processor
■ Digital images are easier to archive than conventional X-ray films. Digital systems generally have an in-built archive facility, with back-up copies of all images kept on CD, DVD or optical discs. This takes up very little physical storage space in comparison with conventional film storage. It is also easier to retrieve images from the digital system, and images are less likely to be misplaced

■ The digital system is equipped with sophisticated image viewing software. Amongst other options, this software allows the viewer to adjust the brightness and contrast of the image, to annotate the image and to take measurements
■ If the digital radiography system is linked to the practice computer network, it is possible for the X-rays to be viewed simultaneously in different locations around the practice. Images can also be sent via email or CD for a second opinion, without the inconvenience of sending away the original films.

Disadvantages

The disadvantages of digital radiography include:

■ The installation of a digital radiography system is expensive. For a completely film-less system, running costs should be lower than conventional radiography because there are no film or chemical costs. However, if hard copies of the images are printed these savings may quickly be lost
■ As digital radiography systems are able to compensate for overexposure, it is easy to unknowingly use higher exposures than necessary. This can lead to an overall increase in staff exposure
■ Although digital radiography should save time on image processing, there is inevitably a period of familiarization with the system, during which image processing and management may take longer
■ The quality of the final image is dependent on the resolution of the viewing monitor. To optimize the image, expensive high-resolution monitors are required
■ Whilst the monitor can display multiple images simultaneously, it is probably only possible to accurately assess up to two images on the screen at once (Figure 11.12). To compare and evaluate more views at the same time, more viewing monitors will be needed

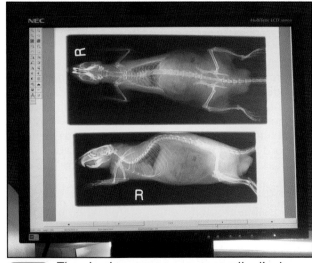

11.12 The viewing screen can generally display two images satisfactorily. Where more images are displayed, it becomes increasingly difficult to assess the images accurately.

- Viewing monitors will also be required wherever there is a need to display the images, for example in the operating theatre and consulting rooms
- Not all systems will display the images 'life-size', which can be frustrating when trying to select the correct size of surgical implants
- The bulky nature of the imaging plates or flat panel detector systems currently make direct radiography challenging to use for intraoral radiography
- The digital radiography system is reliant on a central computer, with potential loss of both image data and the ability to process further X-rays if it crashes. It is therefore essential to back-up all data on a regular basis, and to invest in a comprehensive support package for the system.

Fluoroscopy

Fluoroscopy uses X-rays to create a real-time image of moving structures. The image is displayed on a monitor, with radiopaque structures appearing dark and radiolucent structures appearing light (i.e. the opposite to conventional radiographs). The need for sophisticated and expensive equipment means that the use of fluoroscopy in veterinary medicine is mainly limited to referral centres (Figure 11.13).

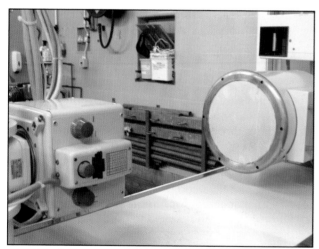

11.13 A fluoroscopy system. The X-rays generated by the X-ray tube (left) are detected by the image intensifier (right) and then displayed on a remote viewing screen.

Basic principles

During fluoroscopy, the X-rays are generated by the X-ray tube in the same way as any routine X-ray examination. However, rather than a single exposure lasting less than a second, it is sometimes necessary to continue producing X-rays for several minutes at a time. This creates potential problems: to personnel due to increased radiation exposure; and to the X-ray tube due to a greatly increased risk of overheating. To minimize these problems, it is important to keep the mA (the 'quantity' of radiation produced) as low as possible. The image detector therefore has to be very sensitive to the low levels of photons passing through the patient. To provide real-time imaging the fluoroscopic image also needs to be generated as instantaneously as possible. The *image intensifier* is an image receptor capable both of detecting and 'intensifying' very low levels of radiation and of translating the photons detected into a visible moving image. This image is displayed on a remote viewing monitor. A C-arm is a mobile fluoroscopy unit, where the X-ray tube and image intensifier are linked by a 'C'-shaped arm.

Image intensifier

The image intensifier comprises an input screen, an electronic 'focusing' system and an output screen, housed within a vacuum chamber (Figure 11.14).

- The *input screen* is a phosphor (caesium iodide), which converts X-rays into light photons in the same way as intensifying screens in conventional radiography. These light photons then strike a photocathode, which responds to the light by releasing electrons.
- The *electronic 'focusing' system* applies a potential difference of 25–30 kV across the vacuum, accelerating the electrons released from the input screen and focusing them on to the output screen at the far end of the image intensifier.
- The *output screen* absorbs the fast moving electrons which strike it, converting their energy back into light. For each electron reaching the output screen, many more light photons are released, therefore amplifying the signal from the electrons. The light creates an image on the output screen: the brightness of this image is also amplified by the fact that the output screen is much smaller than the input screen, 'intensifying' the image into a much smaller area. The image can then be viewed by a television camera and displayed on multiple viewing monitors.

Viewing and recording the image

The image produced at the output screen is viewed by a television camera and displayed as a real-time image on one or more remote viewing monitors. A permanent record of the image can be made using a video recorder. It is also possible to fit an analogue-to-digital converter to digitize the output from the camera, allowing further electronic processing and recording of the image. Instead of producing digital images, older fluoroscopic units use a partially-silvered mirror to direct part of the light from the output screen on to 'spot films' which then record the light image.

Indications

The indications for fluoroscopy include:

- Investigation of dysphagia, regurgitation or suspected megaoesophagus. A barium swallow should be performed, giving the animal liquid or food mixed with barium. Fluoroscopy allows evaluation of swallowing and oesophageal function, observing the passage of contrast medium from the mouth to the stomach

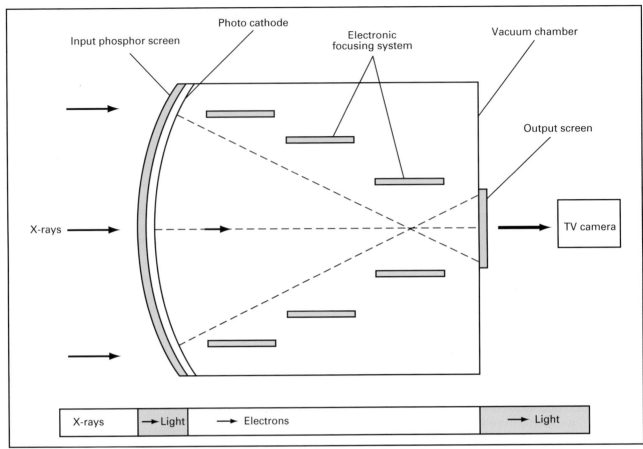

11.14 The image intensifier comprises of an input screen, an electronic 'focusing' system and an output screen, housed within a vacuum chamber.

- Assessment of suspected hiatal hernia or oesophageal reflux. Once the barium has reached the stomach, it is easy to assess the location of the stomach within the cranial abdomen, and to observe whether there is dynamic cranial displacement of the stomach through the diaphragm, or whether there is reflux of the contrast medium from the stomach to the oesophagus
- Observation and removal of oesophageal or tracheal foreign bodies. Fluoroscopy can be used as an alternative technique to endoscopy in guiding the retrieval of radiographically apparent foreign bodies from the trachea or oesophagus
- Fluoroscopy is useful in the observation and monitoring of the stretching of an oesophageal stricture using a balloon catheter
- Dynamic observation of tracheal collapse. Fluoroscopy allows accurate evaluation of the variations in tracheal diameter with the phase of respiration in dogs with suspected tracheal collapse. Dynamic observation of tracheal collapse is also possible with endoscopy and ultrasonography
- Fluoroscopy can be used in incontinence investigations to observe ureteral peristalsis during an intravenous urogram (IVU), and to identify the location of suspected ectopic ureters both during an IVU and during retrograde administration of iodinated contrast media through the urethra

- Portovenography is widely used in the identification of PSS. Contrast medium is injected into a mesenteric vein via a pre-placed catheter. The passage of the contrast medium through the hepatic portal system and the presence of any shunting vessels can be observed using fluoroscopy
- When carrying out myelography, fluoroscopy is occasionally used in difficult cases to guide needle placement for lumbar puncture
- Fluoroscopy can be used to guide the placement of vascular catheters and, at specialist cardiology centres, is used to guide the placement of cardiac catheters for angiocardiography and balloons used for cardiac valvuloplasty.

Safety considerations

It is important to appreciate that there is an increased risk of radiation exposure to personnel involved with fluoroscopic examinations.

- The overall radiation dose used tends to be higher than for single X-ray exposures.
- Fluoroscopy frequently involves the use of a horizontally directed X-ray beam.
- Staff are more likely to be within the controlled area during exposure, especially where interventional procedures, such as catheterization, are being carried out.

To minimize the risk of radiation exposure, it is important that the minimum number of staff necessary are present during the procedure, that all staff wear appropriate protective lead clothing and keep as far as possible away from the X-ray tube. It should be remembered that most scattered X-rays will be directed back from the patient towards the X-ray tube, so it is safer to stand to the side of the tube. The use of fluoroscopy is covered by the Ionising Radiations Regulations 1999 (Figure 11.15).

- Fluoroscopy should not be used as a substitute for conventional radiography.
- All fluoroscopy units must be provided with viewing facilities that do not permit direct viewing of the fluoroscopy screen. The image should be viewed using a remote viewing monitor, ideally located outside the controlled area.
- All guidelines for standard radiography should be followed (see *BSAVA Manual of Practical Veterinary Nursing*).
- Fluoroscopy should only be carried out when clinically indicated, and only by trained personnel aware of appropriate radiation protection methods.
- Potential requirements for additional radiation protection should be discussed with the Radiation Protection Adviser.
- Unless clinically contraindicated, animals should be sedated or anaesthetized for examination, with remote anaesthetic and monitoring equipment used. However, for some examinations, in particular barium swallows, sedation or anaesthesia is obviously inappropriate.
- Vertical X-ray beams should be used wherever possible. Where a horizontal beam is used, particular attention should be paid to the direction of the X-ray beam.
- Screening time should be kept to the minimum possible to carry out the examination.
- At the end of screening, the operator must double-check that the exposure has terminated correctly.
- Screening time and exposure details must be recorded in an exposure book.

11.15 Guidelines for the safe use of fluoroscopy in veterinary practice.

Ultrasonography

The use of ultrasonography in veterinary practice has increased dramatically in recent years and it is now a standard imaging technique in the majority of veterinary centres. Ultrasonography generally provides different, but complementary, information to radiography. For example, ultrasonography is ideal for identifying and evaluating the individual organs in a fluid-filled abdomen; in such a case radiography provides very limited information as on a radiograph the organs will merge with the surrounding fluid, making them impossible to identify. However, whilst radiography is a very useful technique for examining the lungs, ultrasound waves cannot pass effectively through bone or air. This significantly limits ultrasonographic assessment of the normal lung parenchyma, with only the edges of the lung lying between the ribs being available for examination. In the workup of a patient with suspected heart disease, ultrasonographic evaluation of the heart provides essential information about the appearance and function of the heart chambers and valves, while radiography provides information about overall heart size and allows assessment of the lung fields and their major blood vessels.

Basic principles

Diagnostic ultrasonography works by sending high-frequency sound waves into the body tissues and analysing the echoes reflected back. The most important components of the ultrasound machine are the *piezoelectric crystals*, which are contained within the head of the ultrasound transducer (probe). When a voltage is applied to the crystal, its shape is deformed, emitting a sound wave of a characteristic frequency. By applying an intermittent voltage, short pulses of high-frequency sound waves are generated. If the transducer is placed in contact with the body surface, these sound waves pass into the tissues, from where echoes are reflected back. When these echoes return to the crystals, their shape is again deformed, and the echoes are converted into an electrical signal. In this way, the piezoelectric crystals act to both produce the ultrasound waves and receive the echoes generated. The strength of the returning signal and the time elapsed between the initial ultrasound wave and the echo are used by the machine to work out the nature and location of the reflecting tissues.

Physical properties of ultrasound waves

Sound waves are longitudinal waves produced by the vibration of an object:
- **Diagnostic ultrasound waves are produced by the repeated mechanical deformation and consequent vibration of the piezoelectric crystals.**

The frequency (f) of a wave is the number of times that wave is repeated per second:
- **The frequency of the sound wave will be equal to the frequency of the vibrating source of that sound.**

The wavelength (λ) is the distance travelled by a wave in one repetition (cycle):
- **A shorter wavelength provides better image resolution.**

Diagnostic ultrasonography uses sound waves with a frequency in the range of 2–15 MHz. Assuming that the speed (velocity, v) of the wave is constant, a higher frequency wave will have a shorter wavelength:
- **Velocity (v) (m/s) = frequency (f) (cycles/s) x wavelength (λ) (m)**

The velocity of the sound wave depends on the material through which the wave is travelling:
- **Sound waves require a medium for transmission and cannot travel through a vacuum**

▶

- **Ultrasound machines assume a constant speed of sound within the soft tissues of the body, even though there are small differences (Figure 11.16)**
- **Sound waves travel faster through bone and slower through gas.**

The intensity of the ultrasound wave is reduced (*attenuated*) as it passes through the tissues:

- **Approximately 90% of the sound energy is *absorbed* by the tissues and converted into heat. The amount of absorption is directly proportional to the ultrasound wave frequency: the higher the frequency, the greater the absorption and the shorter the distance the wave can travel. High-frequency ultrasound waves therefore cannot penetrate as far as lower frequency waves**
- **The remaining sound energy is either *reflected* or *scattered***
- **The total attenuation is equal to approximately 1 dB/cm/MHz over the round trip distance.**

Tissue	Velocity (m/s)
'Average' soft tissue	1540
Water	1480
Muscle	1585
Fat	1450
Air	330
Bone	4000

11.16 The velocity of sound waves in different body tissues.

Ultrasonographic image

Production

With the transducer in direct contact with the body surface, high-frequency sound waves pass into the body tissues, travelling at an average velocity of 1540 m/s. Different tissues have a different resistance to the transmission of sound waves. This resistance is known as *acoustic impedance* and is dependent on the *density* of the tissue and the *velocity* of the sound wave in that tissue. When a sound wave meets an interface between two tissues of differing acoustic impedance, part of the sound will be reflected.

- If the difference (mismatch) in acoustic impedance is large, most of the sound will be reflected with very little sound being transmitted deeper into the tissues. For example, the impedance difference at soft tissue:air interfaces is so large that the majority of the sound is reflected. In this way, bone and air effectively form a barrier to ultrasound wave transmission.
- If the impedance mismatch is small, only a small proportion of the sound will be reflected, with the majority continuing into the deeper tissues.

- If there are no differences of acoustic impedance within a substance (e.g. pure water), then no sound will be reflected.

If the interface between the tissues is perpendicular to the incident sound wave, then echoes are reflected back to the transducer, where they are detected. Interfaces at an angle to the incident sound wave result in scattered reflections, of which only a few will reach the transducer. Therefore, the strongest echoes will be produced from interfaces with a large impedance mismatch and from interfaces perpendicular to the incident sound wave. The reflected echoes are usually detected by the same crystals. Having emitted a pulse of ultrasound waves, there is an interval in which the crystal waits to receive the returning echoes, before another pulse of sound is emitted. The returning sound waves, characterized by their strength and timing, are converted into electrical signals and displayed on the screen.

Display

A-mode (amplitude mode)

This is the simplest, but least frequently used mode of display. A single beam of ultrasound waves is used and the resulting echoes are displayed as a single line across the screen. As the ultrasound beam encounters interfaces of differing acoustic impedance, echoes are generated. The horizontal axis represents the depth of the interface while the vertical axis indicates the strength of the returning echo. A-mode is most frequently used in ophthalmic examinations to provide precise depth measurements between the different ocular structures (Figure 11.17).

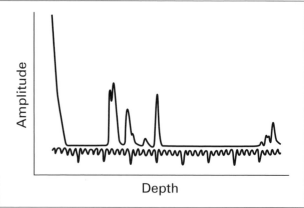

11.17 A-mode ultrasound image.

B-mode (brightness mode)

This is the most commonly used display mode. Multiple ultrasound beams are used to build up a two-dimensional (2D) slice through the patient. The returning echoes are displayed as dots on the screen, with their brightness indicating the strength of the echo. The position of each dot corresponds to the position of the reflecting interface within the patient's body (Figure 11.18). Modern ultrasound scanners display B-mode images in 'real-time'. This refers to the fact that the image is being continuously updated. The frequency at which the image frames are updated

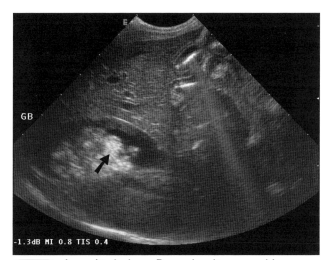

11.18 A sagittal plane B-mode ultrasound image showing echogenic material (arrowed) within the gallbladder.

is known as the frame rate. Where a deeper depth is displayed, the frame rate is inevitably slower as more time is needed for the echoes to return to the transducer. Sagittal, dorsal, transverse or oblique imaging planes through the body tissues may be obtained, according to the position of the transducer on the skin surface.

M-mode (motion mode)

This mode is most commonly used in echocardiography to evaluate the motion of the heart. A single ultrasound pulse is used, as in A-mode. However, the depth of the interfaces imaged is now represented by the vertical axis, and the strength of the echo is denoted by the brightness of the individual dots along the line. The horizontal axis corresponds to time, producing a pencil-thin image along the line of the single ultrasound pulse whose movement over time is recorded (Figure 11.19). Most ultrasound scanners will allow the location of the single line M-mode scan to be selected from a real-time B-mode image.

Echogenicity

For both B-mode and M-mode images, bright echoes represent highly reflective interfaces where a relatively high proportion of the sound waves have been returned to the transducer. Bright areas are described as being *hyperechoic* or *echogenic*. Interfaces of soft tissue with bone or gas will typically appear bright. Areas from where fewer echoes are returned appear relatively dark on the screen and are described as *hypoechoic*. Areas from which no echoes are returned, typically fluids, appear black or *anechoic*. Within the parenchyma of the body organs, the ultrasound waves encounter many small and uneven interfaces which result in *scattering* of the beam, producing lots of weak echoes which are reflected in different directions. Although these echoes are weak, because there are so many of them, some will return to the transducer where they add to the image, creating the parenchymal *echotexture* seen within the organs. Different body tissues have a characteristic echogenicity and echotexture, enabling them to be recognized and abnormalities to be detected.

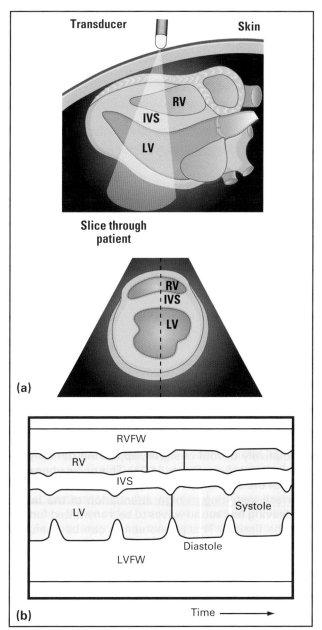

11.19 **(a)** B-mode and **(b)** M-mode images of a transverse section of the heart. Selection of position for M-mode beam is taken from the B-mode image (dashed line). IVS = Interventricular septum; LV = Left ventricle; LVFW = Left ventricular free wall; RV = Right ventricle; RVFW = Right ventricular free wall.

Common artefacts

The aim of all imaging techniques is to represent the structures being imaged as accurately as possible. An artefact is a misrepresentation of reality and, if not recognized as such, this can lead to misinterpretation and misdiagnosis. Unlike radiographic artefacts which are always detrimental to the image, artefacts in ultrasonography can often provide useful clues about the tissues being examined.

Acoustic enhancement

Tissues that are located deep to an area of fluid will appear brighter (more echogenic, Figure 11.20) than adjacent structures. This is due to the fact that fluid causes much less attenuation of the ultrasound beam

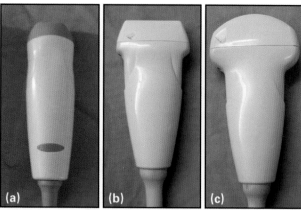

11.25 Transducer probes. **(a)** Sector probe. **(b)** Linear probe. **(c)** Curvilinear probe.

Controls

Different machines vary in their complexity, but all machines have the same basic controls (Figure 11.26):

- *On/off switch.* Some of the more modern machines need to be powered down in the same way as a computer, and simply turning the machine off without following the correct sequence may result in a loss of data
- *Patient ID.* This allows entry of patient details and is important for accurate record keeping
- *Transducer selection.* Where there is more than one transducer connected, this allows selection of the one required
- *Power output.* This controls the voltage applied to the piezoelectric crystals, and therefore the intensity of the sound waves emitted. It should be set as low as possible to optimize the image, as too high a power output will increase background scatter and image 'noise'
- *Time gain compensation.* This allows selective electronic amplification of the returning echoes. Echoes from deeper tissues are weaker because they have travelled further and therefore have been more attenuated. This control allows amplification of these weaker echoes to match the echoes from more superficial tissues, compensating for the attenuation. An organ with evenly echogenic parenchyma, such as the liver, can be used to adjust this control to gain an evenly bright image throughout the field of view
- *Overall gain.* This controls the overall electronic amplification of the signal and is applied uniformly across the field of view
- A *focus* control allows the ultrasound beam to be focused at one or more depths throughout the image, providing optimum resolution at the focal point
- The *freeze* button allows the current image to be frozen on the screen from where it can be analysed, measured, annotated and printed
- Most machines have the capability of *printing* to a thermal printer, providing a permanent record of the examination. Modern machines are also capable of digitally archiving both still images and video clips.

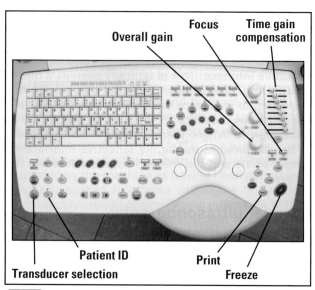

11.26 Ultrasound machine controls.

Patient preparation

- For routine abdominal ultrasonography, animals should be fasted overnight as the presence of gas and food in the gastrointestinal tract can hinder the examination.
- For thorough examination of the bladder, prostate and uterus, and to obtain a cystocentesis sample, a reasonably full bladder is needed. However, if these structures are not of interest, an opportunity to urinate and defecate before examination may make the animal more comfortable and hopefully more cooperative.
- Unless fine-needle aspiration or ultrasound-guided biopsy procedures are being planned, sedation or general anaesthesia are not always necessary. For echocardiographic examination, chemical restraint should be avoided as it will have an effect on heart function.
- An *acoustic window* on the skin surface should be selected for transducer placement, taking into account the fact that the ultrasound beam will not pass effectively through gas or bone.
- The chosen window must be prepared to provide good contact between the ultrasound probe and the skin. The hair coat should be clipped and the skin degreased using surgical spirit. Ultrasound gel is used between the probe and skin to optimize the surface contact and maximize the transmission of sound waves into the patient.
- The animal should be positioned comfortably for the examination. The position selected is operator dependent and it may be necessary to reposition the animal several times during the procedure to facilitate optimal evaluation of different organs.

Techniques

Basic scanning

- Ideally ultrasonography should take place in a designated ultrasonography room (Figure 11.27).
- Once the animal is adequately prepared,

comfortably positioned and effectively restrained, scanning can begin.

- A right-handed ultrasonographer will generally use the right hand to hold the ultrasound probe and the left hand to operate the keypad and machine controls. An effort should be made to keep the machine hand clean of gel.
- Low room lighting is needed to minimize reflections from the screen and to enhance the image.
- As a general rule, the highest possible frequency transducer appropriate for the patient and area being examined should be selected. This will provide the best image resolution but will limit the depth of beam penetration. It may be necessary to change to a lower frequency transducer to examine deeper organs.
- The time gain compensation control should be adjusted to achieve a uniformly bright image across the field of view.
- The ultrasound probe should be held with sufficient pressure against the skin to ensure good contact. However, it should be remembered that too much pressure will be uncomfortable for the patient.
- The area of interest should be scanned slowly and systematically, ensuring that each organ is examined in at least two planes.
- Adjustment of image depth and focal point help to optimize the imaging of different organs.
- It may be necessary to reapply the ultrasound gel several times during the course of an examination to maintain good contact.
- It is good practice to print out or digitally record images of relevant findings during the examination. These can be included with the patient notes and provide a permanent record of the ultrasonography findings. In addition to the images, a written description of the examination and relevant findings should be kept.
- Applications and sites for scanning different organs are summarized in Figure 11.28.

- Wherever possible, ultrasonography should take place in a designated room. Ideally this should be in a quiet area of the practice and not in an area used as a thoroughfare. It is important that the room can be darkened, to allow optimum viewing of the screen. An adjustable dimmer switch on the lights is ideal.
- A sink is required for handwashing before/between examinations and for sterile procedures.
- An X-ray viewer is useful for identifying radiographic abnormalities to be further examined with ultrasonography.
- A table is required for positioning the animal. The majority of animals can be scanned whilst conscious, but require sympathetic manual restraint. The table should be of a suitable height and width for assistants to hold an animal comfortably for up to an hour. For echocardiography, the heart needs to be scanned from underneath the animal. This requires either a permanent cut out area within the table top or an additional platform with a cut out which can be mounted on the table.
- The position of the ultrasound machine relative to the table depends on the person conducting the examination. For a right-handed ultrasonographer, it is easiest to have the machine positioned to the left of the table. The ultrasound machine can then be controlled with the left hand, with the right hand used for scanning. An adjustable stool is ideal for the ultrasonographer.
- Animals are much more amenable to scanning if they are comfortable. A flat cushion or padded ultrasound trough is ideal. These should be washable or have removable covers, which should be changed between patients.
- Clippers, surgical spirit, ultrasound gel and paper towels should all be to hand to facilitate preparation of the animal and removal of the gel when the examination is completed. A scrub kit should also be available to enable sterile preparation for biopsy procedures.
- Facilities for sedation and general anaesthesia, together with a crash kit should be available.
- For carrying out an ultrasound-guided fine-needle aspiration or a Tru-cut biopsy, a range of needles, syringes, slides, blood tubes, urine pots, biopsy needles, sterile blades, sterile ultrasound gel, biopsy pots and relevant laboratory forms will be needed.
- Topical anaesthetics should be provided for ocular examinations.

11.27 The ultrasonography room.

Area/organ	Position of animal	Area to clip	Common indications
Abdomen			
Entire abdomen	Dorsal or lateral recumbency	Ventral abdomen from xiphisternum caudally to the pubis, extending one-third of the way dorsally up the flanks on either side and including the caudal 2–3 intercostal spaces	
Liver	Dorsal or lateral recumbency	Ventral abdomen from xiphisternum to umbilicus, several centimetres to either side of the midline. Ventral half of the caudal 2–3 intercostal spaces in larger dogs	Non-specific liver disease Primary or secondary neoplasia Portosystemic shunts Venous congestion Ascites Jaundice

11.28 Indications and sites for the ultrasonographic scanning of different organs. (continues) ▶

Area/organ	Position of animal	Area to clip	Common indications
Abdomen continued			
Spleen	Dorsal or right lateral recumbency	Ventral and left lateral abdomen from the xiphisternum and along the caudal margin of the rib cage	Primary or secondary neoplasia Anaemia
Kidneys	Lateral recumbency	Just caudal to the rib cage and ventral to the sublumbar muscles on the left, over the caudal 2 intercostal spaces and ventral to the sublumbar muscles on the right	Azotaemia Primary or secondary neoplasia Polycystic kidney disease Hydronephrosis Renal calculi Pyelonephritis
	Dorsal recumbency	In small dogs/cats the kidneys can be examined from a window just lateral to the ventral midline	
Adrenal glands	Lateral or dorsal recumbency	As for the kidneys. The adrenal glands are located just cranially and medially to the kidney on each side	Cushing's disease Neoplasia
Ovaries	Lateral or dorsal recumbency	As for the kidneys. The ovaries are located just caudal to the kidney on each side	Polycystic ovaries Neoplasia
Bladder	Dorsal recumbency	Ventral abdomen from the pubis cranially for several centimetres. To one side of the prepuce in male dogs	Haematuria Cystitis Bladder calculi Neoplasia Cystocentesis
Uterus	Dorsal recumbency	As for the bladder, continuing further cranially if there is uterine distension. The body of the uterus lies dorsal to the bladder	Pregnancy diagnosis Dystocia Pyometra
Prostate	Dorsal recumbency	As for the bladder, continuing caudally to the pelvic brim. The prostate is found surrounding the urethra as it emerges from the bladder neck	Prostatitis Benign prostatic hyperplasia Neoplasia Paraprostatic cysts
Stomach	Dorsal or lateral recumbency	As for the liver. The stomach lies against the caudal liver surface with the fundus to the left of the midline, and the pylorus midline (cats) or to the right of the midline	Vomiting Gastrointestinal motility disorders Neoplasia
Duodenum	Dorsal or left lateral recumbency	As for the right kidney. The duodenum lies along the right body wall superficial to the kidney	Vomiting Gastrointestinal motility disorders Neoplasia
Small intestine	Dorsal or lateral recumbency	Entire ventral abdomen	Vomiting and diarrhoea Weight loss
Pancreas	Dorsal or lateral recumbency	Mid-ventral abdomen from the umbilicus several centimetres cranially and to the right and left of the midline. The left limb of the pancreas is deep to the spleen, the body caudal to the stomach and the right limb between the right kidney and duodenum	Cranial abdominal pain
Large intestine	Dorsal or lateral recumbency	Entire ventral abdomen. The ascending colon is located ventral to the right kidney, the transverse colon caudal to the stomach and the descending colon ventral to the left kidney, running caudally to enter the pelvis dorsal to the bladder	Diarrhoea Constipation Neoplasia
Mesenteric lymph nodes	Dorsal recumbency	Entire ventral abdomen. The mesenteric lymph nodes are found throughout the abdomen, flanking the mesenteric vessels	Generalized lymphadenopathy Primary or secondary neoplasia

11.28 (continued) Indications and sites for the ultrasonographic scanning of different organs. (continues) ▶

Area/organ	Position of animal	Area to clip	Common indications
Abdomen continued			
Sublumbar lymph nodes	Lateral recumbency	Caudal lateral abdomen, ventral to the sublumbar muscles on both sides. The sublumbar lymph nodes are found at the aortic bifurcation	Generalized lymphadenopathy Primary or secondary neoplasia
Testicles	Dorsal or lateral recumbency	Probably not necessary to clip. The transducer is placed directly on the scrotum	Neoplasia Testicular torsion Orchitis
Thorax			
Heart	Lateral recumbency	Right side: ventral one-third of intercostal spaces 3–6 Left side: ventral one-third of intercostal spaces 4–6	Heart disease Screening
Thoracic cavity	Sternal or lateral recumbency	Over area of interest	Pleural or mediastinal fluid Thoracic masses Consolidated lung Diaphragmatic rupture
Head and neck			
Eye	Lateral or sternal recumbency	No clipping required. The transducer is placed directly on the globe. Topical anaesthesia should be used	Lens luxation Retinal detachment Retrobulbar masses/foreign bodies
Larynx	Dorsal or sternal recumbency	Ventral aspect of larynx	Laryngeal paralysis Laryngeal masses
Parathyroid/ thyroid	Dorsal or lateral recumbency	Ventral aspect of neck from larynx caudally for several centimetres	Neoplasia Hyper- or hypoplasia
Musculoskeletal system	Depends on area examined	Over area of interest	Tendon or muscle damage Neoplasia Fracture healing
Superficial structures	Depends on area examined	Over area of interest	Skin masses Mammary masses Foreign bodies

11.28 (continued) Indications and sites for the ultrasonographic scanning of different organs.

Pregnancy diagnosis

Ultrasonographic examination is frequently used in small animal veterinary practice for pregnancy diagnosis. In the bitch, the optimum time to scan is approximately 4 weeks after the last mating. At this stage, the pregnant uterus should contain separate gestational sacs, each containing a fetus, membranes and surrounding fluid. The fetal heart beat should be seen by 25 days after mating, confirming fetal viability. Counting fetuses with ultrasonography can be surprisingly inaccurate, and it is important that the client is aware that any number given is only an estimate.

Fine-needle aspiration and biopsy

- Ultrasound examination can provide valuable information about the internal structure of organs, and is useful in identifying morphological abnormalities. However, to reach a definitive diagnosis, microscopic examination of cells or tissue is required.

- Ultrasonography can be used to guide the placement of a needle or biopsy gun into an area of abnormal tissue to obtain a sample for cytology or histopathology. This is a safer and more accurate technique than blind sampling, and is less invasive than open surgical biopsy. Ultrasonography can also be used to guide needle placement to obtain a cystocentesis sample (Figure 11.29).

- Before a fine-needle aspiration or biopsy procedure of a vascular organ is carried out, it is advisable to check the animal's clotting status.

- The site for sampling should be aseptically prepared. For fine-needle aspiration, the use of gel is best avoided as it can confuse cytological interpretation. Sterile ultrasound gel should be used for aseptic biopsy procedures.

- The needle must be introduced in the same plane as the ultrasound beam, enabling it to be visualized and controlled throughout the procedure.

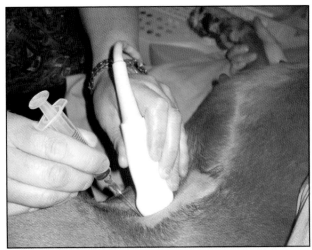

11.29 Obtaining a urine sample via ultrasound-guided cystocentesis.

■ Slides for cytological evaluation should be prepared immediately. The cells are gently smeared across the slide and air-dried. Biopsy samples should be preserved in formalin pots until histological examination.

Computed tomography

Computed tomography (CT) is a cross-sectional imaging technique used to view 2D transverse slices through a patient's body. This technique uses high energy X-rays to acquire the information for the images, and therefore creates a significant radiation hazard for the staff involved in the examination. The availability of CT for veterinary use in the UK is currently very limited.

Basic principles

Veterinary CT should be carried out with the animal under sedation or, more commonly, general anaesthesia. The patient is positioned on a couch, which is moved through a ring (gantry) containing the X-ray source and the X-ray detectors. A survey radiographic image is taken, usually in the sagittal plane, to choose the location at which to obtain the transverse slices. The X-rays used in CT are produced in an identical way to conventional X-rays. As with conventional X-rays, many of the X-ray photons passed into the body will be attenuated within the patient. The CT image produced is a representation of the relative attenuation of the X-rays by the different body tissues.

To build up the image of a slice through the patient, the X-ray tube is rotated 360 degrees around the patient, taking finely collimated exposures at multiple angles around the body (Figure 11.30). Those photons which pass through the body reach detectors located opposite the X-ray source; here they are converted into an electrical signal, the size of which is proportional to the photon energy detected. This signal can be used to work out the amount of energy attenuated by the patient for each of the multiple X-ray exposures taken. To translate this information into a 2D image, the computer divides the tissue slice up into a grid of small blocks (voxels) spanning the width of the slice.

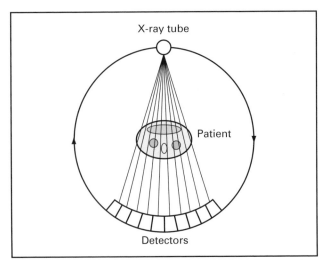

11.30 CT scan. The X-ray tube is rotated around the patient taking exposures at multiple angles around the body.

The attenuation data are then used to calculate a CT number (a measure of attenuation) for each voxel. Each rotation of the X-ray tube will generally provide the information needed to image one slice of tissue. To image subsequent slices, the couch is incrementally moved through the gantry. More recent technology allows continuous movement of the couch, with the X-ray source and detectors effectively tracing a spiral around the patient. The main advantage of this technology, known as helical CT, is the increased speed of image acquisition.

The images are displayed on the viewing monitor, with each three-dimensional (3D) voxel of tissue represented by a 2D pixel. The brightness of the pixels is related to the CT number assigned to that voxel. Water is always assigned a CT number of zero. Tissues which result in less attenuation of the X-ray beam, such as the lungs, have a negative CT number, whilst highly attenuating tissues, such as bone, have much higher CT numbers (Figure 11.31). Although CT numbers cover a range from at least −2000 to +3000, only a limited number of shades of grey can be displayed by the viewing monitor and recognized by the human eye as being discernibly different. The range displayed is referred to as the image 'window'. Two important parameters, the *window level* and the *window width* can be adjusted to optimize the image of the area of interest. The window level refers to the CT number chosen to be in the middle of the displayed grey scale range. The window width refers

Tissue	Approximate CT numbers
Bone	+400 to +1000
Soft tissue	+40 to +80
Water	0
Fat	−60 to −100
Lung	−400 to −600
Air	−1000

11.31 CT numbers of various tissue types.

to the range of CT numbers which are displayed. A wide window displays a wide range of CT numbers. This means that the visual contrast between the shades of grey assigned to different CT numbers will be small. Conversely, a narrow window will display far fewer CT numbers, with much greater contrast. CT numbers which are higher than the selected range will be displayed as white, and those that are lower will be displayed as black.

CT has a number of advantages over normal radiography:

- Because each image is a thin (usually 1–5 mm) slice through the patient's body, there is no confusing superimposition of structures
- CT can detect much smaller differences in contrast between different body tissues than is possible with conventional radiographs
- Using sophisticated software, the CT computer can rebuild sequential slices through the patient into a 3D image. This can be especially useful for assessing complicated fractures.

Indications

CT can provide additional and useful information in a wide variety of small animal cases, and is especially good for imaging bony structures. Common indications for CT include:

- Evaluation of nasal disease
- Evaluation of ear disease (Figure 11.32)
- Evaluation of canine elbow disease
- Detailed assessment of complicated fractures
- Assessment of the location and extent of thoracic masses
- Screening for lung metastases.

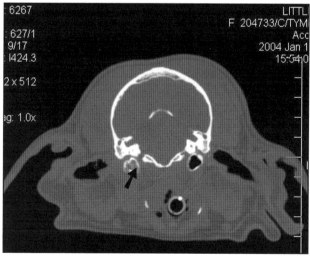

11.32 CT image showing otitis media of the right ear. Note the presence of fluid in the tympanic bulla (arrowed). (Courtesy of G Hammond)

Safety considerations

CT uses high energy X-rays and is therefore a significant radiation hazard. As with all the other imaging techniques involving ionizing radiation, it is covered by the Ionising Radiations Regulations 1999 (IRR99).

- All the requirements for conventional radiography covered by IRR99 automatically apply to CT.
- CT should only be carried out when clinically indicated and never as a substitute for conventional radiography. Scanning should only be performed by suitably trained staff.
- Animals must never be manually restrained. Animals should be placed under general anaesthesia, with remote equipment and monitoring devices used wherever possible.

Magnetic resonance imaging

Magnetic resonance imaging (MRI) is similar to CT in that it produces cross-sectional images of the patient's body. However, unlike CT, it does not use X-rays but powerful magnetic fields to create the image. Although there are no ionizing radiation risks, the magnetic field is a potential hazard for both patients and staff. Due to the increasing number of mobile MRI scanners (Figure 11.33), MRI is currently more widely available to veterinary practices in the UK than CT.

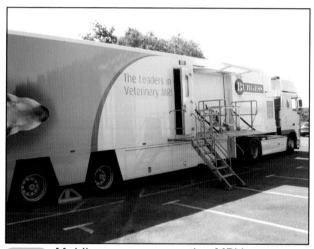

11.33 Mobile scanners mean that MRI is increasingly available to veterinary practices in the UK.

Basic principles

MRI is dependent on the physical properties of electrical and magnetic fields. The most abundant element in the body is hydrogen, whose nucleus contains a single positively charged proton. As with all elements, the protons in hydrogen nuclei are continually spinning. According to the laws of physics, the continual movement of a positively charged proton creates a local magnetic field, and so the hydrogen nucleus is in effect a tiny magnet. Within the body, all these tiny hydrogen magnets are normally pointing in random directions and they cancel each other out. However, when the body is placed within a strong magnetic field, as happens in an MRI scanner, all the magnets (hydrogen nuclei) line up in the direction of this strong field. In higher strength (high-field) MRI scanners, this strong magnetic field is permanently present, although in some lower strength (low-field) magnets, the magnet may be turned off when not in use.

The main magnetic field is generally considered to be oriented in the z-axis. During the scanning procedure, additional magnetic fields are temporarily applied in two different directions (x- and y-axes). The effect of this is to temporarily realign the hydrogen nuclei in the direction of the new magnetic field. When this field is removed, the hydrogen nuclei return to their original position and in doing so they release energy. It is this release of energy which creates a signal characteristic of the tissue type and location. A highly sophisticated computer analyses thousands of these signals, integrating them into the visible image displayed on the screen. By altering the time at which the additional magnetic fields are applied and the time at which the signal is 'read', a different 'weighting' is given to the image which is acquired. These different weightings detect different chemical and physical properties of the tissues. The most commonly used sequences are T1-weighted and T2-weighted sequences.

If T1-weighted and T2-weighted images of an identical tissue slice are displayed side by side, although the anatomy is the same, the shades of grey assigned to the different tissues will be different. T1-weighted images are generally good for depicting normal anatomy. On a T1-weighted image, fat will appear bright, most soft tissues and fluids will be an intermediate shade of grey, and air, tendons/ligaments and compact bone will appear dark. T2-weighted images are generally good for identifying areas of pathology. Areas of fluid, oedema or inflammation appear bright and are therefore more easily identified than on a T1-weighted image, where they may appear similar to the adjacent soft tissues. To highlight such areas of pathology on T1-weighted images, gadolinium is often used as an intravenous contrast agent. Gadolinium can only cross the blood–brain barrier if it is damaged and is often used in the investigation of brain masses. A wide range of differently weighted MRI sequences can be used, each designed to provide additional information about the tissues being investigated.

The actual scanning procedure is in many ways similar to CT. The procedure is carried out with the animal under general anaesthesia. The patient is placed on a couch, which is passed through a gantry (Figure 11.34), allowing the acquisition of images from different parts of the body as they pass through the centre of the magnet.

Advantages

The advantages of MRI over CT include:

- The absence of ionizing radiation
- The ability to obtain slices in any plane (in CT only transverse plane images can be obtained)
- Superior soft tissue imaging, allowing much more soft tissue detail to be seen
- In the UK, increased availability to veterinary practices.

Disadvantages

The disadvantages of MRI over CT include:

- A significantly longer time to obtain images
- Limited use in thoracic imaging due to marked respiratory and movement artefacts. (In humans, this problem is overcome through the use of sophisticated gating software)
- Limited detail of bony structures, especially when assessing traumatic injuries.

Indications

Veterinary MRI is most widely used in the UK for evaluation of brain and spinal disease due to the excellent soft tissue detail which it provides. However, other indications include:

- Evaluation of musculoskeletal disorders. MRI is especially useful in the assessment of joints, where it provides more soft tissue detail than CT (Figure 11.35)
- Evaluation of abdominal masses
- Investigation of retrobulbar disease
- Assessment of nasal disease.

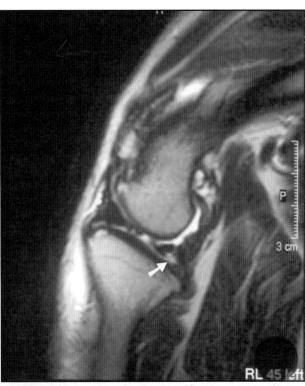

11.35 MR image of a dog's stifle demonstrating a tear through the medial meniscus (arrowed). This injury is most likely to have occurred secondary to cranial cruciate ligament rupture.

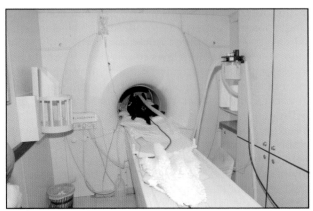

11.34 A patient positioned within the MRI scanner.

Safety considerations

Although MRI does not use ionizing radiation, the strong magnetic field does create a potential hazard (Figure 11.36). Safety concerns include the potential missile effect of any ferromagnetic object (for example, oxygen cylinders, scissors and keys) which comes within reach of the magnetic field. Currently there are no specific legal provisions covering the use of MRI, although electromagnetic exposure is governed by the general provisions of the Health and Safety at Work etc. Act 1974 and the Management of Health and Safety at Work Regulations 1999. A new European Council (EC) Directive covering electromagnetic fields is expected in 2012.

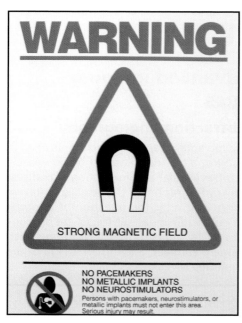

11.36 The strong magnetic field used with MRI creates a potential safety hazard.

Scintigraphy

Scintigraphy (also known as nuclear medicine) uses gamma (γ)-rays released during the decay of a radioactive substance to create an image. Although they are generated in a different way, γ-rays have identical properties to X-rays, and carry the same risks of radiation exposure. In addition, the patient will remain radioactive for some time after the procedure and must be housed and handled safely, with secure storage of all waste material until the radioactivity has dropped to a safe level. Scintigraphy differs from most other imaging modalities by producing images that primarily reflect the *function* rather than the *anatomy* of an organ. Scintigraphic imaging requires specialized equipment, as well as secure facilities to contain the radioactivity, and its availability is generally limited to referral centres.

Basic principles

During a radiographic examination, X-rays are produced outside the body, passed through the tissues, and the pattern of X-ray photons emerging reflects the anatomy of the area under examination. For a scintigraphic examination, the source of radiation is the radiopharmaceutical (the *radionuclide* ± a chemical 'label') which is administered into the body, usually by injection but sometimes by mouth, by inhalation or per rectum, before the examination begins. The radiopharmaceutical releases γ-rays within the body, producing an 'internal' source of radiation. The image is created by the pattern of γ-rays escaping from the body to reach the image detector. This pattern of γ-rays reflects the location of the radiopharmaceutical within the body. This in turn depends on the physiological uptake and concentration of the radiopharmaceutical by the body tissues. Different radiopharmaceuticals with different patterns of tissue distribution can be produced by attaching the radionuclide to chemicals with different metabolic properties. Damage or disease affecting the normal physiological uptake of the radiopharmaceutical by the target organs will be recognized as areas of abnormally increased or decreased radioactivity.

In veterinary medicine, the most commonly used radionuclide is [99m]Technetium (^{99m}Tc), which is obtained from the radiopharmacy in the form of ^{99m}Tc-pertechnetate. This form is chemically similar to iodine: following injection, ^{99m}Tc-pertechnetate is selectively taken up by the thyroid gland in the place of iodine and is used for thyroid imaging. However, if the ^{99m}Tc is attached to a chemical known as methylene diphosphonate (MDP) it will be selectively taken up by bone, and can then be used for bone imaging. [99m]Technetium remains radioactive for approximately 48 hours, and it is necessary to hospitalize patients in a secure area for 48 hours after the [99m]Technetium has been administered.

Detecting and recording the image

The radionuclide is continually undergoing radioactive decay, releasing γ-rays into the patient. Some of these γ-rays will escape from the skin surface, where they can be detected. The simplest technique for measuring the γ-rays is a Geiger counter, which is used as a handheld probe to count the number of radioactive events at different points on the skin surface. This information can then be used to build up a 'map' of radioactivity over the area. A much more sophisticated and detailed way to detect and record the γ-rays is by using a γ-camera.

The γ-camera consists of a large sodium iodide crystal which absorbs the emitted γ-rays and converts their energy into light flashes. Between the crystal and the patient is a collimator: a large lead sheet containing thousands of evenly spaced parallel channels leading through the sheet. Only γ-rays travelling in line with these channels can pass through the collimator and reach the crystal; all the γ-rays striking the lead are simply absorbed. The location of the γ-rays leaving the patient can therefore be accurately mapped as only those travelling in a direct straight line from the patient to the crystal are detected. The light flashes are transferred to many photomultiplier tubes within the camera head, which convert the light energy into an electrical signal. The scintigraphy computer can then analyse the size and the source of the signal, displaying it on the screen in a corresponding location with a brightness related to the number of γ-rays detected from that location.

Indications

- Evaluation of thyroid function and detection of abnormal thyroid tissue, especially in cats suspected of being hyperthyroid (Figure 11.37).
- Bone scanning to detect sources of occult lameness. This diagnostic technique is most commonly used in horses, but can also be applied to cats and dogs. Bone scanning is also a more sensitive technique than radiography for detecting metastasis of aggressive tumours to the skeleton.
- Detection of portosystemic shunts.
- Evaluation of renal function and calculation of the glomerular filtration rate (GFR) for each kidney.
- Evaluation of the ventilation and the perfusion of the lung fields: this can be very useful in investigating the possibility of a pulmonary thromboembolism.
- Evaluation of gastric emptying and intestinal motility.

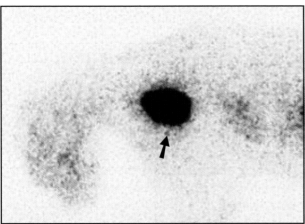

11.37 Scintigraphic image of a hyperthyroid cat demonstrating increased uptake of the radionuclide by the thyroid gland (arrowed).

Safety considerations

The use of scintigraphy in veterinary practice is covered by the Ionising Radiations Regulations 1999, while the holding and disposal of radioactive materials is covered by the Radioactive Substances Act 1993.

- A 'Certificate of Registration' and an 'Authorisation to Accumulate and Dispose of Radioactive Waste' must be obtained by the employer before any work with radioactive materials is begun. The certificate and authorization will refer only to a specified radioactive material (for example ^{99m}Technetium) and will state the upper limit of radioactivity which can be present on the site at one time.
- All work involving the radioactive material must take place in a designated building, room or enclosure, which would generally be considered to be the Controlled Area. Access to the area must be restricted and an adequate number of signs used to indicate the presence of a radiation hazard.

- A copy of the local rules must be displayed in or adjacent to the Controlled Area and should include written arrangements with instructions for handling of the radiopharmaceutical before, during and after its administration to the patient, hospitalization of the patient, disposal of clinical waste (including bedding), decontamination procedures and training of staff.
- To minimize the spread of radioactive contamination, no eating, drinking or smoking should be permitted in the Controlled Area. Washing and changing facilities should be provided and contamination monitors should be available.
- Detailed records must be kept of the quantity and location of all radioactive substances, and should be kept for 2 years.

Other advanced imaging techniques

Digital subtraction angiography

Digital subtraction angiography is a technique used to allow the radiographic visualization of blood vessels following the intravascular administration of contrast media. Digital radiographs of the area of interest are taken before and after the injection of contrast medium. The computer then 'subtracts' the images from each other. The areas of the radiograph which remain the same disappear, leaving an image of the contrast medium filled vessels.

Single photon emission computed tomography

Single photon emission computed tomography (SPECT) is similar to scintigraphy in that it uses photons (γ-rays) emitted by the patient following administration of a radioactive substance to produce an image. However, by using a camera which rotates around the patient's body, a cross-sectional image through the patient is created. These transverse images allow better anatomical localization of abnormal areas.

Positron emission tomography

Positron emission tomography (PET) is similar to SPECT, but instead of emitting photons (γ-rays), the radioactive substance given to the patient emits positrons (which are similar to electrons but have a positive charge). The positron camera consists of a ring of detectors surrounding the patient. This technique is widely used in human medicine for imaging cancer patients. Its use in veterinary medicine is currently limited due to lack of availability and high costs.

Photography

Photography is commonly used in veterinary diagnostic imaging as a way of storing and sharing copies of radiographs. While digital radiography enables convenient storage of digital images, this technology is not yet widely available. In many cases, the use of a digital camera provides a reasonably cheap and effective alternative. To obtain a quality image using digital photography, it is essential that a good quality radiograph is selected and displayed on a viewing box in a darkened room. The area around the radiograph should be masked off. The camera flash should be turned off and the camera supported on a tripod to avoid blurring of the image through camera shake. Manual focusing of the camera tends to produce better results than autofocus. A higher number of pixels and wider grey scale will result in a higher quality image, but will also create a much greater file size. Although the American College of Radiology requires a minimum of 2000 x 2500 pixels with a 16-bit grey scale (65,000 shades of grey) for the digitization of a 35 cm x 43 cm radiograph, in practice acceptable images can be achieved using 1060 x 800 pixels and an 8-bit grey scale (256 shades of grey). This will result in a much smaller file size which can be more easily stored and transferred. Most digital camera images are stored as JPEGs, which only allow 256 grey scales, so a greater image depth (wider grey scale) would be wasted. The use of minimal JPEG compression when storing the images avoids loss of image data.

References and further reading

Barr FJ and Kirberger RM (2006) *BSAVA Manual of Canine and Feline Musculoskeletal Imaging*. BSAVA Publications, Gloucester

Easton S (2002) *Practical Radiography for Veterinary Nurses*. Butterworth-Heinemann, Oxford

Lamb CR (2004) *Digital Photography of Radiographs* EAVDI Yearbook 2004, European Association of Veterinary Diagnostic Imaging

Lavin LM (1999) *Radiography in Veterinary Technology, 2nd edn.* WB Saunders Company, St Louis

Llabres-Diaz F (2006) Practical Contrast Radiography 5: Other Techniques. *In Practice* **28**, pp. 32–40

Morgan PJ and Silverman S (1987) *Techniques of Veterinary Radiography, 4th edn.* Iowa State University Press, Ames

Slatter D (2003) *Textbook of Small Animal Surgery, 3rd edn.* WB Saunders, St Louis

12

Clinical pathology in practice

Mark Pinches

> **This chapter is designed to give information on:**
>
> - The choice and use of external laboratories
> - How to establish and manage a laboratory in the veterinary clinic
> - The key laboratory techniques of microscopy (cytology, haematology and urinalysis)

Introduction

Over recent years there has been an increase in the recognition of the value of clinical pathology to veterinary practice. Most cases that require more than superficial first aid will now undergo some laboratory evaluation. This approach to case management encourages therapeutic intervention that is both prompt and appropriate for the animal, and usually improves the outcome of cases. This in turn provides an increase in satisfaction for both the clients and the practice team. It also increases turnover per case for the practice.

This chapter provides an introduction to the key features of laboratory practice. It comprises three distinct sections. Firstly, it considers when and how to use an external commercial laboratory and also what features to look for when choosing a laboratory. Secondly, it reviews how to successfully set up a laboratory in the clinic and how to go about managing it for best practice. Finally, it focuses on the key laboratory techniques of microscopy, notably urinalysis, haematology and cytology. Cumulatively these sections provide a background to the essential concepts within clinical pathology, a practical guide to laboratory management and an overview of the essentials of microscopy.

External laboratories

External laboratories provide the easiest and most convenient access for veterinary practices to a wide range of diagnostic tests. Most laboratories offer highly competitive pricing structures and provide access to specialist equipment and personnel that would be otherwise out of reach for practices. The following section considers how to make effective use of an external laboratory and how to select a laboratory for the practice needs.

Benefits of using external laboratories

The benefits of using an external laboratory include:

- Competitive pricing
- Quality assurance and quality control
- Quality equipment
- Better training of personnel
- Access to pathologists
- Avoidance of capital investment by the practice.

Competitive pricing

External laboratories make use of large economies of scale to reduce the cost of tests. Generally the cost at an external laboratory will be cheaper than that of a fully costed test performed in-house.

Quality assurance and control

Quality assurance (QA) and quality control (QC) (see below) take a very high priority within most commercial laboratories as the production of accurate and meaningful results is essential for their continued economic survival.

Quality equipment

Laboratories have greater numbers of samples to analyse, so they invest in equipment that is generally more robust and more accurate than that available in practice. For example, most commercial laboratory analysers will cost many times that of an in-house analyser.

Better training of personnel

In commercial laboratories, staff are trained to individual test standard operating procedures (SOPs) and their performance monitored regularly with competence testing (see below). Due to the increased number of samples they analyse, the staff are also more familiar with performing the test in question and are more likely to note unusual or unexpected results that may be the result of an error or indicative of a particular pathology.

Access to pathologists

Specialist personnel can be very useful to clinicians in practice as they are usually both highly trained and familiar with the test or pathology in question. Their insight and experience can be invaluable to clinicians, especially when encountering a diagnostic dilemma for the first time.

Avoidance of capital investment by the practice

Outsourcing diagnostic testing negates the need for a potentially large capital investment by the clinic.

Drawbacks of using external laboratories

The drawbacks of using an external laboratory include:

■ Postal delay
■ Pre-analytical changes during transportation.

Postal delay

In many circumstances samples are submitted through the post. This introduces a 24–48 hour delay before results are received. This may be acceptable in some cases but in others, more rapid assessment may be required. Further, a small proportion of material may become lost or delayed within the postal system leading to further inconvenience and frustration.

Pre-analytical changes during transportation

Pre-analytical changes (see below) are alterations to the physical makeup of a sample, so that analysis produces results that are inaccurate or misleading. Examples include haemolysis of samples, cellular deterioration in fluid analysis, and crystal dissolution or formation in urine.

Choosing an external laboratory

The best approach for a practice to adopt when choosing an external laboratory is to develop a strong and lasting relationship with a single diagnostic facility. The choice of laboratory will be individual to each practice; however, the following should be considered:

■ The commercial laboratory standards that have been achieved by the laboratory in question. There are a number of established standards, which assess laboratory procedures, QA and QC, to which laboratories can apply for accreditation. The accreditation process is rigorous and laboratories that have achieved such accreditation will include some mention within their promotional material. Examples include ISO 9001:2000 and ISO 17025 (the highest currently attainable)
■ Locality. A locally based laboratory may be able to analyse samples with a same day turnaround and provide a convenient courier service with which to submit samples. A larger laboratory may be able to provide 'overnight bags' which guarantee next day delivery
■ The pathology team. Members of the pathology team should be easily accessible and available for consultation. They should be active in continuing education and some members should have obtained board certification
■ Price. Most laboratories have similar pricing structures, although there may be the possibility of a discount for practices with high sample submission numbers
■ Some laboratories specialize in histology, endocrinology or equine samples. These laboratories may be more appropriate for some practices
■ A number of smaller laboratories forward some of their pathology work to specialist or larger laboratories, particularly for highly specialized or unusual tests. This can lead to an increased delay in obtaining sample results for some tests. This may be of concern for some practices.

Appropriate choice of in-house or external laboratory

An external laboratory is most appropriate:

■ For routine and diagnostic analysis where immediate results are not required
■ In situations where specialist pathologist analysis of samples is necessary, e.g. blood film analysis, histology, cytology and bone marrow analysis
■ For tests that require specialist technology, specialist techniques or those that are either particularly labour-intensive or offensive to perform, such as faecal analysis.

An in-house test is most appropriate:

■ In situations where rapid evaluation is required, i.e. emergency assessment
■ When monitoring and assessing change with therapy. (Note: direct comparison can only be made to results obtained from the same analyser. Direct comparison of results obtained from different analysers (i.e. point-of-care analyser *versus* external laboratory analyser) should not be made
■ Some individual tests are best performed in the clinic. These are principally tests in which sample deterioration is rapid and include urinalysis, blood gas analysis and electrolyte analysis.

Key concepts in laboratory medicine

Reference intervals

Reference intervals are values often provided by analyser manufactures to help clinicians determine whether results are 'normal'. These values are calculated by analysing a series of healthy, usually adult animals (n = ≥40). For each analyte a range of results will be obtained from the different animals, reflecting the variation in that analyte value between individuals of the same species. This range of values provides the basis for developing the reference interval – usually the 95% confidence interval, where the highest 2.5% of values and lowest 2.5% of values are removed.

Biological variation

Biological variation is variation in analyte values within or between different individuals. Each individual has a *homeostatic set point* around which normal homeostatic mechanisms cause analyte values to vary. This is known as individual biological variation. In addition, each individual has a slightly different homeostatic set point to another individual. This is referred to as inter-individual biological variation and is reflected in the reference range for each analyte.

Interferences

Interference is the production of inaccurate results due to the analysis of a sample that contains an endogenous substance that has interfered with the biochemical assay. Such substances include fats (lipaemia), haemoglobin (haemolysis) and bilirubin (jaundice). The exact extent of the interference will vary from assay to assay and from analyser to analyser. Good patient preparation (i.e. adequate fasting) prior to sampling can minimize lipaemia, and appropriate sample collection and storage can often minimize haemolysis.

Sensitivity and specificity

The *sensitivity* of a test is the proportion of true positives (i.e. animals with the disease) that are correctly identified by the test.

Example
A test with a high sensitivity but low specificity is that for levels of canine thyroxine (T4). All dogs with hypothyroidism will have a low T4 level, but not all dogs with a low T4 level will have hypothyroidism. Many animals will be ill with other diseases that depress the T4 level.

The *specificity* of a test is the proportion of true negatives (i.e. animals that do not have the disease) that are correctly identified by the test.

Example
A test with a low sensitivity but high specificity is cytology for lungworm larvae. A positive identification makes the disease certain, but not observing the organism means the disease cannot be ruled out.

Accuracy

This is the closeness a result is to the true value of a sample. It is also referred to (or measured) as the bias. This is a measure of systematic error in the test procedure.

Precision

This is a measure of the repeatability of a test and is the closeness of results from a repeatedly analysed sample. It is a measure of the random error in the test procedure.

Centrifuge

There are two procedures for which a centrifuge is required: (a) for spinning microhaematocrit tubes for the assessment of packed cell volume (PCV); and (b) for spinning other fluids either for the preparation of serum or plasma, or for creating sediment plugs from urine or body fluids. Dedicated microhaematocrit centrifuges are available for the former and a variable speed centrifuge will be required for the latter. A number of centrifuges are designed to perform both functions.

Factors to consider prior to purchasing a centrifuge

- What type of samples does the practice require to centrifuge?
- Does the centrifuge fit the tubes used by the practice (i.e. microhaematocrit tubes, ependorff tubes, practice standard blood tubes, large animal tubes)?
- Does the centrifuge fulfil its requirements (e.g. slow spinning for cytology preparations, fast spinning for PCV)?
- Noise and vibration when in use.
- Safety issues (i.e. lock down lid, heat build up).

Regular maintenance requirements after purchase

- Keeping clean.
- Checking for wear.
- Yearly electrical safety assessment.
- Yearly service.

Refractometer

Refractometers are relatively simple devices that can provide a wealth of diagnostic information. They are used for assessing urine specific gravity (SG) and for total protein (TP) estimation of body fluids and blood, and do this by measuring the refractive index of the liquid. The ideal refractometer should compensate for temperature and have both the urine SG and TP scales present. Most refractometers are actually human calibrated refractometers and these slightly overestimate feline urine SG. There are also available some dedicated veterinary refractometers which have a urine SG scale for dogs and large animals and an extra urine SG scale for cats.

When in use

- The prism should be kept clean and wiped clean with a soft tissue following use.
- The refractometer should be periodically calibrated using distilled water (urine SG of 1.000).

Microscope

Microscopes are very useful pieces of equipment. They can be used for examining urinary deposit, blood smears, body fluids and cytological preparations. Ideally two microscopes should be used: one for urine and faeces; and one for cytology. A good quality cytology microscope will cost around £2000. A standard microscope for basic urinalysis and cytology can be purchased for £500. Most microscopes can carry at least four lenses (Figure 12.7).

Lens	Dry/Oil	Use
4X 10X	Dry	Scanning Viewing parasites (e.g. in skin scrapes) Urinalysis
20X 40X	Dry	Urinalysis Some cytology
50X	Oil	Haematology Cytology
100X	Oil	Cytology Haematology Microbiology

12.7 Uses of different microscope lenses.

When in use

- Oil should be cleaned off the lenses when not in use for long periods of time (i.e. over a weekend).
- Dry lenses must not be contaminated with oil or urine. If contamination occurs, the lens should be immediately wiped down and cleaned.
- Replacement bulbs (either hot or cold) should never be handled with bare hands.
- The microscope should be covered and protected from dust when not in use.
- The microscope will require a yearly service.

Glucometer

There is a wide number of portable glucometers available on the market. These are generally designed for home monitoring of blood glucose in humans with diabetes and sold to veterinary practices as a secondary market. As a general rule of thumb glucometers tend to underestimate blood glucose levels, as hypoglycaemia is more serious in humans than

hyperglycaemia. In addition, whole blood glucometers are influenced by the PCV (increase in PCV leads to increasing overestimation of blood glucose) and by factors such as lipaemia, jaundice and haemolysis. After purchase, a series of blood tests should be performed with the glucometer in parallel with the existing glucose assay used by the practice to assess bias (see below). It should be noted that blood should **always** be placed into fluoride oxalate tubes if not analysed immediately. This halts the cellular metabolism that continues in other sample tubes and leads to a reduction in blood glucose levels of around 3% per hour. Regular assessments of accuracy and bias should be made by comparison with a reference laboratory or other test method.

Biochemistry and haematology analysers

There is a wide variety of different analyser types available to the veterinary market. Analysers can either be purchased outright or leased. A maintenance contract will also be needed to service the analyser and repair it when it fails. This contract may or may not include all reagent costs and these, along with QC reagents/procedure costs, should be factored into any cost analysis. It is also very important to understand the capabilities and limitations of each system so that systems are not misused.

There are a number of different factors to consider prior to acquisition. These include:

- The likely sample number throughput and appropriateness of available assays on each system. It should be noted that in general terms >5 samples per day are required to make equipment cost-effective
- The availability of independent medical literature validating the assays for species from which samples are expected to be run
- The analyser type. Wet chemistry analysers are usually the most accurate and offer the greatest flexibility but are also the most temperamental and have the most complex reagent management systems
- The storage requirements of the reagents, and any COSHH issues with the reagents or waste (some analysers may have cartridges that can go in the clinical waste, others may require more complex disposal)
- The speed with which samples are analysed
- The physical size of the analyser (footprint in laboratory) and whether appropriate dedicated space is available
- The time and expertise required by personnel to run the samples. Wet analysers are more accurate and generally cheaper to run but require more training and involvement by personnel
- The flexibility of sample packages (some analysers come with fixed reagent and analyser packages, others can select individual tests)
- The start up time (including the time required to run any QC samples) in the morning or for out-of-hours emergencies
- The plumbing and electrical requirements (some wet chemistry analysers require a distilled water source)

- The availability of QC materials and quality assessment procedures
- The reliable temperature working range. Some analysers perform very poorly if the ambient temperature exceeds 21°C. This may necessitate either relocation of the laboratory to a cooler room or the installation of air-conditioning.

Biochemistry analyser systems

When considering which biochemistry analyser to purchase, the technology that each analyser uses gives some indication as to its likely performance. There are four distinct systems available to the veterinary market:

- Wet chemistry systems
- Dry chemistry systems
- Reconstituted liquid chemistry systems
- Electrochemistry.

Wet chemistry systems

These are often larger systems in which samples are analysed by assessing the colour change in a small chamber into which reagents and the sample are added. A photodetector monitors the colour change and a microprocessor calculates the results. The advantages of this system include greater flexibility, lower reagent cost and higher speed. The disadvantages of this system include greater personnel involvement and complex reagent systems.

Dry chemistry systems

These use dry reagent slides, which are loaded into the analyser. A small volume of the sample is then pipetted on to the slide and reflectometers monitor colour change on the slide. An internal computer calculates the concentration of the analyte and the results are displayed. The advantages of this system include test flexibility and simple reagent (slide) management. The disadvantages of this system include possible accuracy issues, may be labour-intensive when loading the slides, tubing may be prone to blockage, and samples may take some time to be analysed.

Reconstituted liquid chemistry systems

These are similar to wet chemistry analysers but the reagents are supplied freeze-dried in disposable rotors. The sample is mixed with the reagents by internal centrifugation of the rotor. The advantages of this system include simple reagent management and the other advantages of a wet chemistry system. The disadvantages of this system include a reduced flexibility of test choice and a relatively high cost of rotors.

Electrochemistry

These analysers use small disposable cartridges which contain a series of thin film biosensors that measure analytes, such as electrolytes, pH and blood gasses. The biosensor technology limits the variety of analytes that can be tested. The advantages of this system include the use of whole blood and the availability of analytes not usually available by other means. The disadvantages of this system include a short fridge-life of expensive cartridges; wastage of cartridges is often high due to inadequate filling.

Haematology analyser systems

When considering which haematology analyser to purchase, the technology that each analyser uses can give some indication as to its likely performance. There are three types of analyser on the market each employing a different technology:

- Impedance technology (Coulter counter)
- Quantitative buffy coat analysis
- Laser cell counters.

Impedance technology (e.g. Coulter counter)

This relies on a conductivity/resistance measurement to count and size cells. Cell numbers are calculated by passing a small volume of blood, diluted with conducting solution, through an aperture in an electrode. As the cells pass through the aperture they change the electrical resistance of the electrode and are counted. Cell volume and type are determined by the magnitude of change in resistance as the cells pass through the aperture. This technology produces reliable red and white blood cell counts, and accurate mean corpuscular volume (MCV) and haemoglobin (Hb) levels. The differential white blood cell counts are generally not accurate. Manual differential counts and assessment of platelet numbers from a blood smear are recommended with these analysers.

Quantitative buffy coat analysis

This technique is based on the separation of cells following centrifugation. The buffy coat is further separated by a small float. The sample tubes are also coated with a fluorescent dye that further promotes cellular differentiation by the analyser. This technique depends on the clear separation of layers within the buffy coat to be reliable. Generally, results appear acceptable for haematocrit (HCT) and white cell counts in healthy animals. Results become inaccurate if analysis is not carried out as soon as possible after blood collection, or if an unusual haematological pathology is present.

Laser cell counters

These counters use lasers to count the cells. The laser light is reflected at different angles depending on the size and granularity of the cells. These systems appear good at differentiating anucleate from nucleated cells. This technology produces accurate red and white blood cell counts, and accurate MCV and Hb levels. The differential white blood cell counts are slightly more reliable than with impedance counters but manual differential counts and assessment of platelet numbers from a blood smear are still recommended.

A general rule of thumb is to consider that all haematology analysers are simply cell counting machines and cannot provide full and reliable haematological assessment.

To generate full and meaningful results a blood smear must be examined in all situations (see below).

Set up and use

It should be noted that these analysers, although often easy-to-use, are designed to be used by personnel with some training in laboratory medicine. Misuse may lead to inaccurate results and a detrimental impact on patient care. The following points should be considered:

- These pieces of equipment should be installed and calibrated only by qualified personnel
- Analysers should be used according to the manufacturer's instructions
- Reagents must be stored correctly
- Control samples should be run as required
- Service software updates should be uploaded when provided
- Error flags should be noted and appropriate action taken (for example, repeat sample analysis performed, examination of a blood smear)

- Servicing should be performed regularly and also as required (e.g. if control samples are not within range)
- Start up and close down routines should be followed
- Training and assessment of personnel using the analyser should be performed regularly.

Trial period assessment

Most suppliers will allow practices a short period of assessment prior to purchase. During this time users should consider:

- The ease-of-use (daily set up and shutdown, QC procedures, reagent management and error flag reliability)
- The accuracy and precision of results (Figure 12.8).

Assessing accuracy

The accuracy of any given test with an analyser is the closeness of the results it produces to the actual value within the sample. In reality, determining the true actual value within a sample is very difficult as all measuring methods will be subject to some error. The most practical approach for an in-house analyser is to compare the result it produces with those received from an external commercial laboratory (which carries out more rigorous quality control and is hopefully more accurate). It is important when performing this experiment that samples are subject to stringent controls to minimize any pre-analytical changes. It is important therefore to separate the serum from gel or clotted tubes, and where possible to use a courier service so that samples are analysed by the commercial laboratory as soon as possible.

To perform this experiment:

Split a sample into two parts and test one part by the in-house analyser and one part by a commercial laboratory. Perform this with as many samples as possible.

Basic assessment of results

Visually compare the results. How similar are they? Could the same clinical conclusions be drawn from both parts of the sample?

Statistical analysis

Relatively simple statistical analysis is available for this experiment. The use of computer spreadsheets greatly facilitates this method. A worked example is shown below and an excellent review of this approach can be found in Bland and Altman (1986).

Results for analyte A

Commercial (C) analyser result	In-house (I) analyser result	Mean (average)	Difference (C-I)
10	9	9.5	1
12	13	12.5	−1
11	14	12.5	−3
14	13	13.5	1
6	10	8	−4
14	15	14.5	−1
16	14	15	2
19	22	20.5	−3
20	21	20.5	−1

12.8   Assessing the accuracy and precision of results. (continues) ▶

The plots for analyte A are shown below:

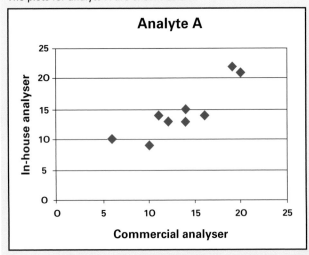

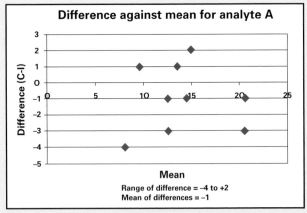

Range of difference = –4 to +2
Mean of differences = –1

Visually, the results show that although there appears to be some agreement (top plot) the in-house analyser generally underestimates analyte A when compared with the commercial analyser (bottom plot). The mean of the differences can be calculated and in this case is –1. Therefore, on average, the in-house analyser underestimates the value of analyte A by –1. The bottom plot also shows that there are some large discrepancies between the two methods: up to a –4 difference at some points, a feature which was not easily apparent when viewing the initial plot.

The practice team should look at these data and determine whether the results produced by the new analyser are acceptable for their use.

Assessing precision (repeatability)

Precision is the closeness of results from a repeatedly analysed sample. If an analyser is imprecise it will never be able to produce accurate results. Guidelines have been suggested (Weiser *et al.*, 2007) (Figures 12.9 and 12.10) which use recommendations produced by the Clinical Laboratory Improvement Amendments (CLIA) to act as a starting point for assessment of analyser precision. These provide useful target ranges for precision, although achieving these is not likely to be possible for most in-practice analysers.

Note: the precision of tests will vary across the testing range, i.e. precision may be tight at low values but very variable at high values. Because of this, for this experiment, the best samples to choose are samples that are close to *clinically important decision levels*. Such levels should be decided by the practice team in advance of the study.

Within run reproducibility experiment

1. Obtain a serum sample with adequate volume.
2. Centrifuge the sample.
3. Draw off the serum and separate into 5 or more aliquots.
4. Analyse each sample one after the other.
5. Tabulate the data, calculate the mean and then calculate the allowable variation around this mean using the CLIA guidelines (see examples below).
6. Compare your results with this range. Do all your results fall within this range? If not, the precision of the analyser has not met the CLIA guidelines and reliable results may not be possible for that analyte.

12.8   (continued) Assessing the accuracy and precision of results. (continues)   ▶

Example 1: basic visual comparison of range

A new in-house analyser has a sample run 5 times consecutively. For urea the results are:

Urea	12	13	14	11	12

From the data:
Mean = 12.4
Maximum value = 14; minimum value = 11

From the CLIA guidelines acceptable variation is ±9% around the mean. Applying this to the mean urea value in this example gives an acceptable range of maximum = 13.5 and minimum = 11.3.

Therefore, for urea, the in-house analyser has a precision that does not meet the CLIA guidelines as 2 of every 5 samples will yield results considered too inaccurate.

Example 2: calculating the coefficient of variation

The coefficient of variation (CV) is the value that the CLIA guidelines use to specify the precision of tests. It is calculated by the equation:

$$CV\% = \frac{\text{Standard deviation}}{\text{Mean}} \times 100$$

From the data (using the same urea results as above):
Mean = 12.4
Standard deviation = 1.14 (calculated using a spreadsheet of the data)

From this the CV can be calculated:

$$CV\% = \frac{\text{Standard deviation}}{\text{Mean}} \times 100 = \frac{1.14}{12.4} \times 100 = 9.2\%$$

The result shows that the CV% of 9.2% is greater than the 9% stipulated by the CLIA guidelines.

Between run reproducibility experiment

The between run experiment is preferred to the within run experiment as it gives the best 'in use' evaluation of precision of the analyser. In the experiment, which should take place over a number of days, the analyser should be used by different personnel, shut down and restarted, and possibly have the reagents changed at some point. All these activities may introduce extra errors that the within run experiment would miss.

1. Obtain a serum sample with adequate volume.
2. Centrifuge the sample.
3. Draw off the serum and separate into 3 (or more if possible) aliquots.
4. Freeze all the samples (–20°C preferred), then defrost and run the samples through the analyser on consecutive days or on any day that the reagents are changed.
5. Evaluate the data in the same way as with the within run reproducibility experiment.

Notes:
- For these experiments the more consecutive samples that are analysed the more reliable is the calculated CV. Most commercial laboratories run a minimum of 20 samples
- This experiment assumes there is no deterioration in the stored sample. Most biochemical analytes are stable when frozen
- The best method for assessing precision is to use daily quality control material. This is generally the approach used in commercial laboratories where such material is available and tested daily. If such material is available, tabulate the data and calculate the CV as outlined above. This method is preferred as quality control material usually does not deteriorate with storage, the analyser is used by a variety of personnel over the test period, and a greater amount of data (over 20 days) can be applied to the CV calculation
- In all cases, the samples should be analysed in the same way as diagnostic samples are run through the analyser (for the most realistic assessment)
- Advanced analysis and more in-depth experimental design for assessing accuracy and precision can be found in Bellamy and Olexson (2000).

12.8 (continued) Assessing the accuracy and precision of results.

Analyte	HCT	MCV	Hb	Platelet	WBC
CLIA guide	±6%	±5%	±7%	±25%	±15%

12.9 Suggested minimum expected precision for haematological laboratory tests (Data from Weiser *et al.*, 2007). Hb = Haemoglobin; HCT = Haematocrit; MCV = Mean corpuscular volume; WBC = White blood cell.

Analyte	Urea	Creatinine	ALT	ALP	Bilirubin	Glucose	TP	Albumin
CLIA guide	±9%	±15%	±20%	±30%	±20%	±10%	±10%	±10%

12.10 Suggested minimum expected precision for biochemical laboratory tests (Data from Weiser *et al.*, 2007). ALP = Alkaline phosphatase; ALT = Alanine aminotransferase; TP = Total protein.

In addition, the trial period should allow assessment of the clinical relevance of the sample results and the problems with interfering substances.

Haemocytometer

This is a very useful inexpensive device that allows cell numbers to be counted. It was originally designed to count erythrocytes and leucocytes in blood samples, but has been superseded by haematology analysers. However, it is still used for erythrocyte and leucocyte counts in samples from birds and reptiles and also for counting cells in body cavity fluid samples from all species. Such fluids (e.g. abdominal fluid, CSF and synovial fluid) are not suitable for running through modern haematology analysers.

Protective equipment

Appropriate protective equipment must be provided to the laboratory staff as part of the health and safety at work legislation. Such protective equipment includes laboratory coats, goggles and disposable gloves.

Urinalysis equipment

The equipment required for urinalysis includes urine dipsticks, a stopwatch, Sedistain® equipment, a microscope and a pH meter (see below).

Bacteriology equipment

A detailed description of microbiological practice is beyond the scope of this chapter. Diagnostic micro-biology is a specialist procedure and is best performed by competent well trained personnel. The standard equipment required includes Bunsen burners, plating loops, growth media (including special media), autoclaves, incubators, Gram stains, a microscope and specific chemical tests for bacterial identification.

Virology equipment

Most virological testing is better outsourced, although feline leukaemia virus (FeLV) and feline immuno-deficiency virus (FIV) tests can be performed in-clinic with relative ease. These include immuno-migration type tests (snap tests or similar) or the plate-based tests, which are more cost-effective and can handle increased sample numbers. Accurate pipettes and stopwatches are required and good staff training is essential.

Miscellaneous equipment

Other essential equipment includes:

- Pipettes – a series of accurate pipettes with disposable tips are required for accurate preparation of samples
- Stains (see below).

Developing a culture of good practice

Appropriate purchasing of equipment is very important; however, the equipment is only as good as the personnel that use it. Misuse can threaten patient care with inaccurate and misleading results. The following section reviews procedures that should be implemented at the outset to help promote good practice within the laboratory.

Key users

Once equipment has been purchased, it is wise to identify a 'key' user. This person should take full responsibility for the machine and be the principal person consulted over matters relating to the equipment. These personnel should:

- Receive the highest training possible in the use of the analysers
- Be comfortable with the methodology and fully understand the limitations and sample requirements
- Be available for troubleshooting, organizing service and repair procedures and for monitoring other users
- Perform the QC
- Write the SOPs for other users.

Standard operating procedures

SOPs are documents that describe exactly how to perform a procedure within the laboratory. The aim of SOPs is to standardize the procedures within the laboratory so that results generated by different personnel can be compared. For example, if one laboratory technician performs an analysis in one manner and another technician in a different manner, the results produced may be so variable as to be misleading to the clinician; SOPs aim to prevent this. SOPs should be written for each procedure carried out in the laboratory and are best written by the person with the most experience of the procedure, or the person who produces the most consistent and accurate results with that assay (usually the key user). SOP instructions should be straightforward and be presented in a stepwise manner so that other personnel can easily follow them. The SOP for each procedure should be filed and be easily accessible for reference by other members of staff who may wish to perform the assay or for those in training. An example of the information required for a useful SOP is shown in Figure 12.11.

Training

Any personnel working in the laboratory should be suitably trained (or work under supervision) both in the procedures they are expected to perform and in the wider laboratory practices. General training should emphasize:

General information

Emphasis on correct patient identification and preparation

Sample requirements for each assay

Collection and handling of samples

How to correctly dispose of hazardous materials

Understanding correct reagent handling, including proper storage and checks for out-of-date material

Individual SOP information

(the purpose of the SOP is to provide a clear simple format for the test which should be followed each time the specific test or procedure is performed)

Clear identification of the procedure or test

Description of the principle behind the test procedure

Description of the capability of the test or procedure (i.e. precision, accuracy, sensitivity, specificities)

Indication of the type of samples that can be used for the test or procedure, including alternative specimens and any samples that can be modified so they become suitable

List of all the materials needed to conduct the test or procedure, including:

- Correct name and order number of the materials
- Name and address of the manufacturers producing the material
- Storage of the materials

Name the equipment needed

Provision of a step-by-step guide to performing the test or procedure – description of how to prepare the samples, materials and the equipment. Inclusion of any appropriate manufacturer's guidelines or product inserts. If necessary, calculations to reach the final results should be described in detail

Definition of when and how the results of the testing are communicated

Provision of details of the quality control procedures for the test or procedure

List of any known or potential interferences which could cause inaccuracies

Definition of the reference and critical values for the specific test. Inclusion of any particular health and safety concerns with regard to the procedure

List of any references concerning the test method, equipment and quality control

12.11 Information for inclusion in a standard operating procedure (SOP).

- Laboratory safety procedures and rules
- COSHH assessments
- Waste disposal and treatment of spillages
- The underpinning scientific principles relating to the procedures
- Individual SOP training.

The SOP should be used as the basis of training for each individual procedure that is performed in the laboratory. In essence, training should aim to make everyone perform the procedure in *exactly* the same way. Training should involve the following steps:

1. Allow the trainee to become familiar with the SOP.
2. Demonstrate the procedure to the trainee.

3. Allow the trainee to perform the procedure under supervision.
4. Allow the trainee to perform the procedure without supervision.
5. Assess the trainee's competence.

Tips for effective training

- *Keep it simple.* Give a solid introduction to the technique and provide short checklists for the trainee to keep afterwards. When putting these checklists together, make them as complete as possible by thoroughly researching instrument manuals, vendor training material, reagent package inserts and QC materials.
- *Keep it real.* Try to simulate real life situations as much as possible.
- *Keep it short and to the point.* Cover the most important points in a brief and easy-to-follow format.

The objectives of complete training include:

- For the trainee to be able to physically perform the procedure with good repeatable accuracy
- For the trainee to be able to adhere to the SOP for the entire testing process from specimen handling and processing to reporting and maintaining laboratory records of patient test results
- For the trainee to be able to recognize critical values and act accordingly
- For the trainee to be able to perform and document QC procedures. (A clear and concise QC protocol must be included in the training and must describe how to respond to out-of-control situations)
- For the trainee to be able to perform routine maintenance, troubleshooting and backup procedures as necessary. If error flags occur, the trainee must also be able to follow established corrective action.

Finally, documentation of training should be made and maintained in the individual's personnel file.

Competency assessment

Adequate competency in a procedure will help ensure reliable test results, which will in turn help maintain patient care. Competency assessment is the endpoint of training, and personnel performing specific procedures should be assessed prior to being allowed to perform the procedure independently. Further yearly competency assessments should be performed to ensure that personnel are still complying with the SOP. Competency assessment is best performed by direct observation. In this manner poor technique can be picked up and feedback given right away by the assessor. The following should be included within the assessment:

- Direct observation of test performance, including patient preparation if applicable
- Monitoring of results recording and reporting

- Observation of the QC procedure (if applicable)
- Observation of any necessary instrument maintenance and function checks
- Questions about troubleshooting
- Questions about the pre-analytical, analytical and post-analytical phases (see below) of the test procedure
- Questions about general procedures such as stocking levels and the ordering procedure
- Re-testing of previously tested samples to assess precision.

Finally, completed documentation and a record of the assessment and outcome should be placed in the individual's personnel file.

Managing a practice laboratory

Managing a practice laboratory takes time and dedication. The key function of the laboratory manager is to take ultimate responsibility for the accuracy of the results that are produced by the facility. There are myriad concerns that have to be monitored and documented on a permanent basis. These include:

- The environment and facilities
- Health and safety
- The equipment
- The personnel
- The results that are generated
- The flow of information through the laboratory
- Customer service
- QA and QC.

Environment and facilities

- Any contamination or pollution to or in the surrounding locality, which may affect the laboratory, should be monitored.
- Power supplies and a good quality water supply should be maintained.
- Adequate ventilation, dust exclusion and optimum temperature ranges for the equipment should be maintained.
- Adequate and appropriate waste disposal facilities should be provided.
- Adequate space to perform the required workload should be provided.
- An attempt to optimize comfort for the personnel should be made.
- Parking, deliveries, sample reception and laboratory security should be considered.

Health and safety

- It should be ensured that staff are following prescribed health and safety procedures and that new staff are fully trained and aware of their responsibilities.
- It should be ensured that risk assessments are up-to-date.
- The accident book should be maintained.
- The laboratory area should be constantly monitored for potential health and safety issues (e.g. using flammable materials such as surgical spirit close to open flames).

Equipment

- It should be ensured that equipment is kept clean and stored properly when not in use.
- It should be ensured that the equipment is installed correctly and that the appropriate resources are available to perform each test safely and reliably.
- It should be ensured that the SOPs are up-to-date, accurate and available for staff.
- Equipment calibration, reliability and servicing details should be monitored and recorded in the equipment log (Figure 12.12) and, if defective, the equipment should be removed from service.
- It should be ensured that the equipment is operated by trained personnel only.
- Validation studies (i.e. repeatability tests or QC data analysis) should be performed as necessary.
- It should be ensured that disposables and reagent levels are monitored and replacements ordered in good time.
- It should be ensured that the reagents are stored correctly and that documentation, including the preparation date, lot number, expiry date and QC checks, are kept and are up-to-date.

Personnel

- It should be ensured that local laboratory rules and health and safety procedures are followed at all times.
- It should be ensured that ongoing training and competency appraisals are completed.
- Training records and individual personnel information should be maintained.

Test results

- The laboratory test log books should be maintained and past results archived. The following data should be included: the date of the test; name/sample identification; type of sample tested; type of assay; equipment used; person performing the assay; test result; and any other information (e.g. sample quality if lipaemic, jaundiced or haemolysed, or duration of colour change).
- It should be ensured that the test results are reported promptly and accurately.
- Critical 'panic' values (Figure 12.13) should be established for each test with the clinicians/ veterinary surgeons. If these critical values are exceeded then the veterinary surgeon should be contacted as a matter of emergency. A guide to the interpretation of basic biochemical abnormalities is given in Figure 12.14.

Information flow

- It should be ensured that procedures for sample reception, identification and recording are in place and are followed.
- It should be ensured that the correct sample is analysed for the requested test and that the results are correctly transcribed and reported to the appropriate person.

Equipment log form

Date ....

BSAVA
BRITISH SMALL ANIMAL
VETERINARY ASSOCIATION

1. Equipment
   • Name:...
   • Type identification:..
   • Serial number:..

2. Manufacturer
   • Name:...
   • Contact person:..
   • Contact address:..
   • Phone number:...
   • Fax number:..

3. Instrument receiving
   • Date:..
   • Condition: New [   ]   Used [   ]   Reconditioned [   ]

4. Current location:...

5. Equipment performance/validation records
   (Mark all tests which were performed and attach the results to the log form)

   • Precision   [   ]
   • Method comparison   [   ]
   • Interference   [   ]
   • Reference interval verification   [   ]
   • Quality control validation   [   ]

6. Maintenance carried out and planned for the future

Date	Action	Reason	Technician	Signature

7. Malfunction, modifications and repairs

Date	Problem	Action	Technician	Problem solved?		Signature
				Yes	No	

8. Predicted replacement date:...

9. Electrical safety check
   • Date:..
   • Performed by:..   Signature:..

12.12   An example of equipment log form.

Erythrocyte appearance	Type	Interpretation
Large blue erythrocyte (see Figure 12.26)	Polychromatic erythrocytes	Seen during regenerative anaemia **Note**: Diff-Quik™ does not stain reticulocytes clearly
Small dark erythrocyte (no area of central pallor)	Spherocytes	Sometimes found in dogs during immune-mediated haemolytic anaemia May be normal feline erythrocytes
Small pale erythrocyte (up to three-quarters of the cell is central pallor)	Microcytic, hypochromic erythrocytes	Seen in iron deficiency. May also become schistocytes as these cells are more fragile

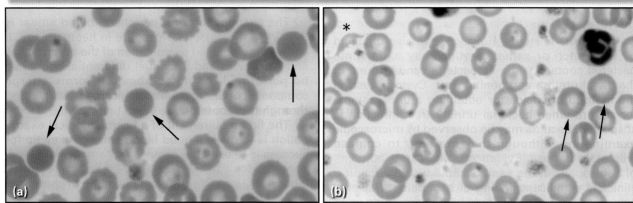

12.27 Alterations in erythrocyte colour and size. **(a)** Spherocytes (arrowed) (Wright's stain; original magnification X1000). **(b)** Microcytic, hypochromic erythrocytes. Normal erythrocytes (arrowed) and a schistocyte (*) are also visible (Wright's stain; original magnification X1000).

Erythrocyte appearance	Type	Interpretation
Erythrocyte has short projections around its border that are regular and similar in size to one another	Crenation or echinocytes	Occurs *in vitro* when slides are dried slowly or if erythrocytes are stored for long periods in high levels of ethylene diamine tetra-acetic acid (EDTA) Very common
Erythrocyte has irregular projections around the cell border that vary in both size and distance around the cell periphery	Acanthocytes	May indicate immune-mediated haemolytic anaemia, haemangiosarcoma or hepatic disease
Fragments of erythrocytes that are in bizarre shapes (see Figure 12.27b)	Schistocytes	May be seen in haemangiosarcoma, iron deficiency or disseminated intravascular coagulation
Target cell, so-called because of the bullseye spot seen in the area of central pallor	Leptocytes	May be seen in strongly regenerative anaemia or in liver disease
Alterations in shape of feline erythrocytes (as described above) are less common due to their smaller size	Changes in shape are often collectively referred to as poikilocytosis	This has been associated with hepatic disease, diabetes mellitus (hepatic lipidosis) and doxyrubicin therapy

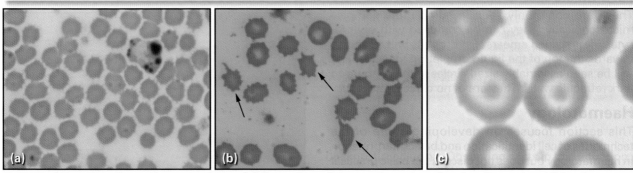

12.28 Alterations in erythrocyte shape. **(a)** Crenation of the erythrocytes. A pyknotic neutrophil is also present (Wright's stain; original magnification X1000). **(b)** Acanthocytes (arrowed) (Wright's stain; original magnification X1000). **(c)** Target cells (a type of leptocyte) (Wright's stain; original magnification X2000).

Erythrocyte appearance	Type	Interpretation
Fine granular basophilic material, often not quite in the same line of focus as the erythrocytes	Stain deposit	None
Similar to lymphocytes with dark nuclei and smooth eosinophilic cytoplasm	Nucleated erythrocytes	Suggests regenerative anaemia if polychromatic cells are also seen. Also seen with serious bone marrow disease (neoplasia), lead poisoning, some serious long bone fractures or a reduction in splenic function (neoplasia and endo- or exogenous corticosteroids)
Single smallish purple/blue spheres within the erythrocyte	Howell–Jolly bodies	These should be removed by 'pitting' in the spleen. Observed when the spleen is overwhelmed (i.e. in very regenerative anaemia), has reduced phagocytic function (following steroid administration) or is not present (i.e. following splenectomy). Cats normally have low numbers of Howell–Jolly bodies as the feline spleen is non-sinusoidal in architecture and has a reduced pitting function
Small colourless areas close to the periphery of the red cell membrane	Heinz bodies	Most commonly seen in cats as feline haemoglobin has an increased susceptibility to their formation (by oxidative damage). May be seen in diabetes, hyperthyroidism, lymphoma, or related to dietary ingestion of oxidants (such as onions and garlic) or to ingestion of paracetamol

Note: some haemoparasites may be seen as erythrocyte inclusions. Most of these are difficult to diagnose without the aid of special stains or confirmatory diagnostic tests. If haemoparasites or anything else unusual is encountered, the smear should be submitted, along with another couple of fresh air-dried smears and an ethylene diamine tetra-acetic acid (EDTA) blood sample, to a local specialist laboratory to examine

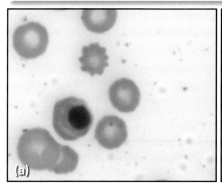 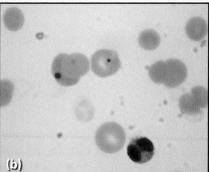 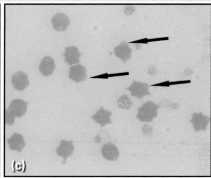

12.29 Internal erythrocyte structures. **(a)** Nucleated erythrocyte (Wright's stain; original magnification X1500). **(b)** Erythrocytes containing Howell–Jolly bodies (Wright's stain; original magnification X1000). **(c)** Heinz bodies (arrowed) are present within most erythrocytes. They appear as pale grey blebs within the erythrocytes or on the erythrocyte membrane (Wright's stain; original magnification X1000).

Evaluation of leucocytes

The evaluation of leucocyte numbers and cytological changes can provide much information about ongoing pathology (Figure 12.30). An estimation of leucocyte numbers can be performed (see Figure 12.17). There should be approximately 10–20 white blood cells per X200 field and the predominant leucocyte should be the neutrophil.

Cell type	Increase or decrease	Interpretation (common causes)
Neutrophil	Increase (neutrophilia)	Inflammation, infection, neoplasia, necrosis, immune-mediated disease, steroid administration, stress, adrenaline
	Decrease (neutropenia)	Overwhelming tissue demand, viral disease (parvovirus)
Lymphocyte	Increase (lymphocytosis)	Adrenaline-mediated excitement, Addison's disease, lymphoma, lymphoid leukaemia or following any antigenic stimulus
	Decrease (lymphopenia)	Stress (secondary to any chronic disease). Other causes include neoplasia, especially lymphoma, chylothorax or lymphangiectasia
Monocytes	Increase (monocytosis)	Infection, necrosis, stress, steroid hormones
Eosinophils	Increase (eosinophilia)	Hypersensitivity reactions (feline asthma, canine atopy, flea allergy dermatitis), neoplasia (mast cell neoplasia, lymphoma), hypereosinophilic syndromes (eosinophilic granuloma complex or pulmonary infiltrate with eosinophils)
	Decrease	Stress, steroids

12.30 Interpretation of alterations in different leucocyte numbers.

Neutrophils

These are slightly bigger than erythrocytes, have clear cytoplasm (neutral staining hence the name) and a lobulated convoluted purple nucleus (Figure 12.31a). There are two important features associated with neutrophils that can illuminate ongoing pathology:

- The presence of immature neutrophils known as a 'left shift'
- The presence of toxic changes within the cells themselves.

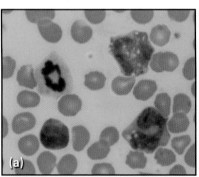

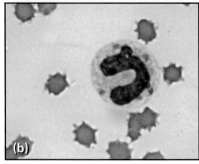

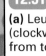

12.31
(a) Leucocytes (clockwise from top left): neutrophil; eosinophil; monocyte; and lymphocyte (Wright's stain; original magnification X1500).
(b) Large toxic immature neutrophil (band) showing Döhle bodies in the cytoplasm (Wright's stain; original magnification X1500).

Left shift

A left shift is a key indicator of active inflammation and is characterized by the presence of immature neutrophils within the circulation (Figure 12.31b). These are called band neutrophils or, if they are even more immature, metamyelocytes. No haematological analyser has been shown to consistently document these cells, so they have to be identified by microscopy. Band neutrophils have nuclei with no segmentation. To identify these cells the narrowest and widest portion of the nucleus should be located: if the indentation at the narrowest part is <25% of the width of widest part, the cell is termed a band. Metamyelocytes appear to have kidney-shaped nuclei and their nuclear chromatin appears paler and less mature.

Toxic changes

Toxic changes within neutrophils are abnormalities that occur due to an increased rate of development within the bone marrow rather than exposure to 'toxins' *per se*. The changes that are seen are variable and have been described as a spectrum of severity. Mild changes include cytoplasm containing Döhle bodies (small blue precipitates) (Figure 12.31b). However, it should be noted that Döhle bodies are also often seen in normal cats. More severe changes include cytoplasmic basophilia and/or vacuolation, whilst the most marked changes include abnormally

shaped nuclei and cellular gigantism. Although 'toxic' changes are commonly associated with systemic toxaemia secondary to bacterial endotoxaemia, there are other causes such as immune-mediated haemolytic anaemia, acute pancreatitis, tissue necrosis, lead toxicosis and cytotoxic drug administration.

Monocytes

These are large blue cells often with pale blue vacuolated cytoplasm and a large U-shaped nucleus (Figure 12.31a). These cells provide phagocytic activity similar to that of neutrophils.

Eosinophils

These have cytoplasm that contains numerous pink staining (eosinophilic) granules with usually a bilobed nucleus (Figure 12.31a).

Lymphocytes

These are generally smaller than neutrophils and have a round dark nucleus with scant amounts of cytoplasm present (Figure 12.31a). Antigenic stimulus causes some lymphocytes to change and become reactive. These reactive lymphocytes are bigger (2–3 times the size of an erythrocyte) and have increased amounts of basophilic cytoplasm.

Other cells

Occasionally, neoplastic cells can enter the circulation and are seen in the blood smear. These cells are often first seen at low power as they are generally much larger than regular leucocytes. They may be a similar size to, or bigger than, reactive lymphocytes but usually have abnormal features, such as altered nuclei shape, visible nucleoli within the nucleus or granules visible in the cytoplasm. Whenever suspicious cells are seen, an experienced haematologist or clinical pathologist should evaluate the smear.

Evaluation of platelets

Platelets (Figure 12.32) are small anuclear cytoplasmic fragments that provide key functions in blood clotting. In healthy animals, platelets circulate in reasonable

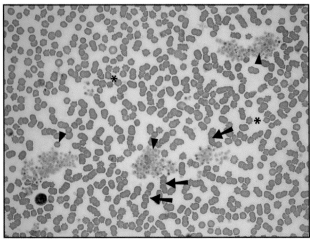

12.32 Platelet clumps (arrowheads). Note also the rouleaux (arrowed) and echinocyte (*) (Wright's stain; original magnification X1000).

numbers with normal levels being 200–500 x 10^9/l. There should be 10–30 platelets per X1000 field of view in the monolayer of a blood smear (see Figure 12.18). Platelet numbers may be normal, decreased (thrombocytopenia) or increased (thrombocytosis) (Figure 12.33). When platelet numbers fall below 40 x 10^9/l, the animal is at risk of haemorrhage and petechial haemorrhages or ecchymoses may be seen. It is possible to determine whether the bone marrow is actively producing platelets by observing large platelets (macrothrombocytes). These are often similar in size to or bigger than erythrocytes. Their identification indicates an increased rate of platelet production (thrombopoiesis).

Response	Platelet number	
	Dogs	*Cats*
Weak	150 x 10^9/l	50 x 10^9/l
Strong	>500 x 10^9/l	>200 x 10^9/l

12.33 Evaluation of platelet response.

Thrombocytopenia

The commonest cause of thrombocytopenia is artefactual, caused by platelet clumping in the blood sample tube. This should be checked for at low power during the blood smear examination by looking along the feathered edge for the large clumps. If no clumps are seen then the reduction in number may be real and associated with pathological mechanisms. These include increased use in severe inflammatory disease and/or disseminated intravascular coagulation or increased destruction by immune-mediated mechanisms.

Thrombocytosis

The commonest causes of increased platelet numbers are reactive processes. These include responses to haemorrhage, exercise, excitement, stress/steroids and splenectomy, or less common causes such as iron deficiency, platelet leukaemia or following fractures. Platelet leukaemia generally causes huge increases in platelet numbers (>1000 x 10^9/l).

Additional tests

Reticulocyte count

The reticulocyte count is the best way of establishing whether anaemia is regenerative. It is easy to perform but requires the use of new methylene blue stain.

1. Place two drops of blood and two drops of new methylene blue stain in an Ependorph tube.
2. Warm gently (37°C) for 15 minutes.
3. Make a smear in the same way as a normal blood smear.
4. Dry and examine at high power. Reticulocytes appear to have blue clumped material in their cytoplasm.
5. Count a minimum of 500 erythrocytes before calculating the reticulocyte percentage.

From this percentage value a reticulocyte count can be made using the total erythrocyte count value from a haematology analyser. This reticulocyte count is the best way to gauge whether the anaemia is truly regenerative.

Cats are unusual in that they have two types of reticulocyte: aggregate and punctate (Figure 12.34). Aggregate reticulocytes are similar to the reticulocyte in other species, so when evaluating cats only the aggregate forms should be counted.

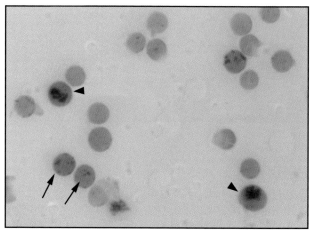

12.34 Aggregate (arrowheads) and punctate (arrowed) reticulocytes visible in a blood sample from a cat (new methylene blue stain; original magnification X1500).

Differentiating agglutination and rouleaux

Differentiating agglutination and rouleaux (Figure 12.35) can have importance in the diagnosis of immune-mediated haemolytic anaemia in dogs. If a question remains over whether an animal is showing agglutination or rouleaux on a blood smear then a *slide agglutination test* can be used to differentiate the two.

Slide agglutination test

1. **Mix one drop of EDTA blood with saline on a glass slide.**
2. **Examine macro- and microscopically for evidence of erythrocyte clumping.**
3. **Progressively add more drops of saline and gently agitate (rock back and forth).**
4. **Repeat the examination of the slide to see whether the cells are separating.**

If rouleaux are present, the plasma matrix is diluted and the cells eventually separate from one another. Dissolution of rouleaux may take up to a 1:5 dilution of the blood sample.

If agglutination is present, the cells remain stuck together despite the dilution.

Note: A positive slide agglutination test is the equivalent of a positive Coombs test.

Rouleaux	Agglutination
Erythrocytes appear to be stacked together on top of one another Normal finding in cats Caused by electrostatic forces Associated with increased levels of immunoglobulin in dogs	Erythrocytes are clumped together like a bunch of grapes Caused by antierythrocyte antibody Most commonly associated with idiopathic immune-mediated haemolytic anaemia

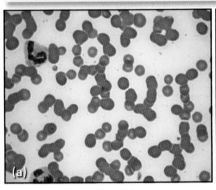 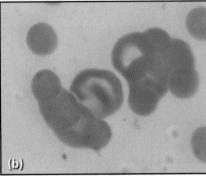

12.35 Differences between rouleaux and agglutination. **(a)** Erythrocytes showing rouleaux (Wright's stain; original magnification X1000). **(b)** Erythrocytes showing microscopic agglutination (Wright's stain; original magnification X1500).

Cytology

Cytology is the study of cellular morphology and cell type patterns. It can be used to examine almost any body tissue or fluid, and findings can be applied very rapidly to the management of cases in the practice. As with all clinical pathology, the quality of sample that is examined directly influences the reliability and accuracy of the results. Therefore, emphasis should be placed on both good sampling technique and correct preparation of samples for cytological examination.

The *BSAVA Manual of Practical Veterinary Nursing* contains details of appropriate techniques for cytological sampling. However, the following general points should be considered:

- Once an aspirate has been collected and the cells are free of their supporting tissues, they are liable to damage. Gentle preparation techniques are recommended
- Any slides should be rapidly air-dried, covered (to prevent dust contaminations) and kept away from moisture
- If possible, at least one of the slides should be stained immediately for a brief examination to note whether any cells are actually present, and if so it should be noted whether they are well preserved. If not, the sampling procedure should be repeated
- A fresh needle should always be used each time a lesion is aspirated. Seeding of neoplastic cells to distant sites is a potential problem, although tracking of neoplastic cells along puncture routes is not a concern
- Good practice dictates that the area be made aseptic beforehand, although complications relating to non-sterile fine-needle aspiration are rarely seen.

Stains

Stains are chemicals that colour different components of the cell. Cellular components with an alkaline component (bases) stain pink (eosinophilic) whilst cellular components with an acid component, such as deoxyribonucleic acid (DNA) stain blue (basophilic). Therefore, the nucleus, which is rich in DNA, stains blue. In addition, if increased ribonucleic acid (RNA) is present in the cytoplasm this will give a blue tinge to the cell (e.g. this occurs when the cell is more active with protein production).

Staining in practice is usually performed using a rapid cytological stain, such as Diff-Quik™. This has a number of limitations, including:

- Variable consistency of staining, as the different solutions have a tendency to change in concentration with use
- Increased cellular debris. As the solutions are reused, more debris (from previously stained slides) accumulates in the solutions
- Poor staining of nuclear features
- Poor staining of reticulocytes.

It is recommended that if a practice wishes to develop cytology beyond cursory assessment, then Leishman stain should be employed. This has better staining characteristics than rapid proprietary stains and, as the stain is not reused, cellular debris does not accrue. Whichever stain is used:

- Stains should be topped up and replaced regularly and the manufacturer's instructions followed for optimal staining
- If, following staining, slides remain clear (under stained) or become intensely blue (over stained) then the staining procedure (i.e. time in stain) should be amended appropriately.

Microscope

The microscope is the key piece of equipment for cytological examination. Cytology requires a magnification of X500–X1000. High optical resolution at high magnification requires the use of oil-based lenses (see the *BSAVA Textbook of Veterinary Nursing, 4th edition* for further details on the use of a microscope).

Basic cytological examination

There are four basic questions to consider during a cytological examination (Figure 12.36):

1. Is this sample of adequate quality to truly represent the tissue/mass/fluid being examined? This is the most important area for the veterinary nurse to consider.
2. Are any of the cells present inflammatory?
3. If the cells are not inflammatory, what category are they?
4. Do these non-inflammatory cells have features of malignancy?

---

1. Place the slide on to the microscope examination stage.
2. Bring the slide into focus at low power.
3. Scan around and identify areas of interest where staining is good (not too heavy or too scant) and cells are not too thick to evaluate. In addition, estimate the degree of blood contamination.
4. Increase the power of magnification on areas of interest and bring into focus.
5. Scan these areas for macro-features, such as tissue clumps, crystals, parasites or foreign bodies. Take note of cellular arrangements in tissue clumps and also any area of interest for high magnification examination.
6. Make an estimate of the number of inflammatory cells if present.
7. Finally, increase to the power for high magnification (X1000) and bring into focus. Identify any cell types present and consider nuclear and cytoplasmic features. In addition, look for background features such as bacteria, protein content or mucin.
8. Repeat this process with a number of slides from the same lesion, especially if the lesion is large. Large lesions may have different degrees of necrosis or inflammation at different points and these will yield different cellular populations.

12.36 How to perform a cytological examination of a slide.

Common artefacts

If any artefacts are seen, a note should be made of them and consideration given as to whether they relate to the sampling technique that has been used, and whether the slide remains useful and representative. Common artefacts are outlined in Figure 12.37.

Cellular structures

The basic cellular structures most commonly used in cytological descriptions are shown in Figure 12.38.

Identification of inflammatory cells

Inflammatory cells are generally easy to identify, and act as good size yardsticks from which to assess the size of other cells. A subjective assessment should be made as to whether they are present in low, moderate or high numbers. High numbers of inflammatory cells indicate the presence of inflammation or infection. Further details on the examination of inflammatory cells is given in Figure 12.39.

Artefact	Description
Heavy blood contamination	Seen as large numbers of erythrocytes, with platelet clumps and a lower number of normal neutrophils (in numbers similar to those seen in a blood smear)
Damage of cells during sample preparation	Slightly damaged cells may be seen as cells that have simply lost their cytoplasmic demarcation and their nuclei are pinker and more fragmented than their intact counterparts. More severe changes can range from cells that have become unrecognizable smudges (three of four times bigger than intact cells) to cells that are completely smeared across the slide
Excessively thick smear	These areas either stain poorly or very darkly. In either case little cellular detail can be seen
Ultrasound gel	Seen as red/purple granular material
Glove powder	Seen as numerous small crystals on the slide

12.37 Common artefacts found on cytological smears.

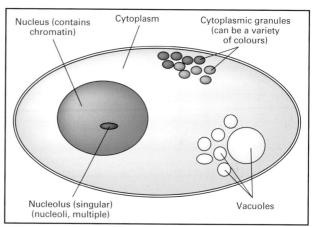

12.38 The basic cellular structures used in cytological descriptions.

Identification of non-inflammatory cell types

Details on the identification and possible interpretation of non-inflammatory cell types is given in Figure 12.40.

Criteria of malignancy

One of the key uses of cytology is the rapid assessment of neoplastic lesions for potential malignancy. This is done by assessing a large number of the cells for a variety of different cellular features, known as the criteria for malignancy (Figure 12.41). If a single population of cells shows more than three or four of these features, then the lesion may be flagged as being potentially malignant.

Although cytology has the potential to rapidly influence the management of clinical cases, misinterpretation or over interpretation of cytological findings remains a potential pitfall. A secondary assessment by a qualified cytologist should always be considered.

Cell type	Description	Interpretation
Neutrophil	Neutrophils are the most commonly seen of all inflammatory cells They should stain fairly uniformly so can be used to gauge how well a smear has stained Normal neutrophils usually have a purple lobulated nucleus with clear cytoplasm In fluids or in thick smears, the nuclei often clump and appear more like lymphocytes Neutrophils should be assessed for 'degeneration'; this is evidence that the cells were in a damaging microenvironment, usually caused by endotoxin-producing bacteria. Degeneration is evidenced by cellular and nuclear swelling (caused by an influx of water): this causes the nucleus to both lose lobulation and appear slightly pinker than usual If degenerate neutrophils are seen, close examination for bacteria either in the background or in the cells themselves is recommended. If bacteria are seen then sepsis is confirmed. (**Note**: if bacteria are seen but no neutrophils, this may be an artefact due to sample contamination and *in vitro* growth)	If 70% of all nucleated cells on the smear are neutrophils it is termed acute inflammation If 85% or more are neutrophils then it may be termed suppurative or purulent inflammation
Macrophage	Macrophages are large fairly pleomorphic inflammatory cells derived from blood monocytes Most commonly they have large amounts of bluish cytoplasm with indented or often kidney-shaped blue nuclei As the cell matures the nuclei become rounder and the volume of cytoplasm increases The cytoplasm often becomes highly vacuolated Macrophages can often be seen phagocytosing a variety of cellular materials	Macrophages increase in number in chronic and granulomatous inflammation Chronic inflammation results in an overall increase in mononuclear cells (>50%). This is usually a combination of macrophages, lymphocytes and plasma cells, with a lower number of usually well preserved neutrophils Multinucleate giant cells may indicate granulomatous inflammation If erythrocytes are seen being phagocytosed this suggests chronic or resolving haemorrhage
Eosinophil	Eosinophils are similar in size to neutrophils They have lobulated (usually bilobed) nuclei and cytoplasm that contains pink granules The staining of the granules may not always be obvious and confusion can sometimes arise with neutrophils that have taken up some eosinophilic stain. In these cases, ruptured cells and the distinct eosinophilic packets should be looked for	High numbers may be associated with hypersensitivity disease, parasitic infections or other eosinophilic proliferations, such as eosinophilic granuloma complex **Note**: an important differential when eosinophils are seen from a cutaneous mass is mast cell tumour. Atypical mast cells should always be looked for in these circumstances

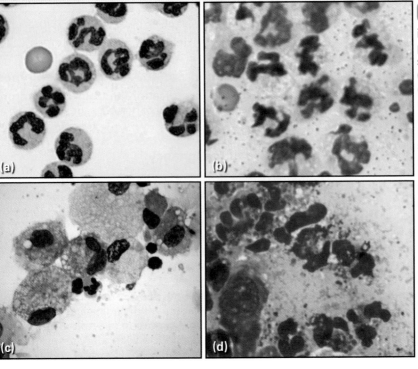

12.39 Description and interpretation of inflammatory cells. **(a)** Well preserved neutrophils (Wright's stain; original magnification X1000). **(b)** Degenerating neutrophils (Wright's stain; original magnification X1000). **(c)** Active macrophages. Note the size of the neutrophil for comparison (Wright's stain; original magnification X1000). **(d)** Numerous eosinophils with numerous pink staining cytoplasmic granules (Wright's stain; original magnification X1500).

Cell type	Description	Interpretation
Round	Round cells usually exfoliate very well during aspiration, meaning that slides are often highly cellular and well spread Individual cells are round in shape The cells usually appear as individuals and do not appear conjoined Cytoplasmic borders are well defined	Examples of round cell tumours include: ■ Mast cell tumours (cytoplasm full of purple granules) ■ Lymphomas ■ Plasmacytomas ■ Histiocytomas
Epithelial	Cells are seen as clumps or sheets as the cells have tight cell-to-cell adhesion. ***Note***: care must be taken not to mistake poor spread of cells for this Individual cells may be seen and they are usually round or polyhedral in shape with well defined margins Nuclei are usually round in shape and will often contain nucleoli Some epithelial cells have large amounts of cytoplasm that may contain granules or large vacuoles Microarchitecture, e.g. acinar formations, may also be noted	Epithelial cells are commonly encountered from preparations obtained from organs, glandular tissues or swabs/washes from tissue surfaces such as the skin, respiratory tract or lower urinary/reproductive tract Differentiating normal from neoplastic epithelial cells is difficult as normal cells may appear fairly pleomorphic (i.e. variable in appearance), especially if inflammation is present
Mesenchymal	Classic mesenchymal cells are 'spindle'-shaped They have tails of wispy ill defined cytoplasm that extend from either pole of the nucleus Their nuclei are often oval and occasionally contain nucleoli Some clumps of spindle cells often contain pink connective tissue matrix	These cells are derived from connective tissue Normally no mesenchymal cells should be harvested during aspiration, although scattered fibrocytes/fibroblasts can sometimes be found in aspirates from almost any tissue Aspirating large numbers of mesenchymal cells with no other cell types is usually an indication of sarcoma. ***Note***: if inflammatory cells are seen, the cells may be fibroblasts. Exercise caution in diagnosing neoplasia

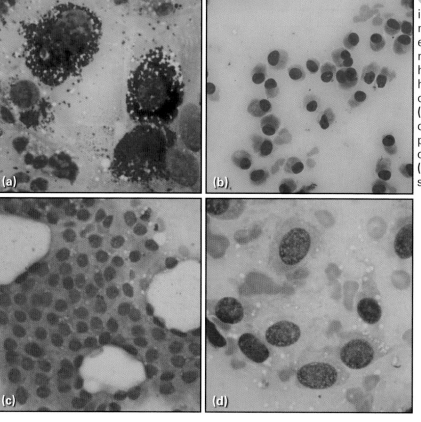

12.40 Description and possible interpretation of non-inflammatory cells. **(a)** Numerous mast cells accompanied by some eosinophils (Wright's stain; original magnification X1500). **(b)** Classic histiocyte round cells from a histiocytoma (Wright's stain; original magnification X500). **(c)** Epithelial cells. Note the clump of benign prostatic cells from a prostatic aspirate (Wright's stain; original magnification X500). **(d)** Mesenchymal cells (Wright's stain; original magnification X700).

Cytological feature	Comments
Increased mitotic activity	Mitotic figures are formed during cell division: chromatin condenses into distinct chromosomes that are then pulled apart as the cell divides Mitotic figures can be seen in any rapidly dividing tissue Finding high numbers unexpectedly is a good indicator of malignancy With some neoplasms, mitotic activity may itself become deranged with chromosomes being pulled asynchronously apart or pulled to multiple different points in the cell; finding this is even more significant
Anisokaryosis (variation in nuclear size)	>1.5 x variation in nuclear size amongst cells is considered significant *Note*: some cell populations have anisokaryosis as a normal feature, e.g. in squamous cells the nucleus shrinks as the cell matures
Variation in nucleolar size, shape and number	Most normal cells will contain a nucleolus but they are often not visible Normal nucleoli are usually small and round and similar in size and number between cells Variable numbers, shapes and/or very large nucleoli are strong indicators of malignancy **Very** significant if seen within the same nucleus
Clumped, coarse chromatin	Normal nuclear chromatin is usually smooth or faintly stippled If nuclear chromatin appears coarse and ropey, this is a good indicator of malignancy
Pleomorphism (variation in cellular shape)	Some variation in cell shape is normal in most cellular populations. Care must be taken not to over interpret this if seen
Anisocytosis (variation in cell size)	Some variation in cell size is normal in most cellular populations. Care must be taken not to over interpret
Increased or abnormal nuclear (N) to cytoplasmic (C) ratio	This refers to the relative amount of space occupied by the nucleus and the cytoplasm within a cell *Note*: some cells such as lymphocytes or basal cells normally have high N:C ratios In epithelial cells or spindle cells, high (nuclei >50% of the cell volume) or variable N:C ratios can be a good indicator of malignancy
Cytoplasmic basophilia	Increased cytoplasmic basophilia suggests increased cellular protein production and metabolic activity It is often a feature of neoplastic cells, but can be seen in dysplastic or hyperplastic cells Interpretation varies according to the cell type being examined
Large vacuoles or granules	This may be a dysplastic change If vacuoles are coalescing or are variable in size then this is a better indicator of malignancy, especially if acini are seen
Multinucleation	Especially if the nuclei are pleomorphic or variably sized
Nuclear moulding	This is where one cell's growth is such that it compresses the nuclei of its immediate neighbour, deforming it out of shape

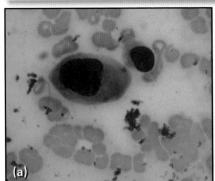
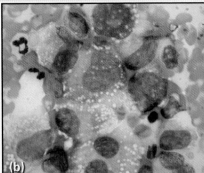
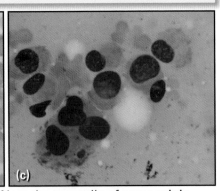

12.41 The criteria for malignancy. **(a)** Anisocytosis and anisokaryosis. Note the two cells of same origin with varying nuclear and cytoplasmic sizes (Wright's stain; original magnification X700).
(b) Clumped, coarse chromatin and marked pleomorphism (Wright's stain; original magnification X700).
(c) Multinucleation (Wright's stain; original magnification X700).

References and further reading

Allison RW and Meinkoth JH (2007) Clinical pathology and diagnostic techniques. In: *Veterinary Clinics of North America: Small Animal Practice* **37 (2)**

Bellamy JEC and Olexson DW (2000) *Quality Assurance Handbook for Veterinary Laboratories*. Iowa State University Press, Ames

Bland JM and Altman DG (1986) Statistical methods for assessing agreement between two methods of clinical measurement. *The Lancet* **327 (8476)**, 307–310

Day M, Mackin A and Littlewood J (2000) *BSAVA Manual of Canine and Feline Haematology and Transfusion Medicine*. BSAVA Publications, Gloucester

Harvey J (2000) *Atlas of Veterinary Haematology: Blood and Bone Marrow of Domestic Animals*. WB Saunders,

Philadelphia

Knottenbelt C (2007) Practical laboratory techniques. In: *BSAVA Manual of Practical Veterinary Nursing*, ed. E Mullineaux and M Jones, pp. 205–228. BSAVA Publications, Gloucester

Osborne C and Stevens J (1999) *Urinalysis: A Clinical Guide to Compassionate Patient Care*. Bayer Company, Kansas

Raskin R and Meyer D (2001) *Atlas of Canine and Feline Cytology*. WB Saunders, Philadelphia

Ward A and Mactaggart D (2007) Laboratory diagnostic aids. In: *BSAVA Textbook of Veterinary Nursing, 4th edn*, ed. D. Lane *et al.*, pp. 317–350. BSAVA

Publications, Gloucester

Weiser M and Thrall M (2007) Quality control recommendations and procedures for in-clinic laboratories. *Veterinary Clinics of North America: Small Animal Practice* **37 (2)**, 237–244

Weiser M, Vap L and Thrall M (2007) Perspectives and advances in in-clinic laboratory diagnostic capabilities: hematology and clinical chemistry. *Veterinary Clinics of North America: Small Animal Practice* **37 (2)**, 221–236

Villiers E and Blackwood L (2005) *BSAVA Manual of Canine and Feline Clinical Pathology, 2nd edn*. BSAVA Publications, Gloucester

13

Practice administration

Sarah C. Hibbert

This chapter is designed to give information on:

- Developing an administrative role in the veterinary practice
- The importance of developing practice policies and protocols
- Record keeping, book keeping and accounts
- The role of computerization within the practice
- Law and legislation for employees
- Considerations for staff recruitment
- Staff support and development
- Marketing and growth of the practice

Introduction

Although veterinary nurses typically enter the profession because of their interest in the clinical care of animals, many soon find themselves involved in the administration of veterinary practices or other small businesses. In this context, it is important to appreciate the difference between administration and management. Administration is concerned with providing the efficient organization of a business. Although management incorporates aspects of administration, it also includes leadership and strategic development, which are not included in most definitions of administration and are not typical roles of veterinary nurses within the practice as a whole. This chapter focuses on the administrative role that veterinary nurses may fulfil within a practice and the understanding of business systems required to appreciate this role.

Administrative systems

Administrative systems are the underpinning elements of a well run practice. They include protocols, policies and standard operating procedures (SOPs), and are basically 'the way we do things' or more formally 'a set of actions'. Formal systems are sometimes thought to be unnecessary and managers are often criticized for contributing to 'system' or 'paper overload'; however, without these systems practices are unable to develop and grow as fast as they should.

A practice without structure is also vulnerable to economic disaster. For example, a practice with no system for stock management (Figure 13.1) could inadvertently prescribe drugs that are out-of-date.

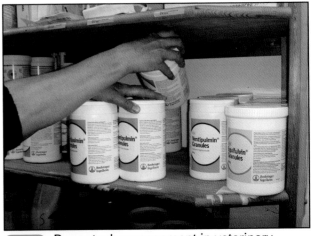

13.1 Drug stock management in veterinary practice.

These drugs could cause severe adverse reactions, leaving the practice liable to litigation and loss of reputation. Practices without formal systems can also expend a lot of energy, time and money troubleshooting short-term problems, so never having the time to plan for the future.

In order for a practice to work at its optimum efficiency, there should be policies covering almost every aspect of the business, both administrative and clinical. A system for ensuring that the office printers are kept clean and well maintained and everyone knows how to change the toner is equally as important as the practice vaccination or worming protocol. Such systems are also required to ensure the practice is compliant with current legislation. For example, HM Revenue and Customs states that financial records are to be kept for 6 years and the Data Protection Act 1988 requires practices to ensure they maintain the confidentiality of any data they hold on file. Other systems, such as the SOP for radiation protection, are issued to the practice which they have a duty to abide by.

Creating a set of practice protocols is a daunting prospect but, like anything else, if broken down into bite-size chunks it becomes manageable. The easiest way to begin is to assess each member of the practice team and ask them to write down their responsibilities. From this list of responsibilities, the activities of the business can be broken down into procedures, and then further down again into tasks, ultimately writing a protocol for each task (Figure 13.2). In addition to the procedures undertaken by individuals there will be some tasks, such as bitch spays, puppy vaccination or stock control, which cannot be assigned to any one person.

Procedure	Task	Protocol
Stock control	Receive stock into practice	Check each item on delivery note has been received Report any discrepancies to wholesaler immediately Mark any discrepancies on the delivery note Submit the delivery note to accounts for matching up with invoice
	Add stock to computer	Record each item received and batch number
	Add stock to shelf	Add stock to shelf in alphabetical order Ensure stock on shelf is in date order
	Remove out-of-date (OOD) stock	Remove any OOD stock from the shelf Obtain authorization for disposal from Head Nurse Record stock as 'OOD' on computer Place OOD stock in dedicated drugs disposal container Add details of drug to dedicated container

13.2 Protocol for drug stock management.

Systems do not have to be elaborate and in fact the simpler they are the easier they are to create, maintain and comply with. Systems in practice are extremely important but it is the compliance with them that makes the difference; without compliance there is no system.

Financial systems

There are two main aspects to business finances: record-keeping and interpretation.

All businesses must keep records of their financial transactions. The main reasons for this are:

- Businesses are required by law to keep all financial documentation for 6 years as this information is required for the accurate completion of tax returns
- Records of all money received, all expenditure made and all goods or services purchased or sold need to be retained for 6 years. The documentation and records that need to be retained are as follows:
  - Cheque book stubs
  - Cancelled cheques
  - Bank paying-in books
  - Bank statements
  - Copies of invoices issued by the business
  - Copies of invoices from suppliers
  - Receipts for all cash purchases.
- Businesses need to know their turnover, i.e. the amount of money they have received in a year from supplying their services. A business with a turnover which exceeds the current threshold is required by law to register for VAT
- This information enables the owners to assess the 'financial health' of their business. If the business wants to take on new partners or investors, or arrange a major bank loan, it is important that it can prove it represents as low a risk as possible to the potential funders. Likewise, if the business is struggling financially it is important to know what is causing the problem so it can be resolved.

Cash book, sales ledger and purchase ledger

The three sets of records needed to start with are:

- The cash book
- The sales ledger
- The purchase ledger.

The *cash book* is the final record of all the money that comes into and goes out of a business; despite its name, the cash book is not restricted solely to transactions made in coins or notes. It is used to record each transaction whether made in cash, by credit card, by cheque or paid directly into the bank. The cash book is divided into two sections: payments and receipts (Figure 13.3).

Management accounts deal with current data and can be prepared for any given period of time. They are not confined to financial information; data may be gathered on employees, sales and clients. For example, a practice may wish to determine how much income each veterinary surgeon contributes to the business, or it may wish to monitor how quickly it pays its suppliers, or how quickly its clients pay their bills. Figures such as these, though valuable, are meaningless unless compared. This comparison of data is called *benchmarking*. Benchmarking allows a business to ascertain how well it is performing in comparison with others. Whilst the veterinary profession now has access to national figures, regional figures and sometimes even local figures, the best comparison that can be made is to the practice's own previous performance as this is the only way of knowing whether or not the business is improving.

Record-keeping

Traditionally all records necessary for the proper functioning of a business were kept on paper but, with the advent of computer technology, there are now many ways of storing data and it is a question of selecting the most appropriate method. However, whether it is done manually or on a computer using specific accountancy software, the principles remain the same.

In order to compare the systems available and make the most appropriate selection, an appreciation of their features is necessary. There are basically two types of data storage available: computerized and paper-based. The advantages and disadvantages of each type are discussed in Figure 13.8.

In veterinary practice with branches in multiple sites, dedicated night staff, mobile clinics and the demands of legislation, computerized record

Feature	Paper-based system		Technology-based system	
	Advantages	*Disadvantages*	*Advantages*	*Disadvantages*
Accessibility	No special training needed Very transportable	Can only be kept in one place	Available to all who need it at a variety of locations	Special training may be required Not easily transportable
Useability	Easy to use and familiar to all age groups No Health and Safety (H&S) implications	Subject to error from reading handwriting and figures Not user friendly to some special needs groups	Special training may be required Can be adapted for personnel with special needs	H&S issues such as repetitive strain injury, eye strain and ergonomics Can result in uneven work distribution as often those who are good at it get the work
Cost	Cheap to purchase	Can be expensive to store	Relatively cheap to store and insure	Generally expensive to purchase and maintain
Confidentiality	Very secure if care taken and very obvious if there has been a breach	Easy to breach as papers often get caught up together or left on a photocopier	User access groups and passwords can be used to maintain confidentiality	If breached can go unnoticed
Retrieval	Input location moveable Self-sufficient	Space-consuming as everything has to be within normal reach levels and multi-location retrieval not possible Can be time-consuming and subject to misfiling	Very quick, accurate and space effective Multi-location retrieval possible, although input and retrieval station fixed	Reliant on power so not self-sufficient
Manipulation	Quick and easy on small projects	Difficult to undertake on larger projects	Excellent on large projects and can capture data for future projects	May require special training and can be time-consuming for small projects
Compatability	Universal acceptance	Time-consuming to distribute	Improving all the time and there is now some standardization	Data can become corrupt in transport Lack of standardization results in programmes working in isolation
Longevity	Probably future proof Ideal for short-term use	Vulnerable to natural disaster, such as fire and flood	Can withstand natural disaster as data can be stored in multiple locations Not easily lost	Not future proof and constantly changing Not ideal for short-term use

13.8 Advantages and disadvantages of paper-based and technology-based storage systems.

management systems certainly have their place. However, there will always be specific instances where paper records remain vital. The key to good record-keeping is knowing and appreciating where each system is best suited and most appropriate.

Information technology

Computers now occupy a vital position in veterinary practice. Patient records, accounting, payroll functions and many diagnostic aids are now routinely computerized. This has given computerized technology an important role in practice but with that importance has come dependence. Life without a computer now causes so many problems and difficulties that an understanding of systems and networks is important.

Networks

A network is two or more computers connected for the purpose of sharing resources. For example, a printer may be connected to one computer but the other computers in the network can also access and use the printer (Figure 13.9).

Most practices have a computer network that is referred to as a client/server network. One of the key points of such a network is that the files and resources are held centrally, on the 'server' and the other computers are 'clients' that can access them. Although

many practices now have a practice management system which is supported by the supplier, the liaison role between practice and supplier is vital. It is helpful to label each piece of equipment with its name and gain a basic understanding of networks and terminology so that when things go wrong, the support desk can resolve problems quickly and efficiently.

Security

Security of both the physical network and the data contained on it is essential. Without this data the practice will very quickly grind to a halt. For this reason it is important to ensure that valuable items such as servers are secured to the floor or kept in purpose built locked cabinets and to ensure that laptops and other computers are secured to desks using specific locking cables. User security is provided by passwords and to ensure that only those trained or authorized can perform certain functions on the network, permissions are granted to each user giving them an access level. Data security is partly provided by user security but in addition antivirus and firewall software help protect the data.

Disaster recovery

Practices using computerized practice management systems to store client and patient data need to be prepared for system failure. Having a good backup

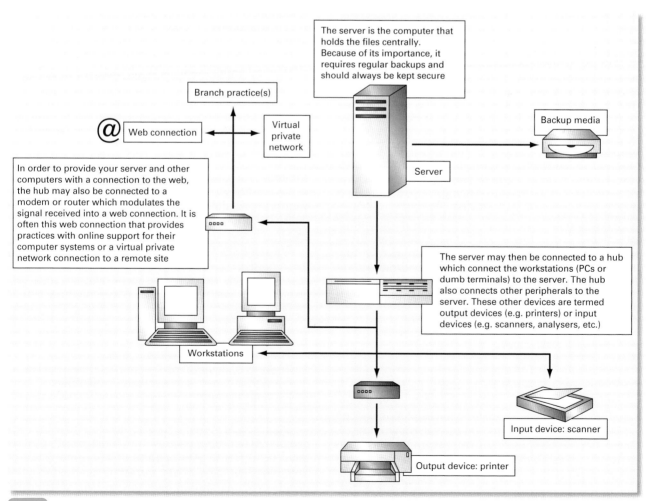

The server is the computer that holds the files centrally. Because of its importance, it requires regular backups and should always be kept secure

Branch practice(s)

@ Web connection

Virtual private network

Backup media

Server

In order to provide your server and other computers with a connection to the web, the hub may also be connected to a modem or router which modulates the signal received into a web connection. It is often this web connection that provides practices with online support for their computer systems or a virtual private network connection to a remote site

The server may then be connected to a hub which connect the workstations (PCs or dumb terminals) to the server. The hub also connects other peripherals to the server. These other devices are termed output devices (e.g. printers) or input devices (e.g. scanners, analysers, etc.)

Workstations

Input device: scanner

Output device: printer

13.9   Computer network in a veterinary practice.

procedure is the only way to minimize data loss or corruption. There are three options for backup: local media backup at the practice; backup to a central server; and online backup to a remote computer system. A full data backup should be taken every night and strict rotation of backup media, if used, ensures extra security. Backup media not in immediate use should be kept offsite or at least in a fire safe for additional protection.

Integrity

A high dependence on computers, and the data contained on them, means that it is important to ensure that the quality of the data is as high as possible. This is called data integrity and can be achieved by adherence to practice protocols, the use of drop down boxes instead of manual field filling, and accurate data input by users. Partially completed fields or incorrectly spelt data can cause problems when searching for records.

Media

Computers are frequently used by more than one user and increasingly work is being undertaken at different locations. The temporary storage of data for transport takes place on media such as tapes, disks, memory sticks, CDs and removable hard drives.

Multiple sites

It is possible to have each branch of a practice linked so that patient and client records can be seen and edited at all sites. Branch linking can happen in different ways. One way is to have the server at the main site and a Virtual Private Network (VPN) between the main site and the branch. A VPN uses encryption to enable signals to be transmitted from one branch to another securely and at the instruction of authorized users only. This method allows the branch access to the server at the main site and consequently avoids the need for data to be transmitted from one site to another. The advantage of this system is minimized data corruption and real-time data sharing at all sites.

An alternative method common for large animal practices, is for the main server database to be replicated on to a mobile terminal such as a laptop. This terminal can be used offsite for limited data input and, when returned to the main surgery, an upload of any changes back to the main server completes the process.

Employment law

Employment law relates to the rights and obligations of individual employees. Over the past 30 years the number of individual labour laws passed has increased considerably, placing a greater burden on employers. The impact on business of this employment legislation is profound, as employing staff is a main component of any business. Businesses have therefore become vulnerable to prosecution and by ensuring that they have tight regulations to protect themselves have incurred increased costs.

In 2007 the responsibility for employment matters was transferred to the Department for Business Enterprise and Regulatory Reform (BERR). Principally employment law covers hours of work, pay entitlement, public holidays and individual employment rights, and these laws have given rise to legislation on many different issues. Legislation is frequently reviewed so, although this information was correct at the time of writing, what follows is only a brief overview and professional advice should be sought before taking any action.

Employment contracts or written statements of employment particulars

It is important to ensure that written contracts take into account the current legislation. Being familiar with any changes and the implications they may have in veterinary practice is essential. The law requires employers to issue to employees a written statement of employment particulars within 2 months of employment. This is not a contract although it may be contained within the body of a contract.

The written statement can be tailored to meet the needs of the business but there is some key information which must be included:

- Name of employer and employee
- Date employment and continuous employment began
- Job location
- Pay
- Working hours
- Holiday entitlements and job description/job title
- Notice periods
- Disciplinary and grievance procedures
- Details of any collective agreements that directly affect the employee's conditions of employment.

This written statement of particulars is the absolute minimum required by law but it is good practice to have a full written contract of employment which addresses further issues as well as the legal minimum. Getting it right at the beginning helps to avoid ambiguity and disputes in the future.

The contract is the start of the relationship between the employee and employer and is legally enforceable. Contracts do not have to be written, they can be verbal or implied, but they exist when three conditions are met:

1. There is an offer of a job.
2. There is an acceptance of a job.
3. There is consideration, i.e. both parties receive something: one receives labour; the other receives money.

Contracts or statements of employment particulars can be changed but as they are binding, both parties have to agree to any change. If agreement is not obtained then 'breach of contract' is deemed to have occurred. Consultation with employees affected by the proposed changes should take place. The changes should be explained in full and consideration must be given to the impact of the proposed changes on the individuals concerned. Full details of the proposed changes should ideally be given in writing, although this is not a legal requirement. Once agreement has been reached the contract or statement of employment particulars can be changed and any new documentation should be issued to the employee within 1 month.

The exception to this is if there are any changes made to the law. These over-ride any clauses in existing contracts that do not comply with them and no agreement is required from the individual parties.

Pay

The National Minimum Wage was introduced in April 1999 by the government and aimed to do two things:

- Provide employees with minimum standards and fairness in the workplace
- Help businesses by ensuring they compete on the quality of their service not on low price facilitated by low rates of pay.

It is a legal right and applies to all workers over the age of 16. Rates change regularly and there are three basic levels:

- Development rate for 16–17 year olds
- Development rate for 18–21 year olds
- Adult rate for those aged 22 and above.

If accommodation is provided free of charge by the employer for the employee, their hourly rate of pay may be reduced but only by the maximum amount stipulated by the regulations. The amount is called 'accommodation offset'. The current rates of pay can be obtained from the government department responsible for employment rights, which is currently the Department for BERR.

Employees have a right to receive from their employers an individual, detailed written pay statement. These are commonly known as payslips and must contain certain information:

- The gross amount of pay
- The amount and details of any deductions
- The amount of net or take-home pay.

It is against the law to deduct anything from the employee's pay without their prior knowledge or consent, and once again any changes to the above should be communicated to the employee in writing.

Dismissal and notice periods

All employees who have been dismissed and have completed at least 1 year's continuous employment are entitled to receive, on request, a written statement of reasons for dismissal within 14 days. The exception to this regulation is if the employee is pregnant or on maternity or adoption leave. In these cases, reasons for dismissal must be given regardless of the length of employment and without request from the employee. Legislation also provides employers and employees with a minimum notice period (Figure 13.10). However, this can be longer for either party if stated in the contract or statement of employment particulars.

Employees with 1 or more years of employment have a right not to be unfairly dismissed and, as the pay awards for unfair dismissal can be substantial, employers are encouraged to follow correct procedures before taking such action. Unfair dismissal is deemed to have occurred if the employer cannot prove that the dismissal was fair. Unfair reasons for dismissal include pregnancy and exercising a statutory right. Fair reasons for redundancy include: the introduction of new systems or technology to the workplace which makes a position unnecessary; the position no longer exists; the need for cost-savings mean staffing levels must be reduced; the business is ceasing to trade or moving location. Selection for redundancy must be fair and employers commonly select on length of employment, employee records on behaviour, performance, experience, skill or qualification, or by asking for volunteers. Employees who think they may have been unfairly dismissed should lodge a grievance with their employer. If an agreement cannot be reached then consulting an independent arbitrator such as the Advisory, Conciliation and Arbitration Service (ACAS) may help. If reconciliation still cannot be attained then the employee may choose to make an unfair dismissal claim to an Employment Tribunal. It is advisable for all parties concerned to keep written records and notes of relevant discussions.

Parental legislation

There is now extensive legislation to protect not only pregnant workers but also their partners and those considering adoption. Once an employee is pregnant they receive greater protection against unfair treatment and employers are obliged to provide benefits such as paid time off for antenatal care, 12 months maternity leave, the right to return to the job held prior to the maternity period and the payment of maternity pay

Length of employment	Length of notice required	
	Employee to employer	**Employer to employee**
1 month	1 week	1 week
2 years	1 week	2 weeks
3 years	1 week	3 weeks
Each year thereafter		1 week's notice per employed year to a maximum of 12 years
20 years	1 week	12 weeks

13.10 Statutory minimum notice periods required by employers and employees.

for those who qualify. There is also a duty to consider the health and safety of the new and expectant mother by assessing the risks in the workplace. In addition to these rights, unpaid parental leave can be taken by either parent during the child's formative years (1–5). Paternity leave, paternity pay, adoption leave and adoption pay are also available to qualifying cases.

It has long been recognized that having a family is a major commitment and involves considerable responsibilities. To help those with young families, legislation has been introduced which means that employees have a right to request flexible working patterns and employers have a duty to take the request seriously.

Statutory sick pay

Not all employees are entitled to statutory sick pay (SSP) but those who meet the qualifying conditions are entitled to be paid SSP for up to 28 weeks for each period of incapacity. SSP is a fixed amount per day as dictated by legislation and so is not directly related to the salary of the sick person; however, they have to be earning a certain minimum amount in order to qualify for the benefit. In order to qualify for SSP the employee must be sick for at least four or more consecutive days and must earn, before any deductions, the current Lower Earnings Limit for National Insurance Contributions as stated by the government.

Antidiscrimination legislation

This is an area of employment law that has seen considerable revision and it now covers all workplaces regardless of their size. Unfair discrimination in employment is wrong and bad for both the individuals and the business. There are a number of Acts which make it unlawful to discriminate (Figure 13.11).

In order to avoid conscious and unconscious discrimination it is a good idea to develop recruitment procedures. Clear accurate job descriptions, carefully worded adverts, appropriate selection methods,

non-discriminatory interview questions which are given to all applicants and above all keeping records for an appropriate period of time, not only help with selection but may also be essential to rely on if the procedures are challenged.

Working time regulations

The implications of these regulations on the veterinary profession are enormous as it has to comply with both the current government legislation on working hours and the responsibilities in the Royal College of Veterinary Surgeons (RCVS) Guide to Professional Conduct to 'make adequate arrangement for the provision of 24 hour emergency cover'.

The basic rights and protections that the regulations provide are:

- A limit of an average of 48 hours a week which a worker can be required to work. Workers can choose to work more if they want to by signing an opt out clause although this too may not be allowed in the future
- A right to 11 hours rest each day
- A right to a day off each week
- A right to a rest break if the working day is longer than 6 hours
- A right to 4 weeks paid leave per year
- A limit of an average of 8 hours work in 24 which night workers can be required to work
- A right for night workers to receive free health assessments.

Compliance with and awareness of all the legislation and the current changes have always been a challenge to any business. Veterinary practice is no exception and the increase in the appointment of Practice Managers and Administrators has largely been because of the need to ensure employees receive their basic rights whilst protecting the interests of the business.

Act	Makes it unlawful to:
Sex Discrimination Act 1975	Discriminate on the grounds of sex including marriage, civil partnership, pregnancy or maternity leave
Race Relations Act 1976	Discriminate on the grounds of race including colour, nationality, citizenship, ethnic or national origins
Equal Pay Act 1970	Make any distinction in pay for men or women who are doing the same or similar work
Disability Discrimination Act 1995	Discriminate against those registered disabled and also those diagnosed with diseases such as HIV, cancer and multiple sclerosis. Employers are duty bound to consider making reasonable adjustments to the workplace for their employment
The Employment Equality (Sexual Orientation) Regulations 2003 and The Employment Equality (Religion or Belief) Regulations 2003	Discriminate or harass someone on grounds of sexual orientation, religion or belief
The Employment Equality (Age) Regulations 2006	Directly discriminate on grounds of age, unless objectively justified Indirectly discriminate unless it can be objectively justified Harass on grounds of age Discriminate on grounds of age in recruitment, promotion, transfer or training, or in the terms and conditions of employment

13.11 Current antidiscrimination legislation.

Human resources

It is often said that people are a business' greatest asset. Considering the financial balance sheet allows comparison of the employment of a veterinary nurse to the purchase of equipment and demonstrates the value of staff (Figure 13.12). Although this is not a realistic comparison, it serves to illustrate just how valuable staff are. When considering the purchase of an expensive piece of equipment, the practice would investigate thoroughly the options available and consider the merits of alternatives; the principle is the same for recuitment.

Recruitment

The recruitment process involves careful planning and the first stage is to consider the position available. Just because a qualified veterinary nurse has left the practice it does not mean that the vacant position needs to be filled by another qualified veterinary nurse. A trainee or a dedicated receptionist may be more appropriate. The staffing mix the practice currently has should be analysed to determine exactly what is needed; a job description for the position can then be developed and a *person specification* written.

Person specification

The person specification describes the essential and desirable knowledge, skills and qualities needed in order to perform the functions of the job to the required standard. It should relate directly to the job description, should not be discriminatory and should contain only the criteria that candidates will be measured against during interview. An example of a person specification for a night staff telephonist is given in Figure 13.13.

Advert

From the person specification and the job description an advert can be written. Advertising is expensive so the balance between the length of the advert and giving sufficient information to candidates to attract the right person must be considered. An example of an advert for a night staff telephonist is given in Figure 13.14.

Selection for interview

It is always a good idea to state a closing date as this makes it clear when the selection for interview will take place. Selecting candidates for interview is

Asset	Cost	Total over 5 years
Purchase of equipment	£20,000	£20,000
Service per annum after year 1	£500	£2000
Total		**£22,000**
Employment of veterinary nurse	£16,000	£80,000
Employer's national insurance contributions	£1385	£6925
Uniform	£75	£375
Continuing professional development	£500	£2500
Total		**£89,800**

13.12 Comparing assets.

Quality	Essential	Desirable	Measured by
Qualifications	Good level of literacy and numeracy and spoken English	GCSE or equivalent in Maths and English	Application form Interview
Experience	Some experience in a customer care environment	Customer care in an emergency or stressful environment	Application form Interview
Specialist training or knowledge	Common sense	Knowledge of the regional area	Interview
Physical	Clear calm voice with good listening skills		Interview
Lifestyle characteristics	Ability to be confined to house for long periods	Flexibility in shift pattern	Application form Interview
Personality	Friendly, confident, calm		Interview

13.13 Person specification for a night staff telephonist position.

Light Sleeper? Earn Money!

Due to retirement we require a new member of staff to join our night service team. Working from home you will be taking telephone calls from clients requesting a veterinary surgeon out of hours and passing the details on to the duty vets. 1:3 rota with full training given. Calm manner, common sense and good telephone message taking skills essential. Knowledge of regional area advantageous.

Closing date 16 August 2008

For an application form contact practice.manager@thisvets.co.uk or telephone 01234 567890

13.14   Advert for a night staff telephonist position.

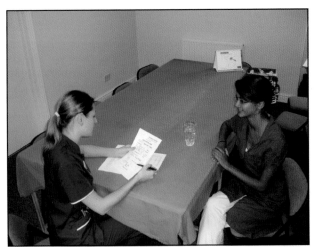

13.15   Interviewing a candidate for the night staff telephonist position.

considerably easier if they have been supplied with an application form. Application forms are easy to create and help to gather only the essential information required, making comparison and selection much easier. Several members of the practice should be involved in the selection process and it is often a good idea to blank out personal details on applications to avoid inadvertent discrimination. In general, 4–6 people should be interviewed per position available but often, for positions requiring specific qualifications, this is not possible.

Candidates should be invited to interview by letter, giving them as much information about the job as possible; it may be helpful to send the job description, stating the salary and any company benefits. Candidates are often nervous on the day of interview so it should be made easy for them to find the practice by giving clear directions in the letter and enclosing a practice brochure. It is also important to inform those applicants who have not been selected for interview, either by stating a date in the advert (e.g. 'Interviews will be held on 16 September 2008, if you have not heard by this date you have been unsuccessful on this occasion') or by writing to them individually. The interview process reflects on the practice so a well managed process helps give a good impression.

Interview

It is crucial that the veterinary practice is prepared for the interview(s). Interviewing is a two-way process: the candidate is assessing the practice as much as the practice is assessing the candidate (Figure 13.15). It should be decided in advance how the interview will be conducted and who will be involved, and ensured that they have enough time to devote to the whole process. Showing the candidate around the practice presents an opportunity to get other members of the team involved. The interview questions should be specific and time should not be wasted finding out information that has already been provided on the application form: the interview is to find out more about the individual and to assess how they would fit into the practice team. Open questions such as 'what

sort of actions would you take in order to cope with a distressed client?' rather than closed questions such as 'can you deal with distressed clients?' should be asked. The interview is also the time to ask about any gaps there may be in employment history or about any inconsistencies on the application form. This is also the time to check when referees can be approached.

The use of an assessment form is a good way of ensuring that each candidate is considered fairly, and can be vital support material if challenged by an unsuccessful candidate. An example of an assessment form for a night staff telephonist position is given in Figure 13.16.

Assessment criteria	Score 1–4	Comments
Communication skills		
Relevant experience		
Specialist knowledge		
Lifestyle		
Personality		
Total score		

13.16   Interview assessment form for a night staff telephonist position.

Selection of the successful candidate

After the interviews and with completed candidate assessment forms and the thoughts of other members of the team, enough information should be available to make the preliminary selection. It is important that the team are involved in the recruitment process as they will be required to provide support to the person in the short term and develop a team working relationship with them in the longer term. Before offering the candidate the position it is essential to obtain references. It is often the person who has had the most jobs for the wrong reasons who is the best at interview!

The interview is the most important yet fault ridden part of the recruitment process. Decisions are often made on instinct and interviewers are observing candidate behaviour in a totally false environment over a very short period of time. One way round this is to offer candidates a work trial. Work trials give candidates the opportunity to relax outside of the interview room and to gain a better understanding of what it is like to work in a veterinary environment. Employers have the advantage of being able to observe the candidate over a longer period of time and better assess their potential and suitability for the position. Work trials often involve offering the candidate travel and subsistence expenses in order to compensate them for their time but this is far outweighed by the benefits of getting the right person in the job.

Once the candidate has been selected, a letter of appointment should be sent to them detailing the start date and salary details and enclosing a Statement of Employment Particulars or a Contract of Employment. A date by which they must accept the offer should also be specified as this date will also be the date to write appropriate letters to the unsuccessful interviewees. Unsuccessful candidates may ask the practice for feedback. The candidate assessment forms will be vital to help provide this information. It is worth remembering that the candidates unsuccessful on this occasion may be the candidates accepted in the future.

Induction of new staff

The process of introducing new employees to the workplace is called induction. If the induction process is carried out well it has the benefit of motivating and engaging the new employee in the team and business. However, if carried out poorly (or not at all) the employee is at risk of becoming disengaged, disgruntled and dissatisfied.

An induction checklist ensures all the necessary information is covered and it is useful to assign times, dates and the people involved. The induction programme will vary for each position. An example of what the induction programme might look like for a night staff telephonist on Day 1 is given in Figure 13.17.

The induction programme may last for 2–4 weeks, or even longer depending on the position, and may also include tasks that the new employee ought to be able to perform by target dates. For example, after 1 week a new employee should be able to answer the telephone, book an appointment and be aware of the practice vaccination protocol. Setting small targets gives the new employee defined goals and objectives and gives confidence to all parties in the employee's progress.

Staff training and development

Training and development of staff should not be something confined only to new employees. In fact, staff who have been employees for many years are often the hardest to motivate. In order to motivate staff, the benefits to them have to be considered. Studies indicate that employees find personal recognition more motivating than money. In particular, interesting work, appreciation for work done, and a feeling of being involved and part of the workplace, are key motivating factors to employees, so it may be a mistake to believe that a disgruntled employee can be motivated by increasing their pay.

Interesting work can only be achieved by ensuring that employees have the opportunity to take on new tasks or revise existing procedures. Additional training may be required but this does not necessarily mean sending employees on expensive external courses. There is often a wealth of skill, experience and knowledge within a practice, which can be shared through in-house training sessions.

Staff appraisal

Appraisals or performance reviews are part of training and development and are an opportunity to assess performance, potential and any training needs. Everyone in the practice should have appraisals, and

Time	Topic	Detail	Personnel	Completed
Day 1				
16:00	Introduction	Meet staff Meet partners Tour practice	Practice Manager	
17:00	Administration	Check received contract Check received job description Complete employee's personal details form P45 or P46 Staff handbook Check uniform Assign mentor	Practice Manager	
18:00	Health and safety	Briefing	Health and Safety Officer	
18:30	Break	Tea with mentor	Mentor	
19:00	Protocols	Rota and duties	Head Nurse	
20:00		Work shadow	Duty Telephonist	
00:00	Shift end	Arrange taxi home	Duty Telephonist	
Day 2				
19:00	Debrief	Feedback and queries	Practice Manager	

13.17 Induction programme for a newly appointed night staff telephonist.

including the partners or directors in the process lends it credence and value. Appraisals are a two-way process: they enable the appraisee and appraiser to exchange valuable information, which should help develop individuals and the practice itself. The objective of an appraisal is to assess, review, motivate and value, so it is inappropriate to use the session to discipline or discuss pay. The session requires preparation, structure and fairness, so many businesses find it easier to provide employees with an appraisal form to complete and return several days before the event. This process ensures the appraiser has time to review the comments and give consideration to the discussion; it also gives the employee an opportunity to give considered responses to things they may otherwise find difficult to verbalize in a meeting.

The appraisal should be held in a quiet location away from any interruptions, allowing at least an hour of dedicated time. Listening skills are vitally important as it is often not what the appraisee *actually* says but the *way* in which they say it which gives a clearer indication of exactly how they are feeling about their work. Promises should not be made that cannot be kept but information given should be acted upon as the whole appraisal process only works if employees recognize that the process is fair and worthwhile.

A record of the discussion should be given to the employee after the event to ensure correct interpretation has been made and a copy should be kept on file. Appraising employees is a learned skill and requires a good listening technique. Many books and articles have been written on the topic and when handled properly, it is tremendously successful in improving performance and motivation.

Employee disputes

Despite best efforts things do sometimes go wrong in practice and the first step to putting it right is to acknowledge the problem. Few people like confrontation and consequently delay addressing sensitive or difficult subjects. However, tackling them when they are in their early stages is far easier than waiting until they become monumental problems. Hoping they will go away simply does not work!

Grievance and disciplinary procedures

Most problems, if tackled sensitively and early enough, can be resolved informally and quickly, but if this does not work there are formal procedures which every employer must follow in an effort to resolve such matters. The Grievance and Disciplinary Procedures came into force in 2004 and both have a standard three-stage process (Figure 13.18).

- A grievance is a concern, problem or a complaint that an employee has raised with their employer.
- A disciplinary issue is a concern, problem or complaint that an employer has with an employee.

Incorrect or clumsy handling of this process can have serious financial and legal consequences for a business so it is sensible to seek legal advice before commencing any such action.

Stage	Process
Step 1	Statement of the problem or issue in writing
Step 2	Hold a meeting to discuss the problem: ■ The employee has the right to be accompanied ■ The employee must take all reasonable steps to attend this meeting The employee will be notified in writing of the decision
Step 3	The employee has a right to appeal if they feel the situation has not been resolved Employer must notify the employee in writing of the final decision

13.18 The standard three-stage process for Grievance and Disciplinary Procedures.

Dismissal

Although effective recruitment, appraisal and staff development procedures help minimize the risk of consistent poor performance, eventually an employer may have to face the difficult task of dismissal. This is a serious course of action and there are steps which should be taken in order to avoid claims for unfair, wrongful and constructive dismissal. Legal advice should always be sought and documentary evidence in the form of accurate employee records is essential.

Exit interviews

Whatever the reason for the termination of employment, exit interviews are an excellent way of gleaning valuable information about why the employee is leaving, how the practice could improve or what it should be aware of. Very often staff terminate their employment because they do not wish to raise grievances or disrupt the status quo and awareness of these covert issues can help retain potentially good employees and keep staff turnover at the most appropriate level.

Exit interviews should be conducted immediately prior to the employee leaving and are designed to obtain relevant information in an environment where the employee has no fear of retribution.

Marketing

Marketing in any business is essential as it is the only way to survive, grow and develop. As the business climate for the veterinary profession becomes more competitive it is imperative that practices aim to satisfy their customers' needs and wants. There are two ways of doing this: one way is to listen to what your customers want and then try and provide it; this is known as being *reactive*. The other way is to be smart enough to anticipate what they need and want, almost before they realize it themselves, so that provision triggers the need or want in the customer; this is by far the most desirable option and is known as being *proactive*.

Veterinary practices are now dealing with a more informed client, one educated via the internet and more aware of value for money with a shop around nature that makes them harder to bond as clients. In addition, pet ownership is changing as lifestyles change and fewer people are able to take on the same commitment of a pet or are prepared to place them higher up the priority ladder and sacrifice part of their leisure time to look after them.

Italian economist Vilfredo Pareto proposed the 80/20 principle, which states that a small proportion of causes, creates a large result; for example, 80% of a veterinary practice's business comes from 20% of its clients. This knowledge is vital when the business is marketed to achieve growth.

There are four main ways veterinary practices can increase their business.

1. Increase the average transaction fee (ATF), i.e. the average amount of money from each of the clients in the 20% bracket. The ATF is calculated by dividing the amount of income by the number of client visits to the surgery.
2. Increase the average transaction volume (ATV), i.e. the number of times the client comes through the door. The ATV is calculated by knowing the ratio of first consultations to second and follow-up consultations.
3. Increase the number of clients overall. Based on the Pareto rule, 20% of clients will regularly visit the practice. If the client base is 1000, then 200 clients will regularly visit the practice; if the client base is increased to 1200, then 240 clients will regularly visit the practice.
4. Achieve better client retention, i.e. stop clients from leaving the practice and going elsewhere for veterinary services.

Determining the needs of clients

Market research helps to determine or anticipate clients' needs and enables the practice to find out how well it is matched to the clients. In marketing, perception is more important than actuality, i.e. although the practice may *believe* it is providing a good service to its clients, it is what the clients *perceive* they are receiving that matters. Ways of finding out what clients perceive and what they want include:

- Surveys
- Focus groups
- Suggestion box
- Informal methods.

Surveys

Surveys can be conducted by telephone, by post or face-to-face, and by questionnaire or by interview. Questionnaires are more structured but interviews allow the questions to change depending on the respondent's answers. More interesting information arises from interviews, but analysing the responses is much harder as the data are qualitative rather than quantitative. Whichever method is chosen, the questions need to be carefully planned. Closed questions encourage a yes/no answer and result in quantitative data. Open questions require a more thoughtful, considered reply and result in qualitative data. The ideal survey contains a mix of both open and closed questions for optimal information gathering. As producing and analysing customer surveys is not an easy job, there are professional companies who undertake to write, conduct and analyse these surveys on behalf of the practice. Distributing, processing and assimilating the results of questionnaires is time-consuming, and professionally administered surveys may be preferred for key marketing decisions.

Focus groups

Focus groups can be very successful, particularly to discuss one specific topic in detail. Large animal practices have traditionally been successful with this method of market research, which involves asking a selected group of clients to a venue, usually providing them with some hospitality, and asking them their opinions, views and thoughts and thereby promoting discussion. As well as providing vital information, it is also highly successful in bonding clients to the practice.

Suggestion box

A suggestion box is a simple, often overlooked, method of finding out what clients want. However, it is a mistake to undervalue it as there are many clients who do not participate in surveys, are not forthcoming on the phone, and are mistrustful of claims of anonymity. However, these clients may be quite happy to drop a discrete note in a suggestion box with a vital clue to meeting their needs and wants.

Informal methods

Informal methods of finding out what clients need or want are also very effective but need good staff training in place to be of benefit. Staff who speak to clients, whether it be face-to-face or on the telephone, can be trained to listen for 'clues'. Off-the-cuff remarks are often delivered to staff at the client interface and if recognized as such can give your business the competitive edge. For example, a client may say in passing 'I'm glad I got an early appointment because I have to get over to the supermarket by noon to pick up the dog food.' A well trained member of staff will pick up on the fact that the client is going elsewhere for dog food, ask what brand is chosen and offer to get it in stock so next time the client only needs to make one trip.

Marketing plans

Marketing is a very powerful tool and consequently can be very effective. However, badly managed it can also be very damaging and there are many major businesses that have suffered at the hands of poor marketing. In order to be effective, marketing has to move with the times and current trends. It should not be assumed that last year's strategy will work this year. The world is constantly changing and marketing techniques have to keep pace with these changes in order to remain competitive.

Planning is an organized way of ensuring that the techniques employed in marketing deliver the desired outcome. A marketing plan is essential in order to deliver a campaign in a structured and well managed manner. It should also be recognized that

14

Nursing clinics

Hayley L. McLeod

This chapter is designed to give information on:

■ Planning and preparation of veterinary nurse clinics

■ Different veterinary nurse-led clinics that have proven success in veterinary practice

■ Considerations within the practice structure prior to offering this service to clients

■ Managing owner expectation and nursing ability with regards to clinic content

■ The marketing and client educational material which could support clinics

Introduction

Veterinary nurses are qualified professionals who have the knowledge and ability to identify debilitating conditions such as obesity, anorexia, ectoparasite infestation, endoparasitic infection, dental disease, arthritis and behavioural problems. It is therefore the duty of care of a veterinary nurse to ensure that owners are educated and supported to a level that prevents the above conditions impinging on their animal's quality of life and causing unnecessary suffering.

Preventive healthcare is not a new concept. For example, human medicine has been screening patients at risk of developing cancer prior to the onset of disease for many years. Veterinary nurses in practice are now starting to run screening and other health-enhancing clinics. Often these clinics have been developed to maintain pace with, and keep ahead of, a demanding marketplace as veterinary practices experience challenges to their role. Nationally there has been a trend towards reduced client numbers, reduced average client spend and, most recently, a change of legislation that has resulted in veterinary products becoming available from other outlets. This has increased the profile of supermarkets, pet shops and internet pharmacies as they recruit custom and increase their market share within the animal health industry.

The veterinary market is constantly evolving and professionals can no longer afford to wait for clients to arrive at the practice or expect them to remain loyal throughout their pet's life (see Chapter 13). There is a greater emphasis on developing new veterinary business than in previous years. An increased focus has been placed on building relationships and bonds with clients during crucial stages of their pet's life, such as during puppy- and kittenhood, the management of senior pets or a long-term illness. Many practices now use computer software packages designed to manage the healthcare of individual pets, which provide a lifestyle map relevant to the animal and specific breed that is to be followed throughout the different stages of development.

The inclusion of veterinary nurse clinics within the practice's scope of service increases the healthcare available to pets, therefore helping the practice to get ahead of the competition. In turn, clients receive accurate advice from knowledgeable and experienced professionals. Providing such a high standard of veterinary care will increase client bonding and thus increase average client spend and satisfaction. This in turn benefits the practice, the client and, most importantly, the pet.

This chapter outlines what veterinary nurses should consider when wishing to develop clinics within the practice.

Planning

Prior to the establishment of clinics it is important to plan the activity, as adequate thought and preparation will go a long way towards ensuring the success of a clinic, and in turn the management of client expectations.

Why does the practice want to set up veterinary nurse-led clinics?

It is important that the practice consider the reasons for developing veterinary nurse clinics in the early developmental stages, as inappropriate motivation may lead to clinic failure and disappointed clients. For example, setting up clinics for senior pets just because the practice has a new blood pressure monitor would not necessarily be a recipe for success. Setting up a clinic because veterinary nurses want to enhance their skills, increase the healthcare services offered to clients or increase practice income is a stronger foundation on which to build.

Who is responsible for the clinics?

It is useful to appoint a named veterinary nurse to take overall responsibility for the management of the clinics. This helps to ensure that all other staff members have a point of contact for questions in relation to any clinic type, thus allowing for better communication and greater success.

Many nursing skills can be developed and practised whilst running clinics, thereby providing an opportunity for both qualified and student members of the team. Some veterinary nurses may have a particular interest and would prefer to work in a specific type of clinic; for example, a veterinary nurse with an interest in the management of diabetes would be the most suitable to run a diabetes clinic, as their interest will ensure the continuation of the service. There are many ways in which practices manage the rota to provide such a service. Often there is a dedicated veterinary nurse who specializes in pet health counselling and runs all the available clinics. Other methods are to employ a rotational system in which all veterinary nurses are contracted to run clinics at given times. Each system has advantages and disadvantages, and can work well, providing veterinary nurse and patient continuity is maintained and they are correctly managed. It is desirable that a veterinary surgeon is available during all consultation times in case there are causes for concern, as an owner would not be happy to leave the surgery with their pet without advice or action appropriate to any findings. The availability of a veterinary surgeon will also allow veterinary nurses to work within their professional restrictions, including taking samples and testing, and will allow for a diagnosis to be made based on the findings.

Level of knowledge

Within general practice there is a variety of abilities and levels of qualification, with many veterinary nurses now being qualified to degree level. It is essential that this knowledge is pooled and shared between staff members to ensure that all clients receive correct and accurate information, while staff are not overstretched in their abilities.

Many pharmaceutical and nutritional manufacturers sponsor veterinary nurses' professional development programmes, which support the development and running of clinics. These often lead to additional qualifications, which help to motivate veterinary nurses and keep their knowledge current and up-to-date. These are therefore highly recommended.

Available resources

The minimum that is required is a proactive veterinary nurse, weighing scales, thermometer, stethoscope, clock with a second hand, urine dipsticks and a means of recording data. Equipment such as blood analysers, refractometers, electrocardiography machines and blood pressure monitors can all help to increase the depth of the examination and the service to the client, but are not essential. However, working with these additional tools may require initial direction from the veterinary surgeon. All members of the nursing team must feel confident to use any necessary equipment and be able to do so comfortably. Lack of training in how to use these instruments may result in an embarrassing situation during a consultation, which could shatter a veterinary nurse's confidence and reduce motivation to conduct further clinics, as well as having a negative impact on client perceptions.

Clinic venue

Consideration needs to be given to the amount of room available. Some practices are purpose built and provide a designated veterinary nurses' consultation room. If this is not available, it will be necessary to discuss with the principal or practice manager the possibility of using other consultation rooms and negotiate a time for their use. This could be disadvantageous as most clients prefer to attend clinics during the evening after work or at weekends.

Appointment times

This consideration links closely to the venue in which the clinic is to be held, as if one consultation room needs to be shared the availability of veterinary nurse consultations will be restricted. This should not deter the practice from developing the clinics, it just means that attendance may be slightly restricted and a more in-depth management strategy may be required to ensure the availability of veterinary nurses, and that consultation times do not overlap.

If there is a designated veterinary nurses' consultation room, there is greater flexibility, and consideration should be given to what times would best suit the clients in order to encourage attendance. Certain times will prove more popular than others and changes can be made to the original plan to ensure client and practice convenience. In addition, choosing a quiet period to allow for more in-depth consultations may be desirable.

Duration of clinics

This is reflective of the caseload; a busy practice with a greater number of clients will be able to allocate less time per consultation. Therefore, as a general rule, in order to perform a thorough consultation, which includes taking an in-depth history, conducting a head to tail examination, feeding back the findings to the owner and answering any necessary questions, an appropriate duration would be a minimum of 20 minutes. This is only a rough guide and variations are commonly seen. It is better to see fewer patients, but have the time to perform a thorough consultation, rather than potentially to miss something clinically significant because of a shorter consultation time.

Clinic protocol

It is important to plan and rehearse an examination protocol for each clinic type. This allows for establishment of a structure and ensures a standard level of care to every patient. In addition, a protocol acts as a reference guide and ensures that veterinary nurses are comfortable with what they are being asked to do. Figure 14.1 provides a reference guide to help plan which examinations are to be included within each clinic.

It is good practice to document findings from every clinical examination; this could be typed on to a computer or written on an examination form. This allows easier health comparisons at subsequent visits, and the owner can be supplied with a copy, which illustrates what has been found and what advice has been given.

Marketing

Marketing is hugely important to ensure the success of veterinary nurse clinics. There are many ways in which clients can be targeted to attend. It is surprising how many clients are able to be recruited from those already registered. Some may already be attending other veterinary nurse clinics; for example, a dental check may prompt a weight management consult. For further marketing ideas, see Chapter 13.

Communication

It is essential that the development of veterinary nurse clinics is communicated to all members of the veterinary team. In general, it will be the veterinary surgeons and receptionists who will be primarily responsible

Health check factor	Considerations
History taking	Dogs should be allowed off leads and cats out of their baskets Ask the owner to comment on gait, appetite, weight, demeanour, sight and skin Ask the owner to compare the animal now as to when it was younger Ask the owner about vaccination, worming and flea protocols
Weight	Ageing dogs are more prone to obesity whereas cats tend to lose weight with age; ask the owner to comment
Head and neck	It is usually easier to stand at the head to examine the eyes, ears and mouth Test the patient's sight by allowing a piece of cotton wool to fall to the floor; due to selectivity the animal will normally catch sight and follow the item Test the menace response by holding the patient's head and using the other hand to quickly move towards the eye; normally the animal will blink in response Place objects on the floor, for example chairs and boxes, and see if the patient is able to navigate around them Make a loud clap away from the animal, the patient should react to the sound by twitching its ears Examine the ear canal using an otoscope Examine the mouth for gingivitis, periodontitis, plaque tartar, odontoclastic resorptive lesions (cats), caries (dogs), fractures, hyperplasia, epulids and other oral masses Run hands down the patient's neck for abnormal lymph and thyroid glands
Thorax	Examine for masses. Lipomas are common in the overweight, ageing patient (investigate any masses) Auscultate the heart on the right- and left-side of the thorax with a stethoscope Record heart rate, rhythm and murmurs
Abdomen	Examine skin and fur for ectoparasites Feel for cutaneous and subcutaneous masses Check the rectum and genitalia for abnormalities
Limbs	Check for swelling and discomfort Examine and clip claws if necessary
Blood tests	Run a basic haematology and biochemistry profile Run a thyroxine (T4) level for feline patients
Urinalysis	Use a dipstick to test for protein, blood glucose, ketones and urine pH. A refractometer should be used to measure specific gravity Test for haematuria
Blood pressure	Monitor blood pressure as hypertension is a common clinical sign of ageing, including chronic renal failure, hyperthyroidism and other endocrine disorders
Diet	Ask the owner to detail a normal day's feed Ask if the patient has any gastric disorders Inform the owner of the lifestage diets if the patient isn't currently being fed such a food stuff

14.1 Health check reference guide to help plan examinations for different clinics.

for promoting the clinics and recruiting clients. They must be familiar with the details and protocols of the clinic if they are to pass this information on to the clients correctly. An ideal time to inform members of the veterinary team about the clinic would be during a practice meeting. Written communication is an alternative if meetings are not regularly attended. Written documentation also provides a reference guide for staff members and acts as a memory prompt.

External communication with the client is also important. It is good practice to call or mail the client with a reminder a week prior to the appointment to maintain compliance, as the appointment may have been booked several months earlier. Generally, if a clinic fails to be a success it is often due to poor communication methods. For this reason a huge amount of consideration should be given to communication during each stage of the development and management of a clinic.

Paediatric clinics

Ensuring that the veterinary practice is like a second home for a new pet is important. The practice needs to become a safe haven, a place where the animal has positive experiences and discovers new lifestyle skills with confidence in a safe environment. For the owners it should pose minimal stress and be a place in which they can obtain advice and learn from the experts in order to ensure that their pet remains fit and healthy throughout its life.

Impressions are made at the first phone call and visit to the practice. It is at this stage that new clients can be introduced to the full spectrum of healthcare advice and support that the practice team is able to offer. It is also an opportunity to differentiate the practice from its competitors and to fill clients with confidence and reassure them that the team cares for their new family member.

During puppy- and kittenhood there is an opportunity to bond clients early with the practice using initiatives that support them at this crucial stage of their animal's development. By addressing the client's needs from the beginning, the practice is able to increase client bonding significantly, and increase the number of visits to the practice throughout the lifetime of the pet.

Vaccination clinics

It is essential that an animal's first visit to the veterinary practice is an enjoyable and memorable experience. Often it has arrived by car, and may have had an unpleasant journey, so time should be allowed for it to relax and have the opportunity for a drink of water. Puppies and kittens showing good, non-fearful behaviour should be rewarded with play, petting and treats. Signs of fear should be ignored at this stage. Rewarding fearful behaviour at the surgery by offering a treat may condition the animal to display fear whilst attending the veterinary surgery in future. This behaviour may become very stressful for the owner and will often result in reduced visits to the practice and poorer overall healthcare compliance.

Ideally, all pets presenting for first vaccinations should be seen by the veterinary nurse prior to the veterinary surgeon's examination. This helps to socialize the pet as they are being handled by two members of the veterinary team. It also allows for the communication of the healthcare advice required for the first few weeks of life. This advice should be accompanied by a puppy or kitten pack so that the owner has a written copy of the advice given on topics such as parasite control. It is important not to confuse the owner by offering too much advice, as they may not understand the recommendations. An ideal opportunity to provide further information is at the second vaccination.

Following the veterinary nurse and veterinary surgeons' examinations the vaccination should be given in a calm manner. The animal will be able to sense the anticipation suffered by the owner and for that reason it is often a good idea for the veterinary nurse to hold the patient at the time of injection. Finally, owners should be encouraged to visit the practice each month to weigh and worm their pet. This will help to build a positive association and reduce the risks of anxiety associated with visiting the practice.

Kitten clubs

Veterinary nurses can play an important role in ensuring that cat owners are fully educated about preventive healthcare, therefore engaging clients with the concept of lifetime care from the start. Although the requirement to socialize a cat is much less than that for a dog, there are still some educational considerations that should be communicated to new owners. This information can be provided in the form of a kitten club.

In addition to vaccination clinics, veterinary nurses could invite new cat owners to an evening meeting aimed to outline the key points of responsible pet ownership. Topics may include advice on endoparasites and ectoparasites, neutering, dental care, insurance and microchipping. With reference to cats' asocial preferences, socialization advice can be discussed with owners who have other pets at home.

Puppy parties

A popular addition to the practice timetable is the introduction of puppy parties (Figure 14.2). These have certainly proved very successful for practices that have spent the time and resources to focus professionally on the opportunity. Puppy parties not only benefit the owner and the puppy, they also have advantages for the practice.

Puppy parties offer an excellent socialization experience for a puppy. They also allow positive associations to be built between the puppy and the practice, allowing the pet to learn important life skills through correct socialization and habituation. For owners they present an ideal opportunity to ask questions and share experiences with staff and other owners, and to ensure that they leave with a better understanding of all the important healthcare issues associated with responsible pet ownership (Figure 14.3).

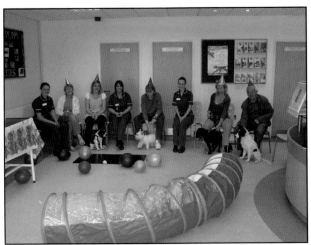

14.2 Veterinary nurses can provide important client education in the form of puppy parties. These are well attended and great fun for the puppies, owners and veterinary nurses.

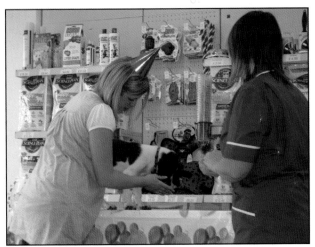

14.3 Puppy parties provide an opportunity to show owners how to handle their pets for a health check.

There is a large amount of work involved in planning and running puppy parties. To ensure their success it is important that there is an organized approach and that all the necessary resources are available. The following are a few considerations that should be given prior thought before inviting the first group of puppy owners:

- Who will host the parties?
- What date and time?
- Party protocol
- Venue
- Marketing.

Who will host the parties?

It is essential that the person running the parties is knowledgeable, interested and able to relate their personal experiences of owning and training a puppy. The host needs to have a thorough knowledge of the subjects that are to be discussed; for example, basic training and elementary behavioural issues, parasite control, vaccinations, canine nutrition, neutering, dental care, insurance, microchipping, grooming and common health problems. An ideal person would be an experienced veterinary nurse. If the host is independent from the practice, it should be ensured that the information given is correct and in line with practice protocols and guidelines.

The host should be polite, approachable and have the ability to manage a group of people, deal with different client social styles and learning habits, and have the confidence to speak clearly and slowly. This will ensure that the structure of the party is maintained and that the experience is an enjoyable one for all concerned.

Ideally there should be a minimum of two hosts per party, so that one can observe the event and provide any extra help and support required. An assistant should have an interest in the animals and appear confident. They may not need to take a particular verbal or educational role, but must be confident to refer clients to the party organizer if they cannot answer questions asked by the clients.

What date and time?

As mentioned previously, the careful timing of veterinary nurse clinics is essential as many owners work during the day and would therefore be unable to benefit from a daytime service. Ideally, puppy parties should be available during an evening or at the weekend to ensure maximum compliance, with all family members being able to attend. Where this is not possible, care should be taken to ensure that all clients are catered for in some way.

Another consideration is whether to host a single party or a series of parties. It should be ensured that the timing fits in with the practice hours and other commitments. Parties should last no longer than one hour per session, which allows plenty of time to cover the important aspects of pet ownership and time for puppy socialization and play.

Party protocol

Once it has been established, it should be ensured that everyone within the practice is aware of the protocol as this will help to prevent failure and disappointed clients. It is particularly important with regard to the age of puppies invited, as the upper age limit will be determined by the youngest recruit. There should be no more than 6 weeks between the youngest and oldest puppies, which should help prevent boisterous, bullying behaviours. These behaviours promote bad socialization and may deter some owners from attending the parties.

The number of parties in any one course can vary from one to four. Inviting the whole family to attend is a good idea. This gives the puppies the opportunity to socialize with people of all ages. Although each practice will be different, as each will have a different amount of space and experience available, below are some guidelines on the basic protocol of a party:

- A maximum of eight puppies should be invited each week
- Puppies should be fully vaccinated or at least have started their course

- Collars and leads must be worn at all times
- Families are welcome by prior arrangement
- A refundable deposit helps to ensure course completion
- Parties may be run as 4-week blocks or individual sessions
- Party bags should be available.

Once the basics have been identified it is important to look at the content and structure of the event. Figures 14.4 and 14.5 give an indication of topics and games that could be included during the party, and Figure 14.6 shows a typical set up.

Venue

Ideally the parties should be held within the practice, to ensure the development of the perception of a safe haven rather than a place of fear. The waiting room out of hours or a meeting and training room would be ideal. However, this is not always possible and it may be necessary to look at alternative venues such as village or school halls or local parks. If other venues are to be used it is important to consider factors such as insurance, toilet and first aid facilities, and car parking. Most importantly the premises must be totally secure for patient safety. Figure 14.7 provides guidance on the venue.

Subject	Advice
Socialization	Why socialization is important Ideas to further socialize the puppies
Fleas	Understanding the nature of flea infestations
Flea prevention	Why preventive treatment is better than waiting for an infestation to arise
Worms	The worm lifecycle and its importance in canine and human health
Worm control	The importance of regular worming
Vaccination	Why we vaccinate The importance of annual health checks and regular boosters
Nutrition	Benefits of balanced commercial lifestage foods
Neutering	Health benefits of neutering
Dental care	The benefits of regular dental care
Insurance	Highlighting the benefits of pet insurance
Microchipping	The importance of being able to reunite owners with lost dogs
Monitoring growth	Weekly checks to ensure puppies are developing at their normal rate, which should be ≤3–4 g/kg of estimated adult bodyweight

14.4 Healthcare topics for a puppy party.

Activity	Benefit
Training	Supports owners with: ■ Socialization ■ Toilet training ■ Teaching the basic commands ■ Explaining the principles of positive reinforcement
Tour of the practice	Raises awareness of the facilities and expertise within the practice If owners are familiar with the practice they are likely to be less concerned about leaving their pet at the surgery should it be necessary in the future
Pass the puppy	Allows the puppy to be exposed to different people and supports the socialization process
Puppy bingo	This involves playing an educational DVD to the clients. The first to circle 10 identified words wins a prize
Fancy dress	If you are able to encourage owners to dress up in big hats and helmets, etc., while playing pass the puppy it will allow puppies to learn about different human presentations

14.5 Puppy party games.

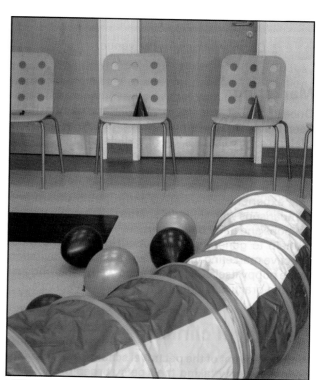

14.6 The ideal set up for a puppy party.

When clients are offered this choice they tend to select the middle level, as they want to take advantage of the service but do not want to be seen to be offering only the basics to their pet. This therefore ensures that a more in-depth preventive healthcare package can be offered.

Conclusion

In summary, there is a great deal of work involved in the development and initiation of nursing clinics; however, they are a hugely rewarding service for both the client and the profession.

They ensure the health and welfare of companion animals and help to ensure the continuation of veterinary practice.

References and further reading

Evans JM and White K (1994) *The Doglopaedia (revised edition)*. Ringpress, Lydney
Jevring C and Catanzaro T (1999) *Healthcare of the Well Pet*. WB Saunders, Philadelphia
Lane D, Cooper B and Turner L (2007) *BSAVA Textbook of Veterinary Nursing, 4th edn*. BSAVA Publications, Gloucester

15

Behaviour

Trudi Atkinson and Francesca Riccomini

This chapter is designed to give information on:

- The role of the veterinary nurse in identifying behavioural problems and communicating with clients
- The most common behavioural problems seen in the cat and dog
- Prevention of common behavioural problems
- Considerations when choosing a cat or dog
- Problems encountered when introducing a pet
- Problems encountered with poor pet management and discipline
- Behavioural referrals

The role of the veterinary nurse

One of the most common reasons for relinquishment and euthanasia of otherwise healthy pets is behaviour which owners, or society, regard as problematic. Veterinary nurses are uniquely placed to make an impact on these distressing statistics as clients frequently feel more at ease with nursing staff, who they often perceive as being less intimidating than veterinary surgeons, and as being particularly interested in the general management of their animals. In addition, veterinary nurse-led clinics provide an ideal scenario in which to discuss the way a dog or cat actually copes with its environment, interacts with its owner or family group, and behaves towards unfamiliar individuals, human or animal, both inside and outside the home.

For the welfare of the animals under veterinary care and to be able to advise on animal behaviour, it is essential for veterinary nurses to have a reliable knowledge of:

- The ethology (natural behaviour) of the species concerned

- The appropriate management of the species
- The relevance of associative learning theory
- The impact of social and physical environments on companion animals.

Combined with awareness of the need to phrase questions in a non-judgmental manner that invites confidence, such knowledge allows veterinary nurses to offer advice and highlight behavioural issues that might otherwise be overlooked or dismissed as unimportant by clients. This opens the way for a detailed discussion and for the individual case to be dealt with in the most appropriate fashion, either through in-house behavioural consultation, or by referral to a trainer or behaviour specialist.

Common behavioural problems

As problem behaviour varies widely, it is essential that each animal's case be viewed individually. Nevertheless, the most commonly encountered behavioural problems tend to fall into a number of categories:

- Aggression
- Fear- and anxiety-based problems
- House soiling
- Separation-related conditions
- Compulsive disorders
- Senior pet conditions
- General control and management problems.

There is no doubt that prevention is better than attempts at resolution once difficulties are encountered. An understanding of causation is also important.

Aggression

Aggression is the most commonly referred problem in dogs and an important reason for behavioural consultation in cats. It is difficult to classify and for practical purposes tends to be described in terms of the presumed underlying motivation and the target towards which the behaviour is directed. It is important to understand that aggression is a normal element of the canine and feline behavioural repertoire. The various stages of behaviour in aggression leading to physical contact are generally recognized by other animals, which respond appropriately if circumstances and human actions allow. Problems occur when:

- People fail to recognize behaviours that can signal impending aggression and/or to understand the underlying cause
- People intervene in an unhelpful or inappropriate manner
- Other animals themselves suffer from behavioural difficulties
- Pets are prevented from adopting an appropriate strategy to defuse the situation
- Pets are placed in artificially competitive situations by unhelpful management practices.

Companion animals that are not prepared adequately for the lives they will lead and environments they will inhabit as pets are particularly at risk of becoming aggressive, hence the emphasis on good socialization and habituation to domestic circumstances. This is not a 'once and for all' phenomenon: care should subsequently be taken to maintain and broaden an animal's experiences.

However, fear-based aggression can also result from negative experiences later in life or from unacceptable pressures with which an individual cannot cope. Therefore, anticipating what these might be, highlighting them for clients and offering pre-emptive and remedial advice when the first signs are observed is an area of general practice that could usefully be expanded.

Fear- and anxiety-based problems

Fear is an adaptive response. However, the anxiety that quickly becomes associated with signs that a fearful stimulus is likely to be encountered, if prolonged or frequently experienced, can threaten an individual's emotional well being. Eventually health and welfare will be undermined. Fear and anxiety can arise in relation to people, other animals, inanimate objects and common environmental stressors. Examples of the latter are those associated with noise, such as traffic, fireworks and storms.

Animals bred from timid parents are most at risk. Not only can young animals learn to become fearful by observation of parental behaviour, but personality traits such as boldness or timidity may also be inherited. Studies have shown for example that kittens sired by a timid tomcat are likely themselves to be timid, whereas those sired by a bold individual will tend to be more confident (Figure 15.1). This would appear to be an inherent trait as generally tomcats play no part in raising the young. Thus, it is inadvisable to breed from timid, nervous animals. However, any pet can develop a problem as a result of one major or numerous minor exposures to an individual stressor or group of related stimuli. The manifestation of such conditions can range from mild to severe with the development of phobic reactions increasingly being seen. A phobia is an abnormally intense fear that is of such magnitude that it interferes with an animal's ability to lead a normal life.

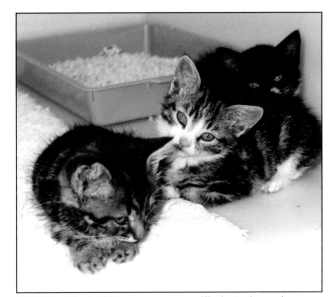

15.1 Timid kittens are more likely to have been sired by a timid tomcat, whereas, confident kittens are more likely to have been sired by a bold individual.

Problems of this type are most commonly identified in dogs, not because they are absent in the cat population but because feline coping strategies, primarily based on flight and hiding, mean that affected cats often defuse their arousal better than dogs so long as the conditions are available for them to do so. Owners are therefore less likely to seek help for their cats, unless they develop more overt and less acceptable problems, such as indoor urinary spraying or over grooming, or the cat's fear and anxiety results in aggression towards people or other pets.

Poor preparation for life and location again underlie many problems of this nature, although accidental exposure to a stressor or particularly stressful experience can also feature in their development. For example, many pets become averse to visiting the veterinary clinic, especially if they have had major problems or are frequent visitors. Dog attacks also put previously sociable pets at risk of developing fearful reactions, which may ultimately become extremely self-defensive and result in aggression towards other dogs. In addition, the influence of modern living conditions, particularly minimalist design styles, both inside and outside homes, is undoubtedly linked with the development of this category of problem behaviour.

The organization of specific clinics aimed at recognizing stressors, such as fireworks, identifying at-risk individuals, and offering preventive advice is an area in which nursing staff can play a crucial role.

House soiling

This is a very common problem for which cat owners seek behavioural advice. In both species, a distinction must be made between failure of house training, its breakdown, and territorial marking behaviour. Resolution is unlikely to be effected unless strenuous efforts are made to understand the motivation, or motivations contributing to the problem behaviour, the causes of which are myriad. They include:

- Unrealistic owner expectations
- Inadequate management in terms of routine and provision of facilities
- Poor house training procedures
- Failure to accurately identify and deal with underlying medical conditions or causal motivations such as fear, anxiety, stress and distress.

Separation-related conditions

This group of conditions is characterized by destruction, house soiling, vocalization, pacing, agitation, vomiting, diarrhoea and hypersalivation, in the partial or complete absence of owners. The evidence must be examined in detail to avoid the common mistake of assuming that all such behaviour results from anxiety related to the loss of a specific attachment figure or human company. Separation anxiety is undoubtedly over-diagnosed and is only one of the potential contributors to this category of observed behaviours, which include:

- Fear of environmental stressors:
  - Internal (e.g. noisy household equipment, boilers, smoke alarms)
  - External (storms, building work, burglary).
- Frustration:
  - Mental (lack of appropriate stimulation, and environmental conditions that do not provide acceptable outlets)
  - Physical (lack of exercise).

Compulsive disorders

Stress, motivational conflict and frustration, which often result from insufficient mental or physical stimulation, underlie this complex class of behavioural problems, which tend to be either locomotory or oral in nature. Although a comprehensive medical investigation is always required prior to any behavioural consultation, it is particularly important with these conditions to rule out, or adequately manage, any concurrent and/or contributory diseases. These conditions, which are not well understood, are increasingly being identified and particularly affect certain canine and feline breeds: for instance, flank sucking in Dobermanns, tail chasing in English and Staffordshire Bull Terriers, light spot and shadow chasing in Border Collies, and wool and fabric sucking in Siamese and Burmese cats. However, this does not preclude their development in other breeds and non-pedigree animals and, as they are often associated with compromised welfare, at-risk individuals need to be identified and appropriate preventative advice given as early as possible.

Senior pet conditions

With the current increase in the number of pets reaching the senior stage, knowledge of the behavioural problems from which they are likely to suffer is increasing. Cognitive dysfunction in the dog has been recognized for some time, and a similar disease has been identified in cats more recently. These are extreme manifestations of brain ageing but the lives of many senior pets, and their owners' enjoyment of them, could be improved and possibly even prolonged with appropriate behavioural support in addition to dedicated medical care.

Veterinary nurse-run clinics (see Chapter 14) offer the ideal opportunity to discuss the importance of maintaining in good order the minds of ageing dogs and cats because, although evidence is still lacking, it is suggested that appropriate mental stimulation can delay the onset of some effects of the negative changes associated with brain ageing. Instigating desirable and necessary management changes ahead of problems developing, when animals have an increased chance of adapting to them, is particularly useful. In addition, identifying the potential changes that may be seen with successful ageing, as well as the more extreme indicators that all is not well, is an increasingly important part of the support required by clients who own senior pets. Otherwise many owners may simply regard minor lapses in memory or changes in sleep patterns, for example, as something to be expected, thus missing an opportunity for early intervention to obtain the best results for their pet.

General control and management issues

A number of behaviours that cause concern to owners of both dogs and cats, and frequently indicate deficiencies in management and provision of a suitable environment, may also be prevented by specifically targeted appropriate advice. Opportunities for discussion of the important issues surrounding avoidance of such problems commonly arise during dedicated clinics or client information sessions, routine consultations concerning other matters, or general conversations, such as those that frequently occur in the waiting area of any general practice.

Problems relating to general control and management

In dogs:
- **Jumping up and mouthing**
- **Poor recall and general obedience**
- **Barking**
- **Destruction, inside and outside the home.** ▶

In cats:
- Destruction, especially by scratching furniture or 'kneading' clothes
- Juvenile behaviours such as sucking hair, clothes and skin of owners.

In both species:
- Attention seeking
- Inappropriate play
- Hyperactivity
- Predatory behaviour
- Roaming
- Food stealing
- Pica, including coprophagia
- Relationship difficulties, i.e. failure to bond or over-attachment
- Problems associated with car travel.

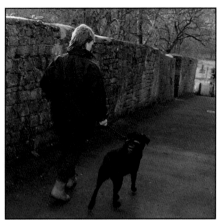

15.2

New owners may believe that they will conscientiously exercise their dog twice daily, but might not maintain such a commitment long term.

- Point out realities and potential problems
- Offer practical knowledge based advice to resolve minor issues before they develop further
- Direct clients towards suitable support, such as good dog walkers and experienced cat sitters
- Suggest appropriate specialist help as an alternative to the well meaning but unqualified advice owners may otherwise follow.

Related issues

In addition to preventing or addressing specifically behavioural problems, the importance of behaviour counselling in helping to manage medical conditions, such as feline lower urinary tract disease (FLUTD) and obesity, is now increasingly being recognized. Once established these disorders are difficult to treat, so efforts at prevention are not only worthwhile but with many pets essential.

Preventive measures

Common contributory themes

Whatever the species, or problem, an individual's behaviour is often influenced by more than one factor. Veterinary nurses are often ideally placed to offer well targeted advice, make suggestions, or alert veterinary surgeons to potential problems, with the result that pre-emptive action can be taken to prevent unacceptable behaviours developing.

Unrealistic owner expectations

Owners frequently have unrealistic expectations of their pets, and sometimes of themselves, for example:

- Expecting a previously free-ranging cat to readily adapt to a restrictive urban area or indoor living
- Introducing a poorly socialized animal to an active family or multi-pet home
- Expecting a social animal to adapt to its owners' busy schedules and frequent absences
- Believing they will conscientiously exercise their new dog twice daily, despite not being temperamentally predisposed to undertake such a commitment (Figure 15.2).

Prevention

Conversations with veterinary nurses provide valuable opportunities to:

Inappropriate choice of pet

By highlighting the potential pitfalls, people may be given sufficient good quality information to prevent them from acquiring an inappropriate pet: for example, acquisition of an unsuitable canine breed for their circumstances and dog-owning experience, or another cat for an already stressed multi-cat home, which is likely to result in problem behaviour, disappointment and possibly compromised welfare.

Unsuitable source of pet

Potential owners often acquire pets whose background has not prepared them to adapt easily to the circumstances in which they are subsequently expected to live. For example, dogs bred in rural locations may or may not experience a domestic environment, but generally encounter a limited range of people and environmental stressors. They are then poorly prepared when relocated to busy urban areas where:

- Human and pet populations are high
- Space is restricted
- Environmental stressors, such as heavy traffic, are myriad
- Exercise opportunities are often inadequate.

Not unusually dogs from working breeds, and whose parents are working stock, are sold as pets to inexperienced town-dwelling owners. Similarly, pedigree cats raised in outdoor cages attended by a single individual are not released for sale until past the socialization period (2–7 weeks of age) when they go to busy homes as part of a family group containing children of varying ages.

Prevention

Some of the most significant contributions of veterinary staff in preventing behavioural problems are therefore to:

- Help people make an appropriate choice of pet
- Direct people to a source that will produce a suitable animal for their needs
- Ensure people avoid obtaining a cat or dog from shops or other unsuitable sources
- Provide sufficient information to ensure that potential owners ask breeders and other suppliers of pets the questions necessary to avoid acquisition of an unsuitable dog or cat for their circumstances.

Breeding animals

Another important opportunity to prevent problem behaviour arises when the veterinary team has access to breeders and pet owners, a position that potentially allows its members to influence both providers and future carers of pets. Many behavioural problems can be avoided by the appropriate choice of pet for individual circumstances. Likewise responsible sale of animals only to those people who are in a position to make a success of the animal's management and the pet–owner relationship is important, as is breeding from behaviourally sound stock.

Homing of animals

Pets are not just obtained from those actively breeding for sale but increasingly from rescue societies. Some involved in this world put considerable effort into their re-homing protocols. The larger and well funded charities, in particular, are often prescriptive about the placement of animals under their care. Unfortunately this is not always the case, especially with small local voluntary groups. It is not always easy to exert influence over those actively engaged in breeding, selling, rescuing and re-homing cats and dogs. This is an area where extreme tact is required, but again veterinary nurses are often well placed to make a positive contribution by subtle intervention of an advisory nature. This is especially the case where close relationships build up between locally based rescue societies and a particular veterinary practice.

Introducing pets into the home

Failure to plan appropriate strategies, inadvertent pressurizing of animals and hasty implementation of integration protocols are often responsible for behaviour problems. These situations may be associated with:

- Introducing another animal from the same or a different species into a household already containing one or more pet
- Moving an established pet to a new home (Figure 15.3)
- Reintroducing a patient into its social group after a veterinary visit.

Moving house with your cat
(A similar regime could be used to introduce a new cat to a home without other pets)

- **Getting ready to move** – make sure that you minimize the impact of the changes in your cat's territory that inevitably accompany packing and moving home. For example, try to store boxes and cases in rooms not generally frequented by your cat or throw a blanket that has acquired your cat's scent over such items to make them smell more familiar if you cannot store them out of its way. In addition, use a recommended synthetic feline pheromone, available from your veterinary surgery in either spray or diffuser form (carefully follow the manufacturer's directions), to help reassure your pet all is well with its environment.
- **Familiarize your cat with its carrier ahead of travelling** – keep the carrier out as part of the furniture for some time before you move. Place a comfortable familiar blanket in it and some treats. Feed your cat nearby or in the carrier and/or play with your cat in its vicinity. Such activities should help to reduce the cat's distress when it needs to be confined in the carrier during the journey.
- **On moving day** – it can be a good idea to book your cat into a cattery for 'moving day'. Cats can become highly stressed and frightened by the general upheaval and commotion caused by moving house. In addition, a cat may try to return to its old home if taken directly from one home to another. Breaking the initial journey with a short spell in a cattery can disrupt the cat's sense of direction and make attempts at return journeys less likely to occur.
- **If you keep your cat with you on moving day** – shut your pet up in a quiet area, for example a spare bedroom or bathroom, from which the removers can be excluded. Make sure the cat has all the facilities it may need: food, water, bed, hiding place such as a cardboard box, litter tray (placed well away from all food dishes), toys and scratching post, which a cat can use as a means of reassurance by 'topping' up its territorial marks. Use of synthetic feline pheromone can also help the cat relax. In addition, you can help your cat cope better by providing something that smells strongly of its favourite person or people. For example, a recently worn T-shirt or old towel that you've slept with in your bed.
- **Transport your pet with care** – and when you reach your destination allow your cat to quietly adjust to the new surroundings by placing it in a refuge area similar to the one you had provided in your old home. If you have the opportunity to set this up ahead of arrival so much the better.
- **Before allowing your cat access to more of the new house** – rub around the skirting boards and furniture with a cloth you've used to wipe its face and flanks so that you transfer its own reassuring odours into the environment. Gradually allow more access once your pet appears relaxed and reasonably settled. Always make sure that your cat's 'sanctuary' is available and that it has lots of easily accessible hiding places to retreat to if feeling anxious or frightened.
- **Take things very slowly** – keep your cat inside until it is completely settled. Then supervise the first few outings, keep them short and make sure it can easily run inside if frightened. Never force your cat outside or leave it there. It must always be able to get inside quickly at any time.
- **You will need to be especially patient if there are a lot of other cats already living nearby** – this can be highly intimidating for 'a new cat on the block' and it may take a while before your cat is confident to venture outside. You can help by providing lots of hiding places, particularly near its exit point to the outdoors and by discouraging the other cats from your garden.
- **In addition** – if you provide a suitable outdoor latrine area near to the door or cat flap this may encourage your cat to start eliminating outdoors once it is settled. Do this by digging over a nearby flowerbed or similar and add some good quality sand, such as is used for children's sand pits, to make it more pleasant for your cat to dig in. Plus, if it is possible, try to construct some sort of shelter so that your cat may be more likely to use this area in bad weather. But even once your cat is using an outdoor toilet it is always wise to retain an indoor litter tray in case it feels too intimidated to go outside or is taken ill.

15.3 Example handout – moving house with your cat.

to approach other providers of pet services, such as dog trainers, breeders, pet shops, kennel or cattery staff, or even friends and family, before consulting the veterinary practice. The veterinary practice may be willing and able to provide help, but unless staff witness a problem behaviour it is easy to remain unaware that a condition exists unless the client informs the practice and requests help.

There are several reasons why even regular visitors to the practice may not mention that their pet has a behavioural problem:

- They may simply be unaware that help and advice are available from the practice
- They may feel embarrassed that their pet is demonstrating behaviour that they are unable to control
- They may feel afraid of possible reactions and may believe that the only 'solution' that the practice may be able or willing to offer, or even enforce, is re-homing or euthanasia
- They may feel fearful of being reported to the authorities, especially if their pet is aggressive or behaving in a way that could be considered a public nuisance.

There are a number of things to consider that can encourage clients to approach the practice with regard to their pets' behaviour:

- Advertising both externally (e.g. in local directories, newspapers) and internally (e.g. waiting room posters, leaflets, postings to clients). Even if the practice does not hold 'in-house' behaviour consultations it can be beneficial for both the practice and clients to advertise the fact that referral to a reputable external behaviourist is available. Clients experiencing behavioural problems with their pets may go to another practice if they feel that they may not be able to obtain a referral or appropriate help from their regular practice
- Enquire about the pet's behaviour at other times. Routine consultations and veterinary nurse-led clinics provide an excellent opportunity to discuss basic behaviour problems and enquire whether the client is experiencing any difficulties with their pet
- Team members should always be non-judgemental and empathetic when dealing with clients, especially when discussing behavioural problems. Pet owners are likely to be less willing to discuss such problems if they feel they may be criticized, disapproved of and/or ridiculed.

Refer or manage in the practice?

Once a behavioural problem has been identified and the client has requested help, it is then necessary to decide if the problem is one that can be treated in-house or if referral to an external behaviourist would be a better option.

The ability to deal with behavioural problems within the practice may mean that the client and their pet are seen sooner, and possibly at less expense, than if the case were referred to an outside behaviourist.

However, if the problem is addressed inappropriately by the practice then improvement in the animal's behaviour is less likely to occur, resulting in the client and their pet requiring referral at a later stage, thereby actually delaying effective treatment and increasing overall cost to the client. It is therefore important to consider a number of factors when deciding whether a case can be managed in-house or if referral would be the more appropriate course of action:

- The relevant experience and expertise of practice personnel
- Time available to deal with the case
- A suitable environment
- Nature of the problem being presented.

Time available to deal with the case

Providing anything other than basic first aid advice without thoroughly investigating the underlying cause(s) of the behaviour is likely to be ineffective and may even result in the development of other, possibly more serious, behavioural problems. Sufficient time is required to obtain the information necessary to correctly identify all the factors influencing a behaviour and give appropriate advice, which may also require the demonstration and teaching of training and handling techniques to the owner. It is advisable to allow approximately 2 hours' consultation time for each case. Follow-up consultations and telephone back-up may also be required, and time must be made available after each consultation to prepare comprehensive written advice for the client.

A suitable environment

Visiting the home environment (Figure 15.5) and surrounding area can often be highly beneficial as an animal's behaviour can be influenced by its environment, sometimes in ways that may not initially seem apparent. This does not mean that successful behaviour consultations cannot be carried out in a clinic environment; however, extra time and provision may be required for the client to give a full and detailed description of their home and surrounding area.

If the client and their pet are to be seen at the practice, sufficient space must be made available to comfortably accommodate the behaviourist, the pet

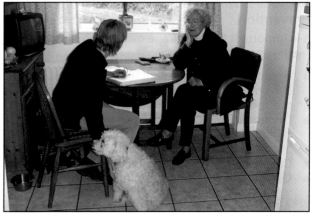

15.5 Visiting an animal's home environment can be highly beneficial for identifying and understanding the cause(s) of a behavioural problem.

with the behavioural problem, other household pets who may be influencing the undesirable behaviour, and all household members who regularly handle and interact with the problem pet. Space must also be made available for the demonstration and teaching of training methods. As well as being spacious, the consulting area needs to be comfortable. It is not reasonable to expect clients to stand or sit on hard chairs for up to 2 hours. Comfort of the animal should also be taken into account; a water bowl must be provided and easy access to outside should the pet need to be taken out to eliminate.

Nature of the problem being presented

The extent and severity of any real or potential risks connected with the behaviour must be considered and, if the risks are great, referral may be the wisest option. Risks to consider should include:

- The possibility and likely severity of injury to people and/or other animals
- Other risks to the owner, such as the threat or probability of eviction or prosecution, domestic or neighbourhood disputes, and financial costs
- Risks to the animal, for example, if the owner is seriously considering re-homing or euthanasia. The risk of potential physical abuse toward the animal if the owner is unable to cope should also be considered
- Risks to the practice and associated individuals, including the potential for physical injury and litigation.

Behavioural case history

As with any medical or surgical intervention, correct identification of all possible underlying causes must be achieved before any specific and appropriate therapy can be offered. It is therefore essential to ask the right questions in order to build up a constructive behavioural case history. In all cases, it is necessary to obtain information that is both specific to the problem behaviour that the animal is exhibiting, and general information which may or may not be relevant to the problem behaviour but is still an essential part of the practical case history.

The general information to be gathered in all cases should include:

- Owner/handler details: name, address, contact telephone number(s), number, age and sex of people and other animals in the household
- Animal details:
  - Species, breed/type, age, sex, neuter status
  - Age obtained by current owners
  - Where obtained from (i.e. kennels/cattery, family home or rescue centre).
- Veterinary history:
  - Surgical and medical
  - Past and present medication, including supplements, alternative or complementary treatments not prescribed by the veterinary surgeon.
- Management details:
  - Diet: what, where and times of feeding, and which household member usually feeds the pet

- Exercise:
  - Dogs: how often, for how long and by whom, and in what environment (fields, off lead or lead walked only?)
  - Cats: does the cat have free or regular access to outside?
- Training (dogs):
  - Past and/or current attendance at training or puppy classes
  - Training methods used
  - Efforts undertaken in an attempt to resolve current problem.

More specific information required is dependent on the nature of the presenting behavioural problem. However, in most cases this will include:

- The intensity and characteristics of the problem
- The context in which the behaviour occurs
- The owner's expectations and abilities.

The intensity and characteristics of the problem

This is essential information in all cases, but is especially important in cases of aggression, where interpretation of the term can range from no more than barking or growling to serious injury. This information is also important in cases of destructive behaviour, where the type of destruction caused by the animal can be a major clue as to the motivation for the behaviour.

The context in which the behaviour occurs

Where and when the behaviour occurs and the events that immediately precede and follow it, including the behaviour of the animal in question and the actions/reactions of other individuals (people and animals), especially the owner/handler, is important information. In cases of aggression this should also include details of who or what the animal is aggressive towards.

The owner's expectations and abilities

The success of any behavioural modification programme can depend greatly on the owner's expectations and abilities. If the owner's expectations are too ambitious they will soon lose motivation and willingness to follow the behaviourist's advice. The behaviourist must also take into account the client's ability to comply with any proposed regime. Time restraints, physical and intellectual ability, and environmental limitations are all factors that must be explored and any behavioural modification programme devised should take such factors into account.

Identification of a referral behaviourist

There have been many schemes claiming to provide training and qualifications in 'behaviour counselling', many of which have no academic verification. So-called qualifications in 'behaviour counselling' can range from a certificate obtained by attendance at a weekend course or completion of a simple correspondence course to University based education at postgraduate or even doctorate level. When a referral is considered, some understanding of the behaviourist's qualification is therefore essential.

Membership of certain organizations may give another indication as to relevant qualifications and experience. The Association of Pet Behaviour Counsellors (APBC) and the UK Registry of Canine Behaviourists (UKRCB) have stringent membership criteria, including evidence of relevant academic achievement, usually at degree or postgraduate level, plus a minimum of 2 years' experience. However, not all behaviour organizations have such rigorous requirements, if indeed any at all for membership. For example, the Companion Animal Behaviour Therapy Study Group (CABTSG) is a reputable body set up to provide a forum for the exchange of views and information, and is open to anyone in the veterinary or related professions with an interest in companion animal behaviour. Therefore, although membership of CABSTG and other similar societies can be of great value to anyone wishing to practice behavioural therapy, it is no evidence of expertise.

Organizations such as APBC, UKRCB and the British Small Animal Veterinary Association (BSAVA) are primarily trade associations and, as with many other professions, certification of veterinary practitioners is governed by an independent body (i.e. the Royal College of Veterinary Surgeons, RCVS). In 2002 an independent certification scheme administered by the Association for the Study of Animal Behaviour (ASAB) was set up to establish and maintain standards of professional qualification and conduct for animal behaviourists. To become a Certified Clinical Animal Behaviourist (CCAB) an applicant has to 'meet requirements of education to Honours Degree standard or higher in a biological or behavioural science, including appropriate elements of zoology, physiology, psychology, clinical techniques and research methods'. Endorsements from referring veterinary surgeons, evidence of at least 3 years' experience in behavioural practice and the provision of case histories to demonstrate the applicant's academic and practical knowledge is also required. Accredited behaviourists also have to continue a level of ongoing practical work and continued professional development (CPD) in order to retain their certification.

Mechanism of referral

It is important that all members of practice staff know to which behaviourist(s) the practice routinely refers and the accepted referral procedure.

An animal's behaviour can often be linked to its physical condition; therefore, most reputable behaviourists will only work on veterinary referral.

The animal will need to be examined by the veterinary surgeon prior to referral to diagnose, rule out or treat any possible underlying medical condition that could be contributing to the problem behaviour. For this reason a referral can only come from a veterinary surgeon and not from any other member of the veterinary team.

The referral procedure may vary, although most behaviourists will require a letter or a completed referral form signed by the veterinary surgeon and a copy of the animal's past medical history. This can be highly relevant, as previous disease, operations or other traumatic events can be influential in the development of a problem behaviour.

Behavioural first aid advice

Whether a case is to be seen in-house or referred to an external behaviourist, there is likely to be some delay between the client requesting help from the practice and the behavioural consultation. For this reason it is essential to be able to offer suitable behavioural first aid advice. Failure to do so may result in a possible worsening of the existing behaviour problem and even the risk of litigation if a serious incident should occur that might have been avoided by the provision of such advice.

It is often the case that clients are most likely to request help when time is at a premium and/or when the members of staff with the most behavioural knowledge are unavailable. An effective way to minimize these limitations is by the use of handouts (Figures 15.6 to 15.10) as very little time is required to present the client with the appropriate information in this form, and handouts can be provided by any member of staff no matter what their level of behavioural knowledge.

However, it is important to ensure that the client understands that the advice offered at this stage is not intended to provide long-term solutions, but to help them cope with the problem in the short term, reduce the likelihood of serious incidents occurring and prevent any exacerbation of the unwanted behaviour. It is essential that they appreciate the need for a full investigation, including veterinary examination to correctly identify the underlying causes and motivations for the behaviour, before more specific and detailed advice can be offered. One way to ensure that the client receives this information is to add a header to this effect to any behavioural first aid handout (Figure 15.6). Clients must also be made aware of their responsibilities as pet owners in regard to the safety and well being of other people and animals, and potential damage to property.

If your dog is aggressive... first aid advice

The following advice is designed to do no more than prevent incidents and to help you manage your dog's aggression in the short term. Specific advice aimed at resolving the problem cannot be given until we have an understanding of *why* your dog is acting aggressively. This can only be achieved through a combination of both behavioural and veterinary investigation. If your dog is aggressive it is advisable to seek help from a qualified behaviourist but only *after* your dog has first undergone a physical examination by your veterinary surgeon.

15.6 Example handout – aggressive dog first aid advice. (Reproduced from the *BSAVA Textbook of Veterinary Nursing, 4th edition*) (continues) ▶

If your dog is aggressive... first aid advice *continued*

If your dog is aggressive to you or other family members:

- **Never leave your dog alone unsupervised with children**. This advice is applicable to *any* dog not just dogs that are known to be aggressive
- **Avoid confrontations and actions that the dog may regard as challenging or threatening.** Do not fight your dog for possessions and avoid prolonged direct eye contact, leaning over or handling the dog in any way that may provoke aggression
- **Keep your distance and avoid unintentional provocation.** Sudden movements or flapping of the hands can provoke aggression, as can moving into the dog's personal space (typically within about two metres of the dog)
- **Defuse any threat of aggression by the dog** by looking away, slumping your shoulders and *slowly* walking away
- **Do not attempt punishment** as this is likely to increase a fearful dog's need to be defensive and aggressive, and an assertive dog may be more willing to rise to the challenge of a confrontation and react with increased aggression
- **Anticipate and avoid any potential situations that may result in your dog becoming aggressive.** For example, if your dog is aggressive around food, do not give it bones or long lasting chews and ensure that it is not disturbed whilst eating meals
- **Keep in mind that a growl is a warning and a normal part of canine 'language'.** If you are doing or about to do something to a dog that causes it to growl, by continuing with that action the dog may feel the need to get the message across with a bite
- **Attach a long lightweight lead to your dog's collar** if it attempts to bite you whenever you try to move it, so that you can lead it away without needing to handle or confront it. *However, it is important that your dog is supervised at all times while the lead is attached.*

If your dog is aggressive to other dogs or people:

On walks

- **Avoid exercising your dog in public places until professional help is obtained**. Every time your dog uses aggression it is likely to learn that it is a successful way to make other people or dogs 'go away' or keep their distance. In other words it will learn that 'aggression works', thereby reinforcing the behaviour.
- **Do not attempt to punish your dog**. This includes pulling back roughly on the lead. Doing so will cause discomfort, even pain, which your dog is likely to associate with the main focus of its attention at the time, i.e. the other dog or person, which will have the effect of increasing aggression in the long run.
- **Do not attempt to reassure your dog or use food treats as a distraction** whilst it is acting aggressively. Doing so may actually reward and so reinforce the aggressive behaviour.
- **Never leave your dog tied up in public places.**
- **Ensure your dog is under your control**, on the lead and/or muzzled **at all times**.

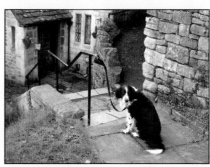

Dogs should never be left tied up in public places.

In or around the home

- **Do not allow your dog to encounter people at the boundary of its territory**, for example at the front door or garden gate.
- **Ensure that all perimeter fences, etc., are secure.**
- **Avoid visitors to the house until professional help is obtained**. If this is not possible, ensure that the dog is securely shut away for the duration of the visit. If the dog cannot be shut away, it should be kept on a lead and/or muzzled whilst the visitor is in the house. Also instruct the visitor to ignore the dog, as direct eye contact or any attempt to approach the dog could provoke an aggressive response. For visits of long duration (a day or more) it may be better to board your dog at kennels while the visitor is in the house. It is only fair to explain to the kennel owner why you need to board your dog and explain that it may be aggressive.

IT IS IMPORTANT THAT YOU ARE AWARE THAT AS THE DOG'S OWNER(S) YOU ARE RESPONSIBLE FOR THE SAFETY OF OTHERS. SHOULD YOUR DOG CAUSE INJURY YOU COULD BE AT RISK OF PROSCECUTION, WITH AN ORDER THAT YOUR DOG IS DESTROYED. DO NOT TAKE ANY UNNECESSARY RISKS.

15.6 (continued) Example handout – aggressive dog first aid advice. (Reproduced from the *BSAVA Textbook of Veterinary Nursing, 4th edition*)

Training your dog to wear a muzzle

- A basket muzzle is the type that is recommended as these muzzles allow dogs to breathe easily and to pant if need be.
- It is important that your dog has positive experiences of the muzzle from the outset by introducing the muzzle gradually and allowing the dog to associate it with something nice.
- Introduce the muzzle when your dog is calm and relaxed. Do not proceed if your dog becomes frightened or aggressive.
- Place a piece of your dog's favourite food in the bottom of the muzzle, and bring the muzzle up to the dog's nose. Hold the muzzle still and let the dog sniff the food – allow the dog to put its nose into the muzzle to get the treat.
- Repeat, placing the food treat further into the muzzle. Try using something soft and slightly sticky such as cheese or meat paste that can be smeared over the inside, so that the dog will take longer to lick it off.
- Once your dog is happy to put and keep its nose in the muzzle do up the strap, praise the dog and then immediately take it off again.
- Keep repeating this exercise, but on each occasion leave the muzzle on for longer, so the dog gradually gets used to wearing it.
- Try not to put the muzzle on at the same time or place every day, or your dog could start to anticipate it. Put the muzzle on and take it off again at different times of the day, and in different locations.
- It is also a good idea to put the muzzle on the dog at 'pleasurable' times, for example, just before play or walks (the muzzle can be taken off during the walk unless this is the time when the dog needs to wear the muzzle).
- Each time the muzzle is put on praise your dog and make a fuss of it.

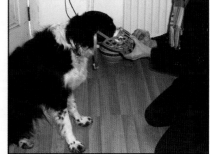

Introducing a muzzle using food treats.

15.7 Example handout – muzzle training.

If your dog is destructive or noisy... first aid advice

- Generally, a dog that is under stimulated is more likely to use up its energy in other ways, such as destructive behaviour or excessive barking. It is important that your dog receives plenty of daily exercise (preferably including at least one good run, or sniff around, off lead) and has plenty to do to keep both body and mind active at home. Engage your dog in short frequent daily reward-based training sessions and/or make your dog work for its food by either providing it in a food ball or stuffed in a tough hollow toy designed for this purpose, or by simply scattering dried food over the floor or out in the garden.
- Provide your dog with safe and enjoyable things to chew, such as chews and toys that are designed to be stuffed with food, thus making them more tempting to the dog.
- Make the toy or chew even more appealing by giving your dog plenty of praise and attention whenever it picks up or chews the toy.
- As much as possible keep things that your dog is most likely to damage out of its reach.
- Do not attempt to punish your dog. Barking, chewing and other destructive behaviours can be due to anxiety. If the dog is punished after the event it will be unable to connect the punishment with the behaviour. Your dog may look as though 'he knows he's done wrong', but that 'guilty' look is actually fear! Punishment can actually increase anxiety and in turn increase the unwanted behaviour. In addition, if you shout at a barking dog, it may believe that you are 'joining in', so you may inadvertently encourage further barking. Also, if it is barking to get attention, trying to tell the dog off will only give the dog the attention it wants, thereby actually rewarding and reinforcing the behaviour. However, be aware that initially your dog may try harder to get your attention and so bark more until it gets the message.
- Likewise if your dog is destructive be careful not to direct its attention on to the damaged items or areas, as doing so may increase its interest in the object and so increase the likelihood that it may return and chew or otherwise damage the area or item again. So, do not clear up any mess that the dog may have made while it is in the same room, or otherwise make a fuss about the damaged items.
- If your dog is on its own territory and barking at people or other dogs going by, try to block the dog's view. Use curtains, blinds, solid fences or simply keep your dog away from the area where it can see passers by.
- Always remember to praise and reward your dog for wanted behaviour and ignore unwanted behaviour.

If your dog is only destructive or noisy when you leave:

- Until professional help is obtained, try to avoid leaving your dog alone. Either take the dog with you when you go out, or ask a friend or family member to act as a 'dog sitter'. Another option is to contact local boarding kennels who may run a day service or otherwise be able to look after your dog for short periods
- Never attempt to punish your dog when you return or clear up any mess while your dog can see you (see above)
- Before you go out, as much as you can, remove anything that might be damaged
- Do not shut your dog in an indoor cage or similar *unless* your dog is accustomed to being caged. Caging a dog that is used to relative freedom can be highly traumatic and may increase or even cause anxiety associated with being left, resulting in other, possibly more serious, behavioural problems. Even if your dog is happy to spend time in an indoor cage, it is not advisable to keep a dog severely confined for periods of more that 3–4 hours
- There are many reasons why a dog may be destructive or bark and howl when left. It is obviously easier to identify the underlying causes if the behaviour can be observed. Therefore, it can be a great help to the behaviourist if you are able to set up a camcorder while you are out to record exactly what your dog does while you are away.

15.8 Example handout – destruction and vocalization first aid advice.

If your dog is not house trained... first aid advice

- **Do not attempt to punish your dog**, even if it appears 'guilty' (that 'guilty' look is actually fear!). The dog will not be able to associate the punishment with the act if the attempt at punishment occurs after the event. The dog may make an association with punishment and the *presence* of urine and/or faeces, but not with the 'act' of going to the toilet. When this occurs the dog may act fearfully as soon as it sees you and before you've even seen any urine or faeces in the house. Worse, the dog may start to eat its own waste to avoid punishment. Even attempting to punish the dog when you 'catch it in the act' is inadvisable as this may simply teach the dog that it is not 'safe' to eliminate whenever you are around. It may then decide that it is safer to 'sneak off' and go to the toilet in another room or behind the sofa rather than relieve itself on a walk or use the garden if you happen to be nearby!
- **Feed your dog a highly digestible dry diet.** If the diet fed to the dog is poorly digested much of it will be excreted as waste, but if the diet is highly digestible there is very little waste, so the dog will not need to go to the toilet so often. Likewise, a diet with a high water content is more likely to produce a full bladder and softer faeces that are not so easy to clean up. *But do not restrict your dog's access to water unless otherwise instructed.* Whatever diet you choose make the change gradually; a change that is made too quickly, even to a better food, may result in an upset stomach or a refusal to eat the new food.
- **Try to keep your dog near to you.** You are more likely to notice when your dog needs to eliminate if your dog is confined to the same room as yourself. Another idea is to attach a bell to your dog's collar so you have more chance of being aware of where it is. Additionally, placing a long lightweight lead to your dog's collar will allow you to lead your dog outside as soon as you suspect it may need the toilet.
- **Take your dog outside as often as possible:** at least once every 2 hours. The most important times are after meals and as soon as it wakes up from a nap.
- **Confine your dog to an area with an easily cleaned floor whenever it cannot be supervised.**
- **Clean soiled areas well to remove residual scent.** The most effective method is to either use a good proprietary 'odour elimination' product or use a 1:10 solution of biological washing detergent. Then wipe over or spray lightly with a spirit, e.g. surgical spirit or even vinegar (always test a small area first). DO NOT USE BLEACH or any bleach-based cleaner, even one that smells of fruit or flowers. Urine degrades to ammonia (bleach), so no matter how nice bleach-based cleaners smell to us, to a dog it will always smell of urine!

15.9 Example handout – dog house training first aid advice.

Feline elimination problems... first aid advice

- **Provide extra litter trays.** Many cats prefer to have one area for urination and another for defecation. If this is the case with your cat, you may find that it urinates in the litter tray but then defecates in a different location or *vice versa*. The simple solution is to provide another litter tray positioned initially in the area the cat uses. If this is an inconvenient place for you, the tray can be slowly and gradually moved to a more suitable location. Be careful not to move the tray too quickly or the cat will simply go back to its previous toileting location.
- **Provide an indoor litter tray even if your cat would normally eliminate outdoors.** Attacks by other cats, being chased by dogs or even bad weather may cause a cat to feel vulnerable and reluctant to eliminate outside.
- **Position litter trays well away from the cat's bed, food and water bowls.** Cats prefer to keep eating, sleeping and toileting areas separate.
- **Position litter trays in a quiet place where the cat is less likely to be disturbed or feel threatened.** Avoid areas close to windows, doorways, household machinery (such as washing machines) and areas frequented by other pets.
- **Avoid the use of scented cat litter or litter that may be uncomfortable for the cat to walk on or dig into.**
- **Clean out any faeces and wet patches once or twice daily and then empty the tray completely and wash it out about once a week.** Cats can be fairly fastidious so may not use an already soiled litter tray.

Scent marking:
The major difference between scent marking and elimination is the position that the cat adopts. When urinating to empty the bladder a cat will usually squat down with its tail stuck out behind, but a cat that is spraying to scent mark will stand up, often with the back legs standing on 'tiptoes' and 'stomping' from one foot to the other with the tail held upright and usually quivering slightly at the tip. The urine is directed backwards on to a vertical surface (although horizontal surfaces are sometimes sprayed as well). The amount of urine that is produced can vary, if the cat has a fairly empty bladder at the time then only a small squirt will be produced, but if the cat has a fairly full bladder then quite a large amount can be deposited.

- **Do not shout at or otherwise attempt to punish your cat even if 'caught in the act'.** A cat may spray indoors because it feels threatened or insecure. Therefore, any attempt at punishment will only increase the cat's insecurity and make matters worse.
- **Keep your cat away from areas where it is most likely to spray.**
- **Clean soiled areas well to remove residual scent.** The most effective method is to either use a good proprietary 'odour elimination' product or use a 1:10 solution of biological washing detergent. Then wipe over or spray lightly with spirit, e.g. surgical spirit or even vinegar (always test a small area first). DO NOT USE BLEACH or any bleach-based cleaner. Urine degrades to ammonia (bleach), therefore using bleach will increase rather than decrease the scent as far as the cat is concerned.
- **Prepare a number of 'food squares' and place them in areas most likely to be scent marked.** Cats are less likely to spray if there is food present, but if you leave bowls of cat food all over the house your cat will just eat it before spraying the area, so you need to prepare some 'permanent' food squares: cut up some fairly rigid cardboard into squares of around 3–4 inches. Then using a strong, safe glue cover the squares with dried cat food. Ensure the glue is completely dry and then place the squares around the house wherever the cat sprays, or anywhere you definitely don't want your cat to start spraying! You can move them around if necessary, sticking them in place with a temporary adhesive.
- **Apply a recommended feline pheromone spray to areas that have been scent marked.** The area should be cleaned of urine, rinsed and dried well first, then repeat the spray daily for at least 1 month or until your cat starts to rub against the furniture instead of spraying. (If you use a biological detergent to clean the area make sure you rinse it away well and allow the area to dry completely or any residue will 'deactivate' the pheromone spray.)

15.10 Example handout – feline elimination problem first aid advice.

Drug intervention

Prescribing medication is the remit of the veterinary surgeon alone and should never be undertaken by veterinary nurses or non-veterinary behaviourists. Even so, it is important that veterinary nurses have a general understanding of how drugs may influence an animal's behaviour, as well as the indications, limitations and restrictions of drug therapy that may be prescribed for the treatment of behavioural problems.

Medication can be a valuable complement to behaviour therapy; however, it is rarely effective as a standalone treatment. Drugs should only be used in conjunction with appropriate behavioural advice and only after a full investigative procedure to identify the underlying cause of the behaviour. Incorrect use of medication, as well as being ineffective and an unnecessary expense for the pet owner, can result in a worsening of the current behaviour problem or the development of other behavioural issues. Even when an appropriate medication is employed, without a concurrent behaviour modification programme the original problem is likely to recur once the medication is withdrawn. Prescribed drugs may have undesirable side-effects on both the animal's physical health and its behaviour. This factor should always be taken into account when medication is considered, particularly with those patients where concurrent disease states are present.

Sedatives

Sedatives have limited use in the treatment of behaviour problems. Sedating an animal masks problem behaviour rather than addressing the underlying cause. For many years acepromazine was the accepted medication prescribed for fears and phobias, especially fear of fireworks and problems associated with car travel. Use of a sedative alone with no anxiolytic properties may actually exacerbate such conditions by producing a situation where the animal, whilst still fearful, is less able to engage in its species-specific coping strategies. In addition, whilst acepromazine is taking effect, it can cause a heightened sensitivity to sound, which may result in an increased startle response. Acepromazine can also

Summary of drug interventions

Whenever medication and/or pheromone therapy is being considered as an adjunct to behavioural modification programmes, due consideration should always be given to the individual patient's health status and the physical and social environments. These should all be constantly monitored for changes, which may affect the animal's well being and relationships, as well as the problem behaviours for which the medication is indicated.

Veterinary surgeons and veterinary nurses should also be aware of the potential behavioural effects of some medications prescribed for medical rather than behavioural reasons, and possible implications should be considered before such drugs are prescribed. In addition, when an animal is presented with a behavioural problem, current and past medication and the possible behavioural effects upon that individual must always be taken into account.

Conclusion

Safeguarding the behavioural welfare of companion animals is as important as providing good quality healthcare. Veterinary nurses have an invaluable part to play in this respect by being aware of how problems may be prevented, being able to recognize potential or developing behaviour problems, and having knowledge of the processes involved in treatment. Being in possession of this information should allow veterinary nurses to set clients 'on the right path' from the start and to offer guidance and support to help maintain the relationships and well being of both pets and their owners.

References and further reading

APBC and CABTSG (2002) *Manual of Behavioural First-Aid*. The Association of Pet Behaviour Counsellors, Worcester

Appleby D (2004) *The APBC Book of Companion Animal Behaviour*. Souvenir Press, London

Bowen J and Heath S (2005) *Behaviour Problems in Small Animals: practical advice for the veterinary team*. Elsevier, Edinburgh

Horwitz D, Mills D and Heath S (2002) *BSAVA Manual of Canine and Feline Behavioural Medicine*. BSAVA Publications, Gloucester

Useful website

Association for Study of Animal Behaviour – Notes on Accreditation
http://www.asab.org

Appendix: Conversion tables

Biochemistry

	SI unit	Conversion	Non-SI unit
Alanine aminotransferase	IU / l	x 1	IU / l
Albumin	g / l	x 0.1	g / dl
Alkaline phosphatase	IU / l	x 1	IU / l
Aspartate aminotransferase	IU / l	x 1	IU / l
Bilirubin	µmol / l	x 0.0584	mg / dl
Calcium	mmol / l	x 4	mg / dl
Carbon dioxide (total)	mmol / l	x 1	mEq / l
Cholesterol	mmol / l	x 38.61	mg / dl
Chloride	mmol / l	x 1	mEq / l
Cortisol	nmol / l	x 0.362	ng / ml
Creatine kinase	IU / l	x 1	IU / l
Creatinine	µmol / l	x 0.0113	mg / dl
Glucose	mmol / l	x 18.02	mg / dl
Insulin	pmol / l	x 0.1394	µIU / ml
Iron	µmol / l	x 5.587	µg / dl
Magnesium	mmol / l	x 2	mEq / l
Phosphorus	mmol / l	x 3.1	mg / dl
Potassium	mmol / l	x 1	mEq / l
Sodium	mmol / l	x 1	mEq / l
Total protein	g / l	x 0.1	g / dl
Thyroxine (T4) (free)	pmol / l	x 0.0775	ng / dl
Thyroxine (T4) (total)	nmol / l	x 0.0775	µg / dl
Tri-iodothyronine (T3)	nmol / l	x 65.1	ng / dl
Triglycerides	mmol / l	x 88.5	mg / dl
Urea	mmol / l	x 2.8	mg of urea nitrogen / dl

Temperature

SI unit	Conversion	Conventional unit
° C	(x 9/5) + 32	° F

Nutrition

	Conversion	
Kilocalorie (kcal)	4.184	Kilojoule (kJ)

Haematology

	SI unit	Conversion	Non-SI unit
Red blood cell count	10^{12} / l	x 1	10^6 / µl
Haemoglobin	g / l	x 0.1	g / dl
MCH	pg / cell	x 1	pg / cell
MCHC	g / l	x 0.1	g / dl
MCV	fl	x 1	µm^3
Platelet count	10^9 / l	x 1	10^3 / µl
White blood cell count	10^9 / l	x 1	10^3 / µl

Hypodermic needles

	Metric	Non-metric
External diameter	0.8 mm	21 G
	0.6 mm	23 G
	0.5 mm	25 G
	0.4 mm	27 G
Needle length	12 mm	1/2 inch
	16 mm	5/8 inch
	25 mm	1 inch
	30 mm	1 1/4 inch
	40 mm	1 1/2 inch

Suture material sizes

Metric	USP
0.1	11/0
0.2	10/0
0.3	9/0
0.4	8/0
0.5	7/0
0.7	6/0
1	5/0
1.5	4/0
2	3/0
3	2/0
3.5	0
4	1
5	2
6	3

Index

Page numbers in *italic* type indicate figures

Abdominal distension *24*
Abdominal surgery, principles 158–9
 (*see also specific procedures*)
Abdominal ultrasonography *241–3*
Acanthocytes *276*
Accredited Prior Learning 2
Accuracy, laboratory tests 258, *261–2*
Acepromazine 325
Acetated polyionic solutions 115
Acetylcholine receptor antibody titre 27
Acid–base disorders 124–6
Acidaemia 125
Acidosis 125
Acromegaly *43*
Activated clotting time 35
Activated partial thromboplastin time 35
Acute pancreatitis *24*
 clinical nutrition 57–8
Acute renal failure *32*, 33, *34*
 fluid therapy 116
Addison's disease *see* Hypoadrenocorticism
Adenocarcinoma *18, 209*
Administration *see* Practice administration
Admission procedures, critical care unit 104, 107
Adoption leave/pay 294
Adrenal glands, ultrasonography *242*
Adrenaline *20*
Adson thumb forceps *149*
Advanced Diploma in Veterinary Nursing 2
Advisory Committee on Dangerous Pathogens 1995, 2000
 256
Aelurostrongylus abstrusus 19
Agglutination test *279*
Aggression 314, *322–3*
Airway disease *18*
 drug treatment *20–1*
Alanine aminotransferase (ALT) *264, 268*
Albumin *264, 268*
Alfaxalone 132
Alfentanil *134*
Alkalaemia 125
Alkaline phosphatase (ALP) *264, 268*

Alkalosis 125
Alveolar bone *176*, 177
Amiloride *17*
Aminophylline *20*
Amiodarone *16*
Amitriptyline 326
Amlodipine *17*
Ammonia in GI disease 23
Anabolic phase 62
Anaemia *34–5*, 37
Anaesthesia
 balanced 132
 for dentistry 188–9
 emergencies 130–1
 epidural/spinal 136–7
 inhalational 133
 intravenous 132
 local/regional 135
 monitoring *3*
  blood gas analysis 143–4
  capnography 141–2
  pulse oximetry 141
  respiratory gases 142–3
 mortality rates *128*
 muscle relaxation 137–9
 scavenging waste gases 131–2
 setting up
  design 128–9
  equipment 129–30
  health and safety 131–2
 for tracheobronchoscopy 205
 ventilation 139–40
Analgesia
 in balanced anaesthesia 133
 critical care unit 111
 epidural/spinal 136–7
 local/regional anaesthesia 135
 nitrous oxide 134–5
 NSAIDs 134
 opioids 133–4
Anaphylaxis in fluid therapy 116
Angiocardiography 228
Angiography 226–8, 248
Angiostrongylus vasorum 19

330

Anionic gap 126
Anisocytosis *284*
Anisokaryosis *284*
Antacids 64
Antibiotic-resistant bacteria 112–13
Antibiotics in surgery 153
Antibody tests
    for anaemia 36
    for musculoskeletal disease 31–2
    for neuromuscular disease 27
Anticonvulsants in behaviour therapy 327
Antidepressants 326
Antiemetic agents 64
Antinuclear antibody 31
Anxiety 314–15
Appetite stimulants 63–4
Arkansas stone *180*
Arrhythmia 13
Arthritis *31*
Arthrocentesis 30–1
Arthrography, shoulder 225
Arthroscopy
    elbow 217
    equipment *199, 201–2, 216–17*
    postoperative care 218–19
    shoulder 217–18
    stifle 218
    tarsus 218
Aspergillosis, serology 19
Aspirin *17*
Assisted feeding *see* Feeding
Atenolol *16*
Atlantoaxial subluxation 168
Atracurium *139*
Atrial fibrillation *16*
Atrioventricular block *14*
Atropine *20, 139*
Automatic analysers 259–64
Azathioprine *24*

Bacteria in urine 275
Bacteriology
    equipment 264
    sample submission 253–4
Balance exercises 82, 100–2
Balance sheet (financial) *289*
Balfour retractor *158*
Balloon dilation of oesophageal stricture 207
Barrier nursing 39, 113
Basal cell tumours 38
Beating massage 77, *78*
Beclometasone *20*
Behaviour
    preventive measures 316–19
    problems 314–16
        approach to 319–22
        drug therapy 325–8
        'first aid' 322–5
    VN role 313 (*see also* Clinics)
Benazepril *17*
Bilirubin *264, 268, 273*
Biochemical testing
    analysers 260
    precision *264*
    sample submission 253
    (*see also specific analytes*)

Biopsy
    bone 31
    bone marrow 36
    GI tract 207
    kidney 213
    liver 23, 213
    lymph node 36
    muscle 27
    nasal 19
    nerve 27
    pancreas 213
    pleural 19
    skin 39
    synovial membrane 31
    thoracic 19
    tracheobronchial 206–7
    ultrasound-guided 243–4
Bladder *see* Urinary bladder
Blindness 41
Blood
    collection 118
    donors 117–18
    gas analysis 143–4
    groups 117–18
    pressure
        anaesthetic effects 132
        arterial 110
        control (physiological) *12*
        measurement 15
        senior pets 310
    products 119
    tests 110
    transfusion 117–19
Bodyweight, decreased/increased, differential diagnoses *10*
    (*see also* Obesity)
Bone
    biopsy 31
    disease *see* Musculoskeletal disease
Bone marrow biopsy 36
Boneplates 171–2
Borrelia burgdorferi 32
Brachycephalic obstructive airway syndrome (BOAS) 164
Bradycardia 13
Bromhexine *20*
Bronchitis *18*
Bronchoalveolar lavage (BAL) 19, 206
Bronchoscopes 196, *197*
Buccal mucosal bleeding time (BMBT) *23*, 35–6
Budesonide *20, 24*
Buffy coat analysis 260
Bulla (skin) *37*
Bupivacaine *135*
Buprenorphine 133, *134*
Burs (dental) *180*
Butorphanol *20*, 133, *134*

Cabergoline 327
Calcium
    gluconate 124
    levels *268*
Cancer
    chemotherapy 50–2
    clinical approach 48
    clinical nutrition 58–9

Cancer *continued*
    common presentations 49–50
    definitions 47
    radiotherapy 52
    (*see also* Neoplasia *and specific tumours*)
Canine pancreatic lipase immunoassay 23
Capnography 141–2
Carbon dioxide, end-tidal 110
Carcinoma *18*
Cardiac disease, clinical nutrition 56–7
Cardiovascular disease
    diagnostics
        blood pressure measurement 15
        echocardiography 14
        electrocardiography 12–14
        radiography 15
    nursing considerations 15–16
    presenting complaints 11–12
    therapeutics 16–17
    (*see also specific conditions*)
Care plans 5, 6–7
    critical care unit 108–9
    feeding 63, 66
    physiotherapy 74, *87–8, 89, 90*
Caries *188*
L-Carnitine 59, 62
Carpus, radiographic positioning *222–3*
Carts for mobility 93
Carvedilol *17*
Cash book 287, *288*
Casts in urine 274–5
Catabolic reaction 62
Catheters
    central venous 120–1
    for parenteral nutrition 68
        maintenance *71*
Cementum 176
Central venous catheters 120–1
Central venous pressure 110
    measurement 121–2
Centrifuges 258
Cerebrospinal fluid *see* CSF
Certificate in Veterinary Practice Management 1
Charging structure, nurse clinics 311–12
Chemotherapy 50–2
Chest physiotherapy 90–2
Chronic pancreatitis, clinical nutrition 57–8
Ciclosporin *24*
Cimetidine *24*
Circulating nurse 146
Clapping massage 77, *78*
Client information 51–2, 311
    on behaviour problems *317, 322–5*
Clindamycin *30*
Clinical notes, critical care unit 108
Clinical nutrition *see* Diets, Feeding
Clinical pathology
    critical values *268*
    laboratories
        external
            advantages 250–1
            best practice 252
            choice 251
            disadvantages 251
            sample submission 252–5

    in-house
        best practice 264–6
        equipment 257–64, 266, *267*
        health and safety 255–7, 266
        managing 266–71
        quality assurance 269–70
        quality control 270–1
    reference intervals 258
    techniques
        cytology 280–4
        haematology 275–80
        urinalysis 271–5
    (*see also specific tests*)
Clinics (nurse-led)
    charging structure 311–12
    client educational materials 311
    equipment 303
    kitten clubs 305
    marketing 304, 308, 310–11
    paediatric 305
    palliative care 309
    planning 303–5
    puppy parties 193–4, 305–8
    senior 194, 309–11
    travel 308
    vaccination 305
    weight management 308–9
Clomipramine 326
Coagulation tests 23, 35–6
Codeine *20*
Cold therapy 80–1
Collection and Disposal of Waste Regulations 1992 *256*
Colloids 116–17
Colonoscopy 209
Comedo *37*
Compulsive behaviours 315
Computed radiography 231
Computed tomography 244–5
Congestive heart disease, drug treatment *17*
Continuing professional development (CE) 8
Contracts 292–3
Contrast studies *see* Radiography
Control of Substances Hazardous to Health Regulations 2002 (COSHH) 50, *256*
Copper, liver toxicosis 23
Coughing *18*
Coupage 77, *78*
Crash box *105*, 106, *131*
Creatinine *264, 268*
Critical care unit
    admission procedures 104, 107
    aim 103
    analgesia 110–11
    care plans 108–9, *111*
    clinical notes 108
    communication with owners 104, 107
    design/organization 103, 104–9
    drugs *106*
    equipment *105*
    infection control 111–13
    owner visits 107
    patient assessment/monitoring 103, 108, 109–10
    patient indications 103–4
    patient physiotherapy 89–92
    patient psychological needs 110

protocols 108
  rounds/shift change 108
  staffing/teamwork 104, 106–7, 108
Cruciate ligament surgery 170
Cryotherapy 80–1
Cryptorchid testicle removal 214–15
Crystalloids 114–15
Crystals in urine 275
CSF collection/analysis 26
CT 244–5
Curette (dental) 178
  sharpening *180*
Cushing's disease *see* Hyperadrenocorticism
Cyclophosphamide *24*
Cystoscopy 211, 215
Cytarabine *30*
Cytology
  examination 280–4
  sample submission 252–3, 254
  staining 280

Dacryocystorhinography 230
Dalteparin *17*
Data Protection Act 1988 287
DeBakey thumb forceps *149*
Delmadinone acetate 326
Dental caries *188*
Dental charts *183*
Dental explorer probes 178
Dental formula 176
Dentigerous cyst *184*
Dentine 176
Dentistry
  anaesthesia 188–9
  anatomy 175–7
  disease
    anatomical/developmental 186–7
    endodontic 188
    feline odontoclastic resorptive lesions (FORLs) *184*, 188
    periodontal 187–8
  examination 181–4
  extraction 190–1
  homecare 192–4
  instrumentation 177–81
  oral hygiene
    mouthwashes 193
    scaling/polishing 189
    toothbrushing 192–4
  orthodontics 192
  postoperative care 192
  radiography 184–6
  root canal treatment 191
  terminology 175
Dermatology *see* Skin disease
Desflurane, MAC *133*
Dexamethasone *20*
Dextrans 117
Dextrose 115
Dextrose saline 115
Diabetes insipidus *42*
Diabetes mellitus
  diagnostics *44*
  management 45–7
    clinical nutrition 58
  nursing considerations 45–7

Diabetic ketoacidosis 47
Diaphragmatic hernia/rupture repair 157–8
Diarrhoea 22
Diathermy *148*
  haemostasis 149
  incision 147
Diazepam *30*
Diets
  for cancer 58–9
  for cardiac disease 56–7
  and dental health 193
  for diabetes mellitus 58
  for enteral nutrition 66
  for food allergy/intolerance 39, 59–60
  for GI disease 61
  for hepatic disease 54–5
  for joint disease 61–2
  for obesity 59
  for pancreatic disease 57–8
  for parenteral nutrition 68–70
  for renal disease 55–6
  for skin disease 60
  for urolithiasis 60
  (*see also* Feeding)
Digital subtraction angiography 248
Digitoxin *17*
Digoxin *16, 17*
Diltiazem *16, 17*
Diode laser 199
Dipstick, urinalysis 272–3
Disability Discrimination Act *294*
Dismissal of staff 293, 298
Dissecting tissue 148
Dobutamine *17*
Dog appeasing pheromone 327
Döhle bodies *278*
Doppler ultrasonography 239
Dorsal laminectomy 167
Drainage
  open peritoneal *163*
  suction *104*
  thoracic 19, 155–6
Duodenoscopy 207
Duodenum, ultrasonography *242*
Dwarfism *31*
Dynamic compression plate *171*
Dysphagia *24*
Dyspnoea *18*

ECG *see* Electrocardiography
Echocardiography 14
Ectoparasite control 40
Edrophonium *139*
  response test 27
Effleurage 75–6, *77*
Elbow
  arthroscopy 217
  radiographic positioning *224*
Electrocardiography 110
  in hyperkalaemia 124
  indications 13
  interpretation 13–14
  senior pets 310
  technique *13*
  telemetry 14

Electrolyte abnormalities 126
Electromyography 26–7
Electroretinography 41
Electrotherapy
    laser 85
    NMES 86
    TENS 86
    ultrasound 85
Elevator (dental) 179
Employment Equality (Age) Regulations 2006 *294*
Employment Equality (Religion or Belief) Regulations 2003
    294
Employment Equality (Sexual Orientation) Regulations
    2003 *294*
Employment law 292–4
Enalapril *17*
Enamel (dental) 176
    dysplasia *187*
End-tidal carbon dioxide 110
Endocrine disease
    diagnostics *42–4*
    nursing considerations 45–7
    presenting complaints *42–4*
    therapeutics *42–4, 45–6*
Endocrine testing, sample submission 254
Endodontic disease 188
Endoscopy
    equipment
        ancillary 198–200
        cleaning 203–4
        flexible endoscopes 195–7
        instruments 200–2
        maintenance 204–5
        rigid endoscopes 197–8
        sterilization 202–3
    procedures
        flexible
            gastrointestinal 207–9
            tracheobronchoscopy 205–7
        rigid
            arthroscopy 216–19
            intestinal 209
            laparoscopy 212–15
            rhinoscopy 209–11
            thoracoscopy 215–16
            urethrocystoscopy 211–12
Endotracheal (ET) tubes 130
Endurance 82
Enteral nutrition
    administration 65–7
    continuous 67
    diets 66
    equipment 64–5
    nursing considerations 67
    plan 66
Eosinophils
    in blood smears *277, 278*
    cytology *282, 283*
Ephedrine *20*
Epidermal collarette *37*
Epidural anaesthesia/analgesia 136–7
Epistaxis 20
Epithelial cells
    cytology *283*
    in urine *274*
Equal Pay Act 1970 *294*

Erosion (skin) *37*
Erythrocytes
    agglutination 279–80
    in blood smears 275–7
    rouleaux *280*
    in urine *274*
Escherichia coli, antibiotic-resistant 112
Etamiphylline *20*
Etomidate 132
Euthanasia 104
Exclusion diets 39
Exercise, therapeutic 81–2, 92, 97–9
    for cats *93*
Exocrine pancreatic insufficiency (EPI) *24*
    clinical nutrition 58
External skeletal fixation 172–3
Extraction (dental)
    complications *191*
    instrumentation 178–9, 190
    techniques 190–1
Eye
    medication 42
    ultrasonography *243*
    (*see also* Ophthalmic disease)

Faeces, sample submission 254
Fat in urine 275
Fear 314–15
Feeding
    assisted
        enteral nutrition 64–7, 71
        parenteral nutrition 67–71
        plan 63
    after dental surgery 192
    (*see also* Diets)
Feline lower urinary tract disease (FLUTD) 33
Feline odontoclastic resorptive lesions (FORLs) 188
Fentanyl *134*
Fibrin degradation products 36
Financial administration 287–91
Fine-needle aspiration, ultrasound-guided 243–4
First Aid Regulations 1981 *256*
Fistulography 229–30
Fluid therapy
    central venous catheters 120–1
    central venous pressure 121–2
    colloids 116–17
    crystalloids 114–15
    in hyperkalaemia 124
    in hypokalaemia 123
    in metabolic acidosis 126
    (*see also* Blood transfusion)
Fluorescein staining, eye 40
Fluoroscopy 233–5
Fluticasone *20*
Food allergy/intolerance 39
    clinical nutrition 59–60
Forceps, for dental extraction 179
Foreign body retrieval
    GI tract 208–9
    tracheobronchoscopy 206
Fractures
    repair 170–3
    tooth *188*
Friction massage 76–7, *78*
Furosemide *17*

Gabapentin *30*
Gait *28*
Gastrointestinal disease
    clinical nutrition 61
    diagnostics 22–3
    nursing considerations 23–4
    presenting complaints 21–2
    (*see also specific conditions*)
Gastrointestinal endoscopy 207–9
Gastrointestinal surgery 161–2
Gastropexy, laparoscopic 215
Gastroscopy
    equipment 196, *197*
    procedure 207
Gastrostomy tube
    advantages/disadvantages *65*
    diets *66*
    placement 208
Gelatin solutions 116–17
Gene's thumb forceps *149*
Genetic testing, sample submission 254
Geriatrics *see* Senior pets
Gingiva *176*, 177
    examination *182*
Gingivitis *187*
Globulins *268*
Glucometers 259
Glucose *264, 268, 273*
    response curves 45–6
Glyceryl trinitrate *17*
Glycopyrrolate *20, 139*
Glycosaminoglycans 62
Gonioscopy 41
Gosset retractor *158*
Guide to Professional Conduct 8

Hacking massage 77, *78*
Haematocrit *263*
Haematology
    analysers 260
    cells 275–80
        (*see also specific cell types*)
    precision *263*
    quality assurance/control 269–70
    sample submission 253
Haematuria *273*
Haemocytometers 264
Haemoglobin *263*
Haemoglobinuria *273*
Haemopoietic disorders
    diagnostics 35–6
    nursing considerations 36–7
    presenting complaints 34–5
    therapeutics 37
Haemostasis during surgery 148–9
Haemostats 148–9
Halothane, MAC *133*
Halstead's principles of surgery 147
Hand hygiene, critical care unit 112–13
Handpieces (dental) 179–80, 181
Harnesses (support) 93, *94*
Head Surgical Nurse 145
Head trauma 29

Health and safety
    in anaesthesia 131–2
    in chemotherapy 50–1
    in CT 245
    in fluoroscopy 234–5
    in laboratories 255–7, 264, 266
    in MRI 247
    in scintigraphy 248
Health and Safety at Work etc. Act 1974 *256*
Health check protocol 304
Heart
    failure 11, 15
    rate
        anaesthetic effects 132
        from ECG 13
    rhythm 13–14
    ultrasonography *243*
    (*see also* Cardiac)
Heat therapy 79–80, 219
Heinz bodies *277*
Hemilaminectomy 167
Henderson–Hasselbalch equation 124
Hepatic disease 22
    clinical nutrition 54–5
Hetastarch 116
Higher education 2–3
Histiocytes *283*
Histiocytoma *38*
Histology, sample submission 254
History taking, behaviour problems 321
Hospital-acquired infections 111–13
House soiling 315, *325*
House training dogs *324*
Howell–Jolly bodies *277*
Hydralazine *17*
Hydrochlorothiazide *17*
Hydrotherapy 82–4
    for cats 92–3
Hygiene, critical care unit 112–13
Hyperadrenocorticism 44
Hyperglycaemia *46*
Hyperkalaemia 124
Hyperparathyroidism *43*
Hypersomatotropism *43*
Hypertension 12
Hyperthermia 11
    differential diagnoses *9*
Hyperthyroidism *43*
    radiotherapy 52
    scintigram *248*
Hypertonia 90
Hypertonic saline 115
Hypoadrenocorticism *43*
Hypoglycaemia 45, *46*
Hypokalaemia 47, 123, 126
Hyposthenuria *272*
Hypothermia 11
    differential diagnoses *10*
Hypothyroidism *43*

Inappetence, differential diagnoses *10*
Inappropriate elimination 315
    cats *325*
    dogs *324*
Infection control, critical care unit 111–13

Index

Inflammation, cytology 281, *282*
Inflammatory bowel disease *24*
Information technology 291–2
Inhalation therapy 20
Injection site sarcoma 50
Instruments *see* Dentistry, Surgery *and specific instruments*
Insufflation 212
Insulin 46–7
Insulinoma *44*
Intensive care *see* Critical care
Intestines, ultrasonography *242*
Intracranial surgery 168
Isoflurane, MAC *133*
Isoprenaline *20*
Isosthenuria *272*
IT in practice administration 291–2

Jejunostomy tube
    advantages/disadvantages *65*
    diets *66*
Joint disease *see* Musculoskeletal disease
Joint replacement surgery 169–70

Ketamine
    anaesthesia 132
    analgesia 135
Ketones *268, 273*
Key users 264
Kidney
    biopsy 213
    ultrasonography *242*
    (*see also* Renal)
Kitten clubs 305
Kneading massage 76, *78*

Laboratory tests *see* Clinical pathology *and specific tests*
Lactated Ringer's solution 115
Laparoscopy
    biopsy 213
    equipment 200–1, 212
    surgical procedures 213–15
Laparotomy 23
Laryngeal disease *18*
    surgery 165
Laryngoscopes 130
Larynx, ultrasonography *243*
Laser physiotherapy 85
Lateral thoracotomy 154
Leash walking 98
Leptocytes *276*
Leucocytes
    in blood smears 277–8
    count *see* WBC count
Leucocytosis 35
Leucopenia 35
Leukaemia 35
Lichenification *37*
Lidocaine *135*
    in heart disease 16
Liver
    biopsy 23, 213
    ultrasonography *241*
    (*see also* Hepatic)

Local anaesthesia 135
Lung
    disease *18, 48*
    lobectomy 157
Luxator (dental) 178
Lyme disease 32
Lymph node biopsy 36
Lymphangiography 230–1
Lymphocytes *277, 278*
Lymphoma *18, 24,* 49

Macrophages, cytology *282*
Macule *37*
Magnetic resonance imaging 245–7
Malnutrition 62–3
Malocclusion (dental) 186–7
Mammary tumours 49
Management of Health and Safety at Work Regulations 1999 *256*
Mandibular fracture, fixation *173*
Marketing 298–301
    nurse-led clinics 304, 308, 310–11
Maropitant *24*
Massage
    benefits *75, 77–8*
    for cats 92
    contraindications 78
    friction techniques 76–7
    percussion techniques 77
    pressure techniques 76
    shaking/vibration techniques 78
    stroking techniques 75–6
Mast cell tumours 49
Mast cells *283*
Maternity leave/pay 293–4
Mayo scissors 148
Mayo–Hagar needle-holders 149–50
MCHC *270*
MCV *263*
Medetomidine, analgesia 135
Median sternotomy 154
Megaoesophagus *21, 24*
Megestrol acetate 326
Melanocytoma *38*
Melanoma *38*
Mepivacaine *135*
Mesenchymal cells, cytology *283*
Metabolic acidosis/alkalosis 125, 126
Methadone *134*
Methicillin-resisitant *Staphylococcus aureus* 112
Metoclopramide *24*
Metzenbaum scissors 148
Mexilitine *16*
Microscopes 259
Midazolam *30*
Monocytes *277, 278*
Morphine *134*
Mouthwash 192, 193
MRI 245–7
MRSA 112
Mucoperiosteal flap *190*
Muscle
    antibodies 27
    biopsy 27

Musculoskeletal disease
  diagnostics 30–2
  nursing considerations 32
  presenting complaints *31*
  therapeutics 32
    clinical nutrition 61–2
  (*see also specific disorders*)
Muzzle training *323*
Myasthenia gravis *26*, 27, 29
Myoglobinuria *273*

Nasal cavity, anatomy 177
Naso-oesophageal tube
  advantages/disadvantages *65*
  diets *66*
National Minimum Wage 293
National Occupational Standards 4–5
National postal guidelines for samples 254–5
Nausea *24*
Needle-holders 149–50
Neoplasia
  cytology 283–4
  respiratory system *18*
  urogenital *34*
  (*see also* Cancer *and specific tumours*)
Neostigmine *139*
Nerve
  biopsy 27
  blocks 135
  conduction velocity 27
Neurological assessment 27–9
Neurological disease
  physiotherapy 87–8
  (*see also* Neuromuscular disease)
Neuromuscular blocking agents (NMBAs) 137–9
Neuromuscular disease
  diagnostics 25–7
  nursing considerations 27–9
  physiotherapy *87–8*
  presenting complaints 25–6
  therapeutics *30*
  (*see also* Musculoskeletal disorders)
Neuromuscular electrical nerve stimulation (NMES) 86
Neurosurgery, principles 166
  (*see also specific procedures*)
Neutrophils
  in blood smears *277, 278*
  cytology *282*
  in urine *274*
Nicergoline *327*
Nitrous oxide
  anaesthesia 133
  analgesia 134–5
NMES 86
Nociception 133
Nodule (skin) *37*
Non-steroidal anti-inflammatory drugs (NSAIDs),
    analgesia 134
Normal saline 115
Notice periods 293
Nursing clinics *see* Clinics
Nursing plans *see* Care plans
Nutraceuticals 62
Nutrition *see* Clinical nutrition, Diets, Feeding
NVQ qualifications 1

Obesity, clinical nutrition 59
Ocular discharge 42
Oesophageal disease 21–2
Oesophageal stricture, balloon dilation 207
Oesophagoscopy 207
Oesophagostomy tube
  advantages/disadvantages *65*
  diets *66*
  placement *67*
Oestrogen 33
Omega-3 fatty acids 59, 60, 61–2
Omeprazole *24*
Operating theatre *see* Surgery
Ophthalmic disease
  diagnostics 40–1
  nursing considerations 41–2
  therapeutics 42
Ophthalmic examination 40
Opioid analgesia 133–4
Opisthotonic posture *28*
Oral examination
  probes 177–8
  procedure 181–4
Oral hygiene 189
  postoperative 192
Orem model *6*
Orthodontic treatment 192
Orthopaedic surgery
  principles 168–9
  (*see also specific procedures*)
Oslerus oslerus 19
Osteochondrosis *31, 218*
Osteomalacia *31*
Osteosarcoma *31*, 49
Otitis media, CT image *245*
Ovariohysterectomy/ovariectomy 214
Ovary, ultrasonography *242*
Oxygen therapy *17,* 19, 20
Oxyglobin 119–20

Packed cell volume (PCV) *268*
Paediatric clinics 305
Pain
  differential diagnoses *10*
  management in bone disease 32
  perception, assessment 29
  relief, physiotherapy 92
Palliative and disease management clinics 309
Pancreas
  biopsy 213
  ultrasonography *242*
Pancreatic disease 22
  clinical nutrition 57–8
Pancreatitis
  acute *24,* 57
  chronic 57
Pancuronium *139*
Panhypopituitarism *42*
Panosteitis *31*
Papilloma *38*
Papule *37*
Parenteral nutrition
  administration 70–1
  calculations *68, 69, 70*
  complications 71

Parenteral nutrition *continued*
    equipment 68
    monitoring 71
    nursing considerations 71
    solutions 68–70
Passive movements 78–9, 95
    for cats *93*
Patent ductus arteriosus (PDA) ligation 156
Paternity leave/pay 294
Pelvic, radiographic positioning *221–3*
Pentastarch 116
Percussion 77, *78*
Percutaneous endoscopic gastrostomy (PEG) tube
    placement 208
Percutaneous endoscopic jejunostomy (PEJ) tube
    placement 208
Pericardectomy 156–7
    endoscopic 216
Pericardiocentesis 16
Periodontal disease 187–8, 189
Periodontal ligament 176
Periodontal probes 177, *180*
Periodontitis *187*
Periosteal elevator 179
Peritonitis, septic 162–3
PET scan 248
Pethidine *134*
Petrissage 76
Phaeochromocytoma *44*
Pharyngeal disease *18*
Phenobarbital
    in behaviour therapy 327
    for seizures *30*
Pheromones in behaviour therapy 327
Phosphate *268*
Photography 248–9
Physiotherapy
    assistance devices 93–4
    for cats 92–3
    indications 74
    in intensive care
        chest care 90–2
        pain relief 92
        plan *90*
        positioning 90
        progressive exercise 92
        ROM maintenance 92
        swelling control 92
    legal considerations 73
    in neurological disease 87–9
    postoperative 87
    preoperative 87
    for seniors 89
    techniques
        cold 80–1
        electrotherapy 84–6
        exercise 81–2, *93*
            balance/proprioception 82, 100–2
            strengthening 82, 97–9
        heat 79–80
        hydrotherapy 82–4, 92–3
        massage 75–8, 92
        passive movements 78–9, *93*, 95
        stretches 79, 96
    in veterinary practice 73–4

Pimobendan *17*
Plaque
    (dental) 187–8
    (skin) *37*
Platelets
    in blood smears 278–9
    count *263, 268, 270*
Pleural effusion, drainage 19
Pleuritis *18*
Pneumonia *18*
Poikilocytosis *276*
Polishing (dental) 189
Polychromasia *275*
Polycythaemia *35*
Polydipsia, differential diagnoses *10*
Polyphagia, differential diagnoses *10*
Portal hypertension 161
Portosystemic shunt ligation 160–1
Portovenography *160,* 226–7
Positron emission tomography (PET) 248
Possey rectractor *158*
Postural drainage *90–1*
Postural reactions 28
Posture in neurological disease 28
Potassium
    bromide *30*
    levels *268*
    supplementation 123
Pounding massage 77, *78*
PPE (personal protective equipment) 51, 112, 113, 264
Practice administration
    employment law 292–4
    human resources 295–8
    marketing 298–301
    systems 286–7
        financial 287–91
        IT 291–2
Prazosin *17*
Precision, laboratory tests 258, 262–3
Prednisolone *24, 30,* 40
Pregnancy diagnosis, ultrasound 243
Preoperative physiotherapy 87
Proctoscopy 209
Profit and loss statement *289*
Progesterone 33
Prokinetic agents 64
Propentofylline 327
Propofol *30*
Propranolol in behaviour therapy 327
Proprioception exercises 82
Prostate, ultrasonography *242*
Prostatic wash 33
Proteinuria 273
Prothrombin time 35
Protocols, critical care unit 108
Pulmonary oedema 11
Pulp (dental) 176
Pulse 15
    oximetry 110, 141
Puppy parties 193–4, 305–8
Purchase ledger 288
Pustule *37*
Pyometra *34*
Pyothorax *18*
Pyrexia 10–11
    differential diagnoses *9*

Quality Assurance Agency *2–3*
Quality assurance in clinical pathology 250, 269–70
Quality control in clinical pathology 250, 270–1
Quinidine *16*

Race Relations Act 1976 *294*
Radiography *4*
    contrast
        angiography 226–8
        arthrography 225–6
        dacryocystorhinography 230
        lymphangiography 230–1
        sialography 228–9
        sinography/fistulography 229–30
    dental 184–6
    digital 231–3
    positioning 220–5
    thoracic 15
Radiotherapy 52
Ramipril *17*
Ranitidine *24*
RCVS Veterinary Nursing syllabus 4–5
Recruitment of staff 295–7
Recumbency, nursing plan *11*
Reference intervals 258
Refractometers 258–9
Registered Veterinary Nurse (RVN) 7
Regurgitation 21–2
Rehabilitation *see* Physiotherapy
Renal disease
    chronic *34*
    clinical nutrition 55–6
Renal failure, acute *32*, 33, *34*
    fluid therapy 116
Reporting of Injuries, Disease and Dangerous Occurrence
    Regulations (RIDDOR) 1995 *256*
Respiratory acidosis/alkalosis 125
Respiratory disease
    diagnostics 19
    nursing considerations 19–20
    presenting complaints 17–18
    therapeutics 20–1
    (*see also specific conditions*)
Respiratory gas monitoring 142–3
Respiratory rate, anaesthetic effects 132
Resting energy requirement (RER) 64
Reticulocytes 279
Retractors *158*
Rheumatoid factor 31
Rhinitis *18,* 20
Rhinoscopy 209–11
Risk assessment *257*
Rocuronium *139*
Roles 3–4
ROM (range of motion) 78, 92
Root canal treatment 188, 191
Ropivacaine *135*

Salbutamol *20*
Sales ledger 288
Sample submission to laboratories 252–5
Scalers (dental)
    hand 178
    mechanical 179, 180–1
Scalpel use 147
Schirmer tear test 40
Schistocytes *276*

Scintigraphy 247–8
Scissors 148
Scrubbed nurse 146
Sebaceous adenoma/carcinoma/hyperplasia *38*
Sedatives, use in behaviour problems 325–6
Sediment, urinary 273–5
Seizures 29
Selegiline 326
Self-regulation 7–8
Senior pets
    behaviour problems 315
    clinics 194, 309–11
    physiotherapy 89
Sensitivity, laboratory tests 258
Separation anxiety 315
Septic peritonitis 162–3
Sevoflurane, MAC *133*
Sex Discrimination Act 1975 *294*
Shaking massage 77, *78*
Shoulder
    arthrography 225–6
    arthroscopy 217–18
    radiographic positioning *224*
Sialography 228–9
Single photon emission computed tomography (SPECT)
    248
Sinography 229–30
Sinus arrhythmia 13
Sinus bradycardia 13
Sinus tachycardia 13
Skin
    disease
        diagnostics *38*, 39
        nursing considerations 39
        presenting complaints 37–9
            tumours *38*, 49, 50
          therapeutics 39–40
            clinical nutrition 60
    rolling massage 76, *78*
Slings (support) 93, *168*
SOAP scheme *111*
Sodium
    bicarbonate 126
    levels *268*
Sotalol *16*
Specificity, laboratory tests 258
SPECT 248
Spherocytes *276*
Spinal anesthesia/analgesia 137
Spinal reflex assessment 28–9
Spinal surgery 166–8
Spindle cell sarcoma 49
Spine, radiographic positioning *220*
Spironolactone *17*
Spleen, ultrasonography *242*
Splenectomy 159–60
Splenic torsion *159*
Squamous cell carcinoma *38*, 49
Squamous cells in urine *274*
SSRIs 326
Staff
    appraisal/performance review 297–8
    dismissal 293, 298
    grievance/disciplinary procedures 298
    recruitment 295–7
    training/development 297

Standard operating procedures (SOPs), laboratories 264, *265*
Staphylococcus aureus, methicillin-resistant 112
Staplers *157, 159*
Statutory sick pay 294
Sterilization
    dental instruments 180, 181
    endoscopes/instruments 202–3
Stertor *18*
Stifle
    arthroscopy 218
    MRI 246
    radiographic positioning *225*
Stock
    checking, critical care unit 106
    management, drugs 286–7
Stomach, ultrasonography *242*
Strengthening exercises 82, 97–9
Stretching physiotherapy 79, 96
Stridor *18*
Stroking massage 75, *77*
Sucralfate *24*
Sulcular lavage 189
Supraventricular tachycardia *14*
Surgery
    advanced procedures
        abdominal 158–63
        neurosurgery 166–8
        orthopaedics 169–74
        thoracic 153–8
        upper respiratory tract 163–6
    antibiotics 153
    dental *see* Dentistry
    Halstead's principles 147
    laparoscopic procedures 212–15
    minor procedures
        diathermy 147–8
        haemostasis 148–9
        scalpel incision 147
        scissors 148
        suturing 149–53
        tissue handling 149
    team 145–6
    theatre management 145–6
Surgical veterinary nurse 4
Suturing
    materials 150
    needle-holders 149–50
    patterns 150–3
    skin wounds 152–3
Suxamethonium *139*

Tachycardia 13, *14, 16*
Target cells *276*
Tarsus
    arthroscopy 218
    radiographic positioning *223–4*
Teamwork
    in critical care unit 104, 106–7, 108
    in physiotherapy 73–4
    in surgery 145–6
Telemetry, ECG 14
Temporomandibular joint, radiographic positioning *221*
TENS 86, 92
Terbutaline *20*

Testicles
    cryptorchid, removal 214–15
    ultrasonography *243*
Tetanus 29
Thermotherapy 79–80
Thiopental 132
Third-degree heart block *16*
Thoracic drainage 19, 90–2
    (*see also* Thoracostomy tubes)
Thoracic surgery, principles 153–4
    (*see also specific procedures*)
Thoracocentesis 19
Thoracoscopy 158
    equipment 200–1, 216
    procedures 216
Thoracostomy tubes
    hygiene 112
    maintenance 155
    placement 155
    removal 156
Thrombocytopenia 279
Thrombocytosis 279
Thromboembolism 15
Thumb forceps 149
Thyroid gland, ultrasonography *243*
Thyroxine levels *268*
Tonometry 41
Tooth/teeth
    anatomy 175–7
    cleaning 189, 192–4
    eruption times *176*
    (*see also* Dentistry)
Total elbow replacement 169
Total hip replacement 169
Total protein (TP) *264, 268*
Toxicity of local anesthetics 135
TPN *see* Parenteral nutrition
Tracheal disease *18*
Tracheal lavage 19
Tracheobronchoscopy 205–7
Tracheostomy 165–6
Training practices 1
Transcutaneous electrical nerve stimulation (TENS) 86
Travel clinics 308
Triadan numbering system *184*
Triage 9
Tumours *see* Cancer, Neoplasia *and specific tumours*
Tuohy needle *136*
Tympanic bulla, radiographic positioning *221*

Ulcers
    gastrointestinal *24*
    skin *37*
Ultrasonography
    artefacts 237–9
    Doppler 239
    equipment 239–40
    image production 236–7
    interpretation 237
    ocular 41
    patient preparation 240
    pregnancy diagnosis 243
    principles 235–6
    techniques 240–4
Ultrasound physiotherapy 85

Unilateral arytenoid lateralization 165
Upper respiratory tract surgery, principles 163–4
   (*see also specific procedures*)
Urea *264, 268*
Urethral sphincter mechanism incontinence (USMI)
   211–12
Urethrocystoscopy 211–12
Urinalysis
   equipment 264
   techniques 271–5
Urinary bladder
   function assessment 29
   ultrasonography *242*
Urinary catheters, hygiene 112
Urinary incontinence *34*
Urinary tract infection in diabetes mellitus 46
Urine
   appearance *271–2*
   dipstick analysis 272–3
   protein:creatinine ratio 32
   sediment analysis 273–5
   specific gravity *271–2*
Urogenital disease
   diagnostics 32–3
   nursing considerations 33
   presenting complaints 32
   therapeutics *34*
Urolithiasis 33, *34*
   clinical nutrition 60–1
Uterus, ultrasonography *242*

Vaccination
   clinics 305
   for skin disease 40
Vaginal examination 33
   endoscopic 211

Vecuronium *139*
Ventilators 130, 139–40
Ventricular premature contractions *16*
Ventricular tachycardia *14, 16*
Verapamil *16*
Vesicle *37*
Vessel ligation 149
Vestibular syndrome *28*
Veterinary Nurses Register 7–8
Veterinary Surgeons Act 1966 73
   Schedule 3 Amendment Order 2002 146
Vibration massage 77, *78*
Virology
   equipment 264
   sample submission 254
Vitamin supplementation 56, 57
Volume overload 116
Vomiting 21–2, *24*
von Willebrand factor 36
von Willebrand's disease 37
VPMA 1

Water deprivation test 32–3
WBC count
   critical values *268*
   precision *263*
   technique *270*
Weight management clinics 308–9
Wheal *37*
Wheelbarrowing 98
'Wind-up' pain sensitivity 133
Wounds, hygiene 112
Wringing massage 76, *78*

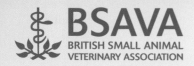
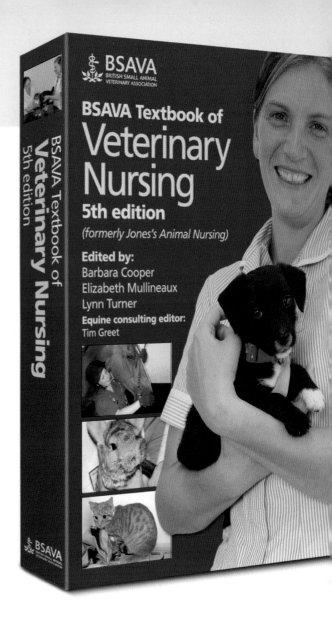

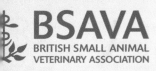
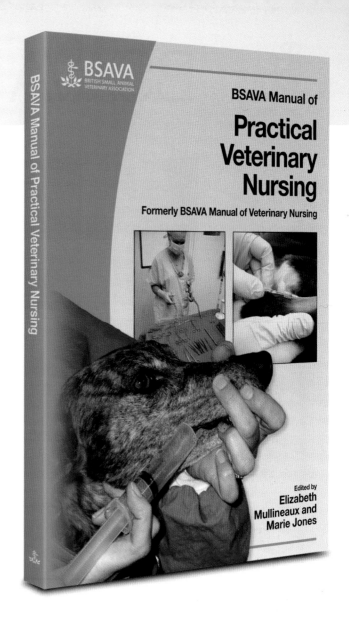

SAVA Manual of

Practical
Veterinary
Nursing

rmerly BSAVA Manual of
terinary Nursing)

dited by Elizabeth
ullineaux and Marie Jones

Manual can be considered a practical
ompaniment to the more theoretical *BSAVA Textbook*
eterinary Nursing (Jones's'). The Manual has been
en to cover the practical requirements of the National
cupational Standards for traineee veterinary nurses and
rovide additional practical support for qualified
rinary nurses during their first years of practice.

a must have for student veterinary
rses and animal nursing
sistants. Both practical and easy to
ow, it is an incredibly useful
source... an essential reference
l for daily use in practice...
VS.CO.UK

PUBLISHING INFORMATION
Published 2007
416 pages
Soft cover
Extensively illustrated
ISBN: 978 0 905214 91 7

Price to non-members: £59.00

MEMBER PRICE:
£39.00

BSAVA Manuals

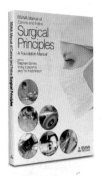
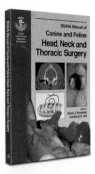
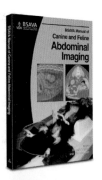
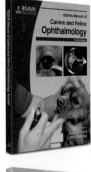
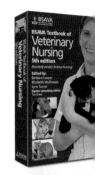
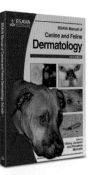

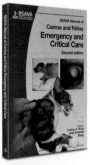
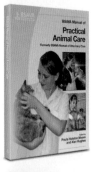
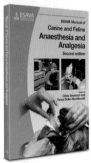
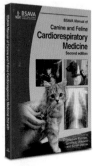
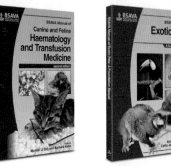

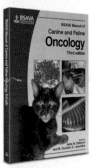
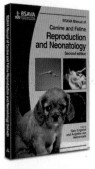
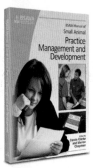
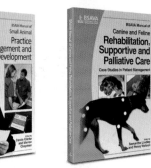
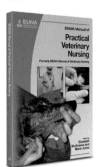
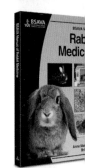

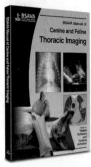
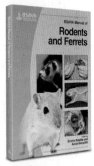
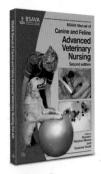
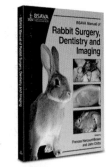
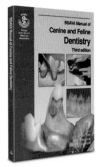
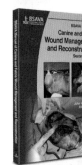

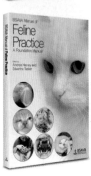
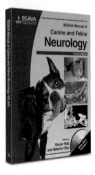
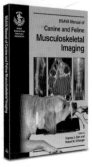
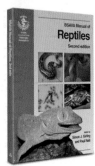
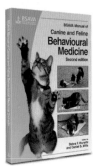
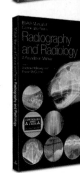

Tel: 01452 726700   Fax: 01452 726701

Email: administration@bsava.com   Web: www.bsava.com